'This book brings together the wisdom and collective knowledge of experts in the application of the principles of dramatherapy, exploring how dramatic enactment addresses embodiment within the context of trauma. However, this volume and its editor go far beyond that—they bring to light the integrative potentials of dramatherapy, theatre, and performance in all its depth and complexities. Setting a new standard for how psychotherapy can envision the treatment of traumatic stress, the book expands our knowledge of just how creative and expressive methods can be applied to resolving the body's experience of trauma. More importantly, this book provides readers with a framework for establishing a pathway to re-sensitizing the body to narratives that are at once resilient, reparative, and restorative.'

Cathy A. Malchiodi, PhD, *Author of* Trauma and Expressive Arts Therapy: Brain, Body, and Imagination in the Healing Process

'*Trauma and Embodied Healing in Dramatherapy, Theatre and Performance* offers a wealth of new insights into the different ways traumas are experienced and understood. Parallel to these windows offered into its *manifestations* and *causations* are opportunities to access ground breaking knowledge and research into an exciting variety of health related *responses* to trauma. The considerable strength of this volume is its interdisciplinarity. It illuminates the many values of new perspectives that are being developed by fascinating dialogues focused on the health potentials of embodiment and somatic approaches. We see the benefits of a range of innovative interactions between diverse traditions and perspectives: from dramatherapy to performance, from cognitive studies to play, from actor training to neuroscience. Context is thoughtfully engaged with, as we gain access to research undertaken in various cultures and countries. I strongly recommend this book as essential reading for those involved in training, practice and research in psychology, psychotherapy, the arts and the arts therapies.'

Phil Jones, *Professor of Children's Rights and Wellbeing, Institute of Education, University College London's Faculty of Education and Society*

'*Trauma and Embodied Healing in Dramatherapy, Theatre and Performance* offers a timely and important contribution to the growing understanding of embodied work with survivors of trauma. The inclusion of both clinical and theatre/performance-based chapters is exciting, generative and germane. With its international and multidisciplinary perspectives and descriptions of culturally-sensitive practices, this book will spark needed conversations and further research – particularly in the field of drama therapy – on the vital role of the body as an outlet for expression and an inroad to healing.'

Renée Emunah, PhD, RDT-BCT, *Founder/Director, Drama Therapy Program, California Institute of Integral Studies. Author of* Acting for Real: Drama Therapy Process, Technique and Performance *(1994, 2020), Co-Editor of* Current Approaches in Drama Therapy *(2nd and 3rd editions), and* The Self in Performance

'The writing is immediate, visceral and urgent in ways which capture and convey what it is to be with embodied, somatic experience. Similarly, the chapter authors mine their insights and understandings from the inside out. Their relational and often moving accounts coalesce into a rich and expansive narrative. This results in a body of work which provides a compelling intersectional and intercultural take on new, diverse and relevant approaches in healing the multifarious wounds of trauma.'

Bryn Jones, MA, HCPC, *Dramatherapist, Clinical Supervisor and Lecturer in Drama (MA Drama and Movement Therapy) at the Royal Central School of Speech and Drama (University of London)*

'This much needed book highlights ways of thinking somatically in dramatherapy and theatre about trauma. It provides a wide range of international perspectives and powerful encouragement for further research in this area. There is an enrichment of perspectives through the cross-fertilisation of theatre and dramatherapy. The chapters illustrate intersecting global North and South perspectives. They provide wonderful examples of dramatherapy as an intercultural space in the embodied healing of trauma and oppression. Literature on the use of the body in the healing of trauma through integration with other somatic approaches remains scarce. This book opens the way for further collaborations.'

Ditty Dokter, PhD, *self-employed dramatherapist (HCPC) and group analytic psychotherapist (UKCP). Former MA Dramatherapy course leader at various universities, doctoral research supervisor and lecturer at Anglia Ruskin University (UK) and Codarts (Netherlands). Co-author with Nisha Sajnani of* Intercultural Dramatherapy: Imagination and Action at the Intersections of Difference *(Routledge, 2023)*

'We know that the actor's body is not just a biological machinery that the actor's mind can master. It has a say in the ways we construe the world and take decisions, it stores positive and negative emotions, and it "keeps the score" of our traumas. Focussing on the latter issue, this book has all it takes to be a milestone. It shows how the embodied nature of drama can help unfreeze the traumas dwelling in our bodies, and how the gentle and respectful approach of dramatherapy can offer us a chance to heal them.'

Salvo Pitruzzella, *author of* Drama, Creativity, and Intersubjectivity: Roots of Change in Dramatherapy *(Routledge, 2017). Member of Honour of the European Federation of Dramatherapy*

'This book makes an important and exciting contribution to the fields of dramatherapy, theatre, performance, and actor training in relation to imaginatively embodied and somatic approaches to the healing of trauma. Jean-François Jacques has brought together a dynamic mixture of multimodal and interdisciplinary approaches to embodied healing practice in this publication. The authors present varied and creative perspectives on the use of embodiment in theoretical contributions to the field of trauma, clinical practice, practice research projects, participatory arts projects, approaches to actor training, directorial and pedagogic practices, and play texts. Importantly, this publication explores cross-cultural perspectives and considers race and systemic racism, ethnicity, social class, gender, sexuality and disability in relation to trauma, healing and embodiment. The authors all situate their varied approaches to embodied healing from trauma as relational and explore this in their respective socio-historical contexts. Some chapters explore detailed case studies of individual clients or participants, others explore group or community contexts. A number of authors share personal experiences and healing journeys, and some chapters explore the collective experiences of trauma, for example the intergenerational experiences of enslavement and systemic racism. In addition, this book addresses the under-explored potential of the embodied methods and principles developed by theatre practitioners such as Michael Chekhov, Jacques Lecoq, Augusto Boal and Susana Bloch for dramatherapy, generating a timely dialogue between these different disciplines. The contributing authors detail an inspiring use of creatively embodied healing techniques including a use of: play; games; gesture work; images; body sculpting; mask work; drawing; poetry; dance; vocal work; myths; metaphors; archetypes; embodied and written storytelling; autobiographical practice; creative historiography; and participatory performance making. This book will be a valuable resource for those working in the fields of dramatherapy, theatre, performance and actor training who are interested in the growing use of embodiment in the treatment of trauma.'

Dr Cass Fleming, *Co-Director of The Chekhov Collective UK and Senior Lecturer, department of Theatre and Performance, Goldsmiths, University of London*

'This collection of essays offers readers a thoughtful exploration of the specific ways in which the imaginative, embodied practice of drama therapy responds to the somatic reverberations of trauma. At once poetic and instructive, it is a must-read for students and experienced practitioners.'

Nisha Sajnani, PhD, *Director of the Program in Drama Therapy, New York University*

Trauma and Embodied Healing in Dramatherapy, Theatre and Performance

This edited volume explores the singularity of embodiment and somatic approaches in the healing of trauma from a dramatherapy, theatre and performance perspective.

Collating voices from across the fields of dramatherapy, theatre and performance, this book examines how different interdisciplinary and intercultural approaches offer unique and unexplored perspectives on the body as a medium for the exploration, expression and resolution of chronic, acute and complex trauma as well as collective and intergenerational trauma. The diverse chapters highlight how the intersection between dramatherapy and body-based approaches in theatre and performance offers additional opportunities to explore and understand the creative, expressive and imaginative capacity of the body, and its application to the healing of trauma.

The book will be of particular interest to dramatherapists and other creative and expressive arts therapists. It will also appeal to counsellors, psychotherapists, psychologists and theatre scholars.

J. F. Jacques, PhD, HCPC, is an independent dramatherapist, somatic practitioner, clinical supervisor, educator, researcher, artist and author with more than 20 years of experience in private practice, and in the statutory and voluntary services in the UK.

Trauma and Embodied Healing in Dramatherapy, Theatre and Performance

Edited by J. F. Jacques

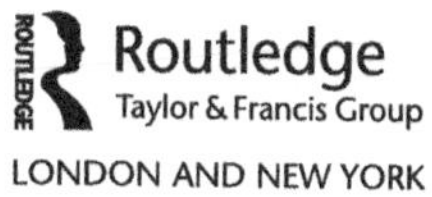

LONDON AND NEW YORK

Designed cover image: © iStock/Dusan Stankovic

First published 2024
by Routledge
4 Park Square, Milton Park, Abingdon, Oxon OX14 4RN

and by Routledge
605 Third Avenue, New York, NY 10158

Routledge is an imprint of the Taylor & Francis Group, an informa business

British Library Cataloguing-in-Publication Data
A catalogue record for this book is available from the British Library

Library of Congress Cataloging-in-Publication Data
Names: Jacques, Jean-François, 1970- editor.
Title: Trauma and embodied healing in dramatherapy, theatre and performance / edited by Jean-François (J.F.) Jacques.
Description: Abingdon, Oxon ; New York, NY : Routledge, 2024. |
Includes bibliographical references and index. |
Identifiers: LCCN 2023041128 (print) | LCCN 2023041129 (ebook) |
ISBN 9781032344836 (hbk) | ISBN 9781032344829 (pbk) |
ISBN 9781003322375 (ebk)
Subjects: LCSH: Drama--Therapeutic use. |
Psychic trauma--Treatment. | Generational trauma--Treatment.
Classification: LCC RC489.P7 T724 2024 (print) | LCC RC489.P7 (ebook) |
DDC 616.89/1523--dc23/eng/20231205
LC record available at https://lccn.loc.gov/2023041128
LC ebook record available at https://lccn.loc.gov/2023041129

ISBN: 978-1-032-34483-6 (hbk)
ISBN: 978-1-032-34482-9 (pbk)
ISBN: 978-1-003-32237-5 (ebk)

DOI: 10.4324/9781003322375

Typeset in Times New Roman
by SPi Technologies India Pvt Ltd (Straive)

I dedicate this book to Susan and Célestin, my life forces,
and to those who left us but whose memories stay with us.

Contents

Illustrations

Figures

Tables

Acknowledgments

The writing of this book has been marked by events pertaining to its subject. I wish to express my deepest gratitude to all of those who have showed support, affection and sympathy throughout the process of writing and editing.

I also wish to thank my editor at Routledge, Grace McDonnell, for her ongoing guidance, understanding and flexibility with what remains one of the most rewarding and demanding experiences in my life thus far.

Lastly, this book would not have been possible without the dedication and talent of all the contributors. I cannot thank them enough for their commitment and generosity to share their ideas and to break new grounds in the exploration of trauma and embodied healing.

About the Editor

J. F. Jacques, PhD, is a dramatherapist, somatic practitioner and clinical supervisor in private practice. He is originally from Belgium but has been living in the UK for the last 25 years. He worked for more than 13 years as a specialist dramatherapist in a community adult mental health service in the NHS. He holds a PhD in autobiographical performance and meaning from Anglia Ruskin University (Cambridge, UK) where he is also associate lecturer on the MA programme in Dramatherapy. His current areas of research focus on therapeutic theatre, autobiographical performance, trauma, shared meaning, aesthetics, embodiment, intersubjectivity, otherness and inbetweenness. He is a published author in the field of creative therapeutic practice and has presented at conferences nationally and internationally. Most recent papers include *Aesthetics of Connection in the Performance of Lived Experience* (2022), *Investigation into the Production of Meaning in Autobiographical Performance in Dramatherapy* (2020), and *A Relational Approach to Trauma, Memory, Mourning and Recognition through 'Death and the Maiden' by Ariel Dorfman* (2017). At the time of writing, he is in the last stages of completing a professional training in Somatic Experiencing®. He also trained in the Chekhov acting technique with Sinéad Rushe. He is co-editor of the *Dramatherapy* journal. Besides his work as a dramatherapist, he is an interdisciplinary artist and the director of the Theatre of Lived Experience, a visual, performance and literary arts practice aimed at opening public and creative spaces of dialogue.
www.jfjacques.com / www.theatreoflivedexperience.com

Contributors

Noha Bayoumy is an assistant lecturer at the Department of English Language and Literature, Faculty of Arts, Ain Shams University, Cairo, Egypt. At the time of writing, she was a PhD candidate at the School of English, University of Sheffield. Her project is entitled: *The Performance of Trauma in Contemporary Drama: Philip Ridley, Debbie Tucker Green and Nora Amin*. Her research interests include the intersections of trauma theories, theatre studies, memory and performance.

Ailin Conant is a Japanese-American director with a background in Lecoq pedagogy and physical theatre. Her South East-based devising company, Theatre Témoin, is a 1 Degree East and Without Walls Portfolio company. She has worked freelance for various companies including the RSC, the Royal Court, the Bush Theatre, New Earth, and Theatre 503, and has created work with refugees, ex-combatants, and survivors of trauma and conflict in Gaza, Lebanon, Sweden, Rwanda, Israel, Kashmir, Northern Ireland, and the USA. She is a twice-recipient of the Wellcome Trust People Award and is currently finishing a practice-as-research PhD at East 15, University of Essex. www.ailinconant.com / www.theatretemoin.com

Laura Facciponti Bond is a Full Professor of Drama and Interdisciplinary Studies at UNC Asheville teaching acting and emotional expression (US). She specializes in somatic education and its relationship to evidence-based emotional effector patterns (EEP). After 20 years of practice-research collaborating with Feldenkrais® practitioners, and research psychologist Susana Bloch, an original EEP researcher, she founded the Emotional Body® method. She develops specialty lessons for expanding expressive capabilities and somatic resiliency. She is the author of *TEAM For Actors: A Holistic Approach to Embodied Acting* and *The Emotional Body: A Method for Physical Self-Regulation*. Professor Bond is a recent recipient of the

Ruth Paddison Distinguished Professorship for promoting interdisciplinary connections between fields. During this time, she has been training in the consent-based practice of Theatrical Intimacy Education, and a year-long professional's training for a certification in *The Kinēsa® Process*, a Feldenkrais®-Inspired Movement System for Pain Relief and Heightened Physical, Emotional and Spiritual Wellbeing.

Shruti Garg (they/she) are a HCPC UK Registered Dramatherapist, queer affirmative therapist, theatre artist and a comic based in India. Currently they are pursuing training in trauma focused therapy from TISS, Mumbai. Shruti works with individuals and groups with varied concerns like grief, childhood trauma, anxiety, depression, adult neurodivergence, C-PTSD, and distress caused by systemic marginalisation. They specialise in working with queer/trans individuals and training healthcare professionals to be queer affirmative through uniquely designed embodied-experiential-play based workshops. As the founder of Raasta India and an Executive Member of Drama Therapy India, they aim to create more opportunities for the application of creative arts therapies across different spaces in India.

Craig Haen, PhD, RDT, CGP, LCAT, AGPA-F has a private practice working with children, adolescents, adults and families in White Plains, NY. He is cofounder and Training Director of the Kint Institute, which offers post-Masters clinical training in the arts and trauma treatment in New York City. He is a Fellow of the American Group Psychotherapy Association, where he serves as a founding member of the Diversity, Equity & Inclusion Task Force and co-chair of the Community Outreach Task Force. In these roles, he has coordinated responses to mass trauma events internationally for the past decade and co-authored the organization's public statements on human rights issues. He received the Social Responsibility Award in 2021 in recognition of this work. He is an independent scholar whose most recent book was *Creative Arts-Based Group Therapy with Adolescents*, with the late Nancy Boyd Webb.

Christiana Iordanou, PhD, is a HCPC registered Dramatherepist with more than 15 years clinical experience with children, adolescents, and adults in several public and private mental health settings. She is a Lecturer in Developmental Psychology and Mental Health at the University of Kent, UK. In 2018, she completed her PhD in Psychology with a fully funded scholarship from the University of Lancaster. Her research focused on the use of drawing and dramatization as memory aids in children's eyewitness testimony. She has written numerous research articles, case studies, and book chapters on topics such as the use of artistic means in children's eyewitness recall, dramatherapy with sexually abused children, and online supervision. She is co-editor of the British Association of Dramatherapists peer-reviewed journal *Dramatherapy*.

Danai Karvouni is an HCPC registered Dramatherapist, certified NARM Therapist and a Creative Clinical Supervisor trainee. She is originally from Greece where she initially studied Psychology and Clinical Psychopathology. She currently lives and practises in the UK. Her passion for working with trauma was developed whilst working in the NHS as a Senior Creative Arts Therapist in a trauma-informed prison treatment service for offenders with personality related difficulties. Following this, she worked as a Dramatherapist in a community Complex Post Traumatic Stress Disorder (C-PTSD) service, promoting trauma-informed practice across the Trust. She currently works as a Specialist Psychological Therapist offering support to staff and service users within community forensic services in the NHS. She is also an Associate Lecturer at Anglia Ruskin University teaching on the Masters programme in Dramatherapy and has a private practice. She is interested in theatre, yoga and clowning.

Sarah Mann Shaw is a supervisor, dramatherapist and psychotherapist in private practice in the UK. She has extensive experience of working with the impact of trauma, abuse and early attachment disruption with children and young people alongside statutory, charity and private agencies. She also supervises therapists who work in these fields. She has written chapters for the *Routledge International Handbook of Dramatherapy* (2016), *Arts Therapies in International Practice Informed by Neuroscience and Research* (Routledge 2021), and *Space, Place and Dramatherapy* (Routledge 2023). She has two articles published in the *Dramatherapy* journal, 'Metaphor, Symbol and the Healing Process in Dramatherapy' (1996), and 'The Drama of Shame' co-written with Di Gammage (2011). She has a particular interest in the interplay between neuroscience, embodied experience and the therapeutic relationship.

Jessica Mayson is an HPCSA-registered drama therapist working in Cape Town, South Africa (MA, University of the Witwatersrand). She works with individuals and groups, with children, adolescents and adults in community-based and private practice settings. Her particular focus is on supporting her clients navigate the impact of trauma, build resilience and process challenging transitions. In her practice, Jessica is committed to offering socially just creative spaces where parts of self and community can be understood, find expression and integration.

Angelo Miramonti, PhD, is a professor of Community Theatre at the Fine Arts University of Cali (Colombia), a lecturer in Trauma and Psychosocial Support at the Technical University of Würzburg-Schweinfurt (Germany), and a registered drama therapist in Italy. He is the founder of the 'Arts for Reconciliation' research project, using theatre for conflict transformation. He is experienced in using drama, poetry, myths and dance to conduct groups with former combatants and people affected by armed conflicts and natural disasters. He coordinated rehabilitation programs for child soldiers in Uganda and Congo with international NGOs and child protection programs with UNICEF. He is conducting anthropological research on spirit possession in Senegal and transcultural therapy for migrants in Italy. He authored several articles and four books on the therapeutic dimension of possession cults in Senegal and the use of arts in peacebuilding.

Roanna Mitchell is a performance-maker and movement artist, and Senior Lecturer at the University of Kent where she specialises in psychophysical performance practice. She is also co-director of The Chekhov Collective UK, the leading UK practice research centre exploring contemporary uses of Michael Chekhov's technique in the arts and beyond. From 2010 to 2018 she worked closely alongside Susie Orbach as artistic director and project coordinator of the charity AnyBody UK. She has created/directed/movement-directed performance internationally, including collaborations with Richard Schechner in India and the US. Roanna has published on actor-wellbeing, body activism, Chekhov technique in actor-movement and dance, and dialogues between theatre training and therapy. Her recent work focuses on applications of psychophysical performer training techniques in community and mental health settings, especially in relation to supporting survivors of Borderline Personality Disorder diagnosis.

Shiu Hei Larry Ng, RDT, NADTA is a registered drama therapist and a certified Feldenkrais Method® practitioner living and practising in Hong Kong. He also completed professional training in Satir Transformational Systemic Therapy and is now studying Neuro-Dramatic-Play under Dr Sue Jennings, and the Therapeutic Spiral Model of Psychodrama. As an artist, he was trained in Physical and Devising Theatre (Lecoq approach), Corporeal Mime (Decroux system), and specializes in mask. He learnt mask design and making from Donato Sartori, Matteo Destro and Renzo Sindoca. He is also a playback theatre practitioner who completed all four levels of training, with more than ten years of on-going experience of practice. He has been working through different kinds of applied theatre modalities to serve a wide range of population in the community. He is also graduated in philosophy and drama education.

Margie Pankhurst is passionate about the transformative healing which stems from embodied creativity, acceptance and curiosity with a deep belief in people's innate ability to find relief when the right environment is available to them. She qualified as a drama therapist through the MA programme at Drama for Life, Witwatersrand, South Africa. She works in many environments including children and adults in formal mental health facilities, people who lived on the street, NGO's and private practice.

Greta Sharp (they/them) is a transqueer disabled artist, writer and researcher who works across multiple disciplines, mainly publications, workshops, collage, and academic research. Their research is located in the intersection between transqueer identities and disability, focussing on the voice and embodied forms of healing within community in relation to the natural world. For the past couple of years, Greta has been exploring their personal relationship with the sea as a survivor whose trauma is located in their bodymind with sounds, sights and smells of the British seaside. Their exploration into the voice expands on research into queer spirituality, being in the sea as a form of resourcing and co-regulation, relating to the sea as a trans AFAB (assigned female at birth) person, and crip care and access.

Emma Westcott has been using body awareness techniques within her psychotherapy practice for over 30 years. Her training as a Movement and Drama Therapist at Sesame in 1989 was followed by her becoming an Integrative Arts Psychotherapist at the Institute for Arts in Psychotherapy and Education. Her subsequent development benefited enormously from supervision within clinics with renowned psychotherapists Anthony Ryle and David Livingstone Smith. She has worked as a psychotherapist in a variety of settings: residential psychiatric care, schools, a Borderline Personality Disorder and Psycho Sexual Clinic in the NHS, and the Priory group. Over the last 20 years she has been in private practice working increasingly with adults with a history of trauma. The experiential and embodied practice that underpinned her earliest training has been the cornerstone of all her clinical work as the crucial pathway to connection in the clinician/client relationship and in the client's compassionate and integrating relationship with Self. Her work is particularly informed by many years of Jungian Analysis and by the discoveries of neurobiology. She has lived and worked in London and Spain, and now runs a private practice in Suffolk, UK.

Foreword

Cathy Malchiodi

The fields of expressive arts therapy and creative arts therapies have long known that the body plays a role in mental health and wellness. Long before the formal practice of psychotherapy emerged, humans turned to arts-based expression as a way of transforming difficulties when confronted by crisis, tragedy, or loss. As a species, we have been turning to the healing rhythms and synchrony of the arts to confront and resolve distress for thousands of years. These actions emerged not only as individual forms of reparation, but also through social engagement, capitalizing on connection with others and community as agents of healing. In recent years, nonverbal approaches including an emphasis on the body's response to trauma, have emerged as accepted and effective methods to address and resolve traumatic stress.

Embodiment is a term that is now ubiquitous in the field of mental health. The word embodiment refers to a tangible or visible form of an idea, quality, or feeling. It is the personification, incarnation, or manifestation of a way of being or characteristic, such as "she is the embodiment of hope" or "their musical performance embodied joy and exuberance."

In contemporary psychotherapy, the term embodiment has taken on a slightly different meaning. Many therapists are now familiar with the idea that the "body keeps the score" (van der Kolk, 2014) or the "body remembers" (Rothschild, 2000). "Our issues are in our tissues" (author unknown) is another phrase often used by body-based practitioners (yoga, massage, and others) to describe the importance of physical awareness. Psychotherapists generally see embodiment as a capacity that supports a healthy relationship with our bodies, emphasizing the importance of observing and noticing one's internal felt sense, also known as interoception.

These ideas influenced the definition of embodiment and what has become known as *embodied practices*, particularly within the field of traumatic stress. These practices underscore the importance of increasing connections between interoception (the felt sense) and exteroception (external sensations and experiences). Embodiment implies that the central focus for emotional repair, transformation, and recovery is through becoming aware of our physical being through the senses. It is a way to include the body as a focus for health and well-being through self-appreciation and self-acceptance of what we physically sense and feel in the moment (Malchiodi, 2020). This perspective also proposes that embodiment is not just a one-time event but is an ongoing practice of establishing a relationship with one's body. It involves various mind-body awareness approaches to sustain attention to how one's body responds and feels in the present moment. Body-based awareness is a form of "somatic intelligence" that increases an individual's understanding of self, others, and the world.

As a trauma specialist, I believe the kinds of cognitions, emotions, and somatosensory experiences we want to make "stick" with clients when using art-based approaches are key to eventually helping them imagine new narratives, post-trauma. In other words, if we do not eventually help individuals move away from distress, we leave them with thoughts, feelings and sensations that will not support new narratives of pleasure, confidence and hope. This premise also emphasizes that somatic approaches re-sensitize body and mind and develop the capacity for positive emotion through engagement with the body (Malchiodi, 2022). Within the field of expressive arts, dramatic enactment in the form of dramatherapy is an approach that uniquely integrates multiple pathways for imagining novel and reparative stories and restoring health and well-being in the body as well as the mind.

Why is dramatherapy an embodied approach? I think there is one obvious answer to this question—it helps individuals find reparation through *performative change*. That is, individuals are engaged in a multi-layered, action-oriented process that taps many levels of expression. Whether improvisation, role play, theatrical reading, or actual performance on stage, dramatic enactment generally integrates movement, gesture, sound, voice, playfulness, visual experiences, and storytelling. Dramatic enactment provides the opportunity to try out new narratives not only through language, but through embodiment of a character.

In years of work with survivors of interpersonal violence, disasters, or war, I have witnessed individuals who are literally haunted by a theater of sensations in their own bodies, unable to control how those sensations impact them in multiple and adverse ways. Dramatherapy addresses the complex sensory and somatic issues that traumatic stress causes and that are not easily ameliorated by more cognitive forms of intervention. Landy (2005) explains this as the "doubleness of all human life." In other words, when enacting a role, the individual has to be more than one entity simultaneously, to play one's own role and the pretend role. I believe this dynamic naturally allows people to experience and act out multiple perspectives, not only in the mind, but also through the body.

This book brings together the wisdom and collective knowledge of experts in the application of the principles of dramatherapy. Each chapter introduces, explores, and illuminates one or more aspects of how dramatic enactment addresses embodiment within the context of trauma. However, this volume and its editor go far beyond that—they bring to light the integrative potentials of dramatherapy, theatre, and performance in all its depth and complexities. These intersections are the foundations of why these approaches are resonant with somatic practices and body-based strategies.

Trauma and Embodied Healing in Dramatherapy, Theatre and Performance sets a new standard for how psychotherapy can envision the treatment of traumatic stress. It expands our knowledge of creative and expressive methods and just how they can be applied to resolving the body's experience of trauma. More importantly, this book provides readers with a framework for establishing a pathway to re-sensitizing the body to narratives that are at once resilient, reparative, and restorative.

Cathy A. Malchiodi, PhD
Author, *Trauma and Expressive Arts Therapy: Brain, Body, and Imagination in the Healing Process*

References

Landy, R. (2005). *Drama therapy: Concepts, theories and practices* (2nd ed.). Jessica Kingsley.

Malchiodi, C. A. (2020). *Trauma and expressive arts therapy: Brain, body, and imagination in the healing process*. Guilford Publications.

Malchiodi, C. A. (2022). *Handbook of expressive arts therapy*. Guilford Publications.

Rothschild, B. (2000). *The body remembers*. Norton.

van der Kolk, B. (2014). *The body keeps the score*. Penguin.

Introduction

Interdisciplinary Perspectives on Trauma and the Body

J. F. Jacques

This book is located in a long philosophical, artistic, and scientific tradition that has claimed the wisdom of the body, its inherent knowledge, and its creative potential for expression, change, and healing. The German philosopher Friedrich Nietzsche was one of the precursors who recognised the innate capacities of the body to inform and reflect our deepest feelings, needs, intentions, and desires. As he wrote, 'The body is a great reason, a manifold with one sense, a war and a peace, a herd and a herdsman' (Nietzsche, 2005, p.30). Nietzsche suggests the possibility (or imperative) to think about the body in psychophysical dynamics terms to overturn the supremacy of reason and the mind (Voigt, 2019). He indicates that the body is also a stage of conflicts that bears the imprint of life experiences, such as trauma, that can shatter its own integrity. The physiological body holds a duality as a lived and living entity or, as Kirsten Voigt writes (2019), 'as shaped and shaping, as exposed to forces and exerting them, in its growth and vulnerability'. It is in that duality that reside its sufferings but also its source for life, vitality, and rejuvenation, as it will be explored in the following pages.

This edited volume aims to explore the singularity of embodiment and somatic approaches in the healing of trauma from a dramatherapy, theatre and performance perspective.

The book brings together voices from international scholars, researchers, practitioners, and clinicians in the field of dramatherapy, theatre and performance, to better understand how these different approaches offer unique and unexplored perspectives on the body as a medium for the exploration, expression, and resolution of chronic, acute, and complex trauma, as well as collective and intergenerational trauma in different cultural contexts.

The links between traumatic experiences and the body are now well documented and researched. Established authors and clinicians in the fields of neuroscience, somatic psychotherapy, and psychology have contributed to significant advances in the understanding of how the body and the nervous system respond to, internalise, store, and speak the trauma. The somatic of trauma translates ways in which the body retains emotions and traumatic memories cut off from cortical and verbal processing. The work of healing

DOI: 10.4324/9781003322375-1

consists in supporting the body to self-regulate as well as working through the sensorimotor imprints of the trauma towards psychosomatic integration.

The somatic of trauma tells us that if the trauma is locked in the body, the body is also the key that can unlock the legacy of the traumatic event(s). As primarily a form of embodied therapy using the emotional and cognitive capacity of the body, dramatherapy offers additional opportunities to think somatically about trauma. From its origins, dramatherapy has underlined the centrality of embodiment as being a core therapeutic factor of change. As Jones (2005) observed, 'embodiment offers a perspective on experience that allows the client to bring or access material physically, to explore bodily experience through the body within the therapy space' (p.257).

Recent studies looking at establishing communal conceptualisation of core therapeutic factors in dramatherapy have shown the centrality of embodied processes in clinical practice. Frydman et al. (2022) describes embodiment as 'a physical, vocal, or emotional inhabiting of the body, attending to sensations, touch, the spectrum of physicalized expression of emotions, thoughts, reactions, impulses, and inner experiences' (p.8). According to this research, embodiment accounts for 15.8% of therapeutic change in dramatherapy alongside six other factors. In another study, de Witte et al. (2021) also identified embodiment as a specific factor producing therapeutic benefits and contributing 'to client experiencing a felt awareness' (p.15).

Yet, literature on the use of the body in the healing of trauma in dramatherapy, the integration with other somatic approaches, and the similarities and differences between these remain scarce. The unique contribution of dramatherapy to the field of trauma from an embodiment perspective largely remains to be explored and conceptualised. A number of very recent studies providing a systematic review and meta-analysis of published empirical research in dramatherapy and drama-based therapies have not allowed to clearly show the moderating effect and therapeutic effectiveness of specific interventions (i.e. embodiment, body-based, or somatic) on particular diagnostic categories (i.e. post-traumatic stress disorder or complex trauma). For example, a paper reviewing the literature on empirical dramatherapy research (Armstrong et al., 2019) does not cite any specific studies on embodiment and trauma. A more recent systematic review of 30 studies looking at the evidence of the effectiveness of drama-based therapies on mental health outcomes (Orkibi et al., 2023), does not allow to clarify the links between specific therapeutic factors in dramatherapy, such as dramatic embodiment, and changes in outcomes. Another recent research (Constien & Junker, 2023) aimed at compiling a comprehensive database of dramatherapy literature produced between 2000 and 2021 and comprised of a total of 345 journal articles, found eight publications with the keyword 'embodiment' (2.32%) and seven with the keyword 'trauma' (2.02%). The analysis doesn't specify the number of publications with both keywords. Lastly, in a research reviewing 24 dramatherapy interventions published between 2007 and 2017, Feniger-Schaal and Orkibi (2020) do not report studies that explicitly name trauma or show interventions specifically based on embodied approaches.

This volume is therefore hoping to address a significant gap in the existing literature to explore and rigorously investigate the links between dramatherapy, trauma, body, and healing. As such, it largely responds to the observations made by Johnson and Sajnani (2014) that, 'we have an obligation to continue to refine and develop more sophisticated and targeted approaches to trauma within drama therapy, and to find ways of empirically testing our work' (p.20).

Although this volume is, in its majority, about embodied approaches in dramatherapy theory, practice and research, and their contributions to the field of trauma, it is nevertheless located at the intersection of other embodied practices in the disciplines of theatre and performance that reflect traditions exploring the physicality of the body and its expressive and artistic capabilities, but that also have a particular interest in the various forms and presentations of trauma. Indeed, it seems now accepted and even recommended that any effective interventions to heal trauma embrace a multimodal and interdisciplinary approach.

The intersection of dramatherapy and body-based approaches in theatre and performance on the fabric and potential of the body to translate, generate, and rework emotional states and memories also remains largely under researched. The link between these disciplines offers additional fertile grounds to further explore and understand the creative, expressive, and imaginative capacity of the body, and its application to the healing of trauma. The works of Chekhov, Lecoq, Grotowski, Meyerhold, Artaud, or Copeau for instance provide additional opportunities to discover the language and history of the body, its emotional expressiveness through physicality, gesture, and movement, and its potentiality for healing and repair. The emphasis on kinaesthetic and embodied relational practice can also significantly contribute to a better understanding of the links between embodiment, trauma, and the arts.

Based on this brief overview, the aims of this volume are threefold:

- to explore the unique contribution of dramatherapy as an embodied therapeutic modality to the field of trauma healing;
- to advance an interdisciplinary dialogue between the fields of dramatherapy, theatre and performance on physicality, trauma, and healing;
- to identify strategies of embodied healing based on specific processes and mechanisms within dramatherapy, theatre and performance.

As the book is based on the concepts of trauma and embodiment, it seems important to provide brief definitions to enable the reader to understand its premise. Throughout these pages, trauma will describe the long-lasting physiological, emotional, and cognitive effects of life situations that threatened the safety, integrity, and survival of the human body. Embodiment is a term that, as Niedenthal and Maringer observe, 'carries a fair amount of baggage' (2009, p.122). For the purpose of clarity, embodiment will describe a process of awareness of the body from the inside and outside as belonging in the world, how this is experienced and how it can lead to change (Shapiro, 2020).

The contributions in this volume are from a diverse range of practitioners, scholars, researchers, and clinicians in the fields of dramatherapy, theatre and performance. The book reflects a wide, international, and intercultural perspective on the intersections of the body, trauma, healing, and theatre, with contributions from a variety of cultural and social backgrounds, traditions, and practices in these fields.

The first part of the book presents several original theoretical contributions to the field of trauma and embodied healing from dramatherapy and theatre perspectives. The second part constitutes a brief literary interlude at the intersection of trauma, body, healing, and society. The third section covers a range of innovative practices and research in dramatherapy, theatre and performance to further understand what these perspectives effectively add to the existing knowledge on trauma and the body.

In Chapter 1, Craig Haen introduces the original concept of the imagined body to describe how the pairing of imagination and embodiment in dramatherapy can be profoundly curative for people who experienced trauma. Haen presents this unique contribution of dramatherapy to trauma treatment by discussing the theoretical underpinnings of this approach and its application to practice. He argues that the integration of imaginative and embodied practices transcends the shattering effects of traumatic experiences on the body by supporting memory reconsolidation and counteracting procedural adaptations.

In Chapter 2, Laura Facciponti Bond writes from a theatre perspective about the method of the Emotional Body®, a trauma-informed practice based on the relationship between physicality and emotions, and aimed at developing emotional regulation and increasing the expressive capabilities of the body. Bond explains how she developed the method after many years of research into somatic awareness, expression, and self-regulation. Bond shows how the method helps identify expressive emotional patterns in the body but also enables the creation of new patterns for greater fluency, flexibility, and agency. She also discusses the therapeutic applications and benefits of the method in relation to trauma healing.

In Chapter 3, Shiu Hei Larry Ng describes an original therapeutic framework based on Lecoq's pedagogical sequence of working with masks to facilitate the healing of traumatised bodies in an Asian context. Ng discusses four types of masks used in Lecoq's teaching and their applications to address different aspects of trauma. He argues for a reversed sequence that corresponds to the different stages of trauma healing whilst also discussing how the different masks can effectively support the indirect and embodied processing of trauma. Ng concludes by acknowledging the intercultural issues of working with masks from a specific theatre tradition.

In Chapter 4, Christiana Iordanou examines the impact of online working, which became common practice following the Covid-19 pandemic, on engaging with the body in dramatherapy with traumatised children. She argues that the shift to a two-dimensional space is simply different without precluding the advantages of face-to-face work. Iordanou critically discusses the adjustments required by the inherent distance in online working and the additional opportunities that it creates for sensory and bodily practices.

In Chapter 5, I introduce an outline of an original integrative psychophysical approach for the healing of trauma mainly based on the teaching of the actor and director Michael Chekhov and the notion of physical gesture. I provide an overview of psychophysicality as described in neuro- and cognitive science, in a range of acting traditions and techniques in theatre, and in trauma-focused somatic therapies. I conclude by critically considering the originality and limitations of the model, and how it provides additional resources to enable and support the embodied healing of trauma.

In Chapter 6, Margie Pankhurst and Jessica Mayson present the outline of an original dramatherapeutic approach based on embodied and symbolic play to meet the needs of children in South Africa who experience multifaceted trauma as a result of ongoing developmental, relational, socio-economic, and historical maltreatments. They critically discuss the benefits of an embodied approach to meaningfully heal the traumatic wounds of young boys, whilst also recognising the limits imposed by the structural inequalities in postcolonial contexts.

In Chapter 7, Danai Karvouni discusses the outlines of an original framework integrating dramatherapy with the NeuroAffective Relational Model (NARM) to treat developmental trauma. She critically discusses the limitations and strengths of both embodied approaches before suggesting an integrative developmental framework for theory and practice. Karvouni argues that an integrative model of embodied healing provides safer and more effective ways of working with development trauma, and essential resources to ensure the wellbeing of the therapist.

Chapter 8 constitutes a transition between the theoretical, and practice and research perspectives. As such, it is at the intersection between questions pertinent to trauma healing that are addressed in both sections. In this chapter, Noha Bayoumy discusses the play *Theatre of Crime*, by the Egyptian writer Nora Amin, to bring the focus to the way in which the individual embodied experience of trauma resulting from the sexual violence against women cannot be considered without acknowledging the context in which it happens and the structural forces of oppression that contribute to it. Bayoumy argues that healing from trauma requires embodied action where the body becomes a tool for resistance and subversion. She also discusses how, as Amin suggests, theatre can be an essential space for collective embodied healing through resistance and the call for social justice.

In Chapter 9, Sarah Mann Shaw discusses the creation of a theatre piece in individual dramatherapy with an adopted child to help process early trauma. Her chapter integrates perspectives from neuroscience, theatre, and dramatherapy to show how theatre making can effectively support embodied healing. She argues that theatre provides a container for the safe exploration and expression of traumatic experiences held in the body. Mann Shaw particularly describes ways in which embodied metaphors can safely assist a young person to develop a sense of autonomy and control, and the ability to connect with themselves and others.

In Chapter 10, Roanna Mitchell discusses how psychophysical approaches in theatre, especially those based on Michael Chekhov's teaching, can effectively contribute to relational repair, more specifically for survivors of a diagnosis of borderline personality disorder. Mitchell presents the outlines of an artist-led project to argue about the radical potential of acknowledgement in the healing of trauma. She suggests that to believe is to heal as too often trauma survivors are denied the true nature of their experiences. Mitchell shows how creative embodied expression embedded in the art form of theatre can contribute to relational thirdness that she envisages as the cornerstone of healing.

In Chapter 11, Emma Westcott intentionally focuses on the hands and provides a detailed discussion on how that part of the body can be a vehicle for the expression of traumatic imprints. She discusses four case studies that each illustrate how paying attention to the implicit language of the hands, in dramatherapy practice, can help bring coherence and meaning to the experiences of traumatised individuals. Westcott argues that hands provide a portal through which clients can connect with their felt experiences in ways that can be profoundly healing.

In Chapter 12, Greta Sharp provides a personal testimony on the power of the voice in the healing of developmental trauma. Sharp draws on Polyvagal Theory research to discuss how the voice can effectively regulate and heal the nervous system. They also argue for environmental, performance, and community healing practices whereby the traumatised body can find containment and safety.

In Chapter 13, Ailin Conant explores different modes of meaning making in theatre practice that respond to personal and collective traumatic events. Conant argues that the complexity of trauma requires multimodal interventions that enable the creation of new meanings and restore coherence to the traumatised body. She presents the outcomes of a practice-as-research project created in collaboration with first responders who worked through the Troubles in Northern Ireland. She introduces excerpts from the performance to illustrate the benefits and limits of embodied aesthetic forms and processes in theatre practice that engages with trauma histories.

In Chapter 14, Shruti Garg describes a mythopoetic approach to trauma based on personal experience. Garg provides a poignant self-reflective account on the role of myths, dreams, symbols, and embodied rituals in the healing of developmental trauma. Garg suggests that a mythopoetic language provides an effective container for the indirect expression of thoughts, emotions, and memories that may elude consciousness as a result of trauma. They also argue for culturally sensitive practices that acknowledge the power of myths and stories in the healing of trauma, whilst avoiding assumptions and generalisations that may deny individuals from finding their own healing path.

In Chapter 15, Angelo Miramonti presents a participatory research project with Afro-Colombian youth exploring how the enactment and embodiment of historical documents can contribute to the healing of the intergenerational trauma of enslavement. Miramonti explores how the legacy of historical trauma keeps finding an expression in present-day systemic racism and violence in Colombia. His research shows how performance in dramatherapy based on the embodiment of archives enable the integration of collective memory. He argues that the multidimensional trauma of Afro-descendants requires a multimodal therapy that acknowledges the belonging of individuals to an intergenerational and collective body in a way that resonates with other chapters.

The reader will not fail to notice a number of threads that run through the different chapters and add to the understanding of trauma and embodied healing from a dramatherapy, theatre and performance perspective:

- First, different contributions illustrate a number of embodied, multimodal, and non-verbal strategies grounded in the art form of theatre, and their applications in trauma healing. These include psychophysical gestures, dramatic embodiment, enactments, masks, the emotional body, the voice, and embodied play.
- Second, authors show how embodied imagination contributes to the repairing and creation of new neural pathways in body physiology and the brain.
- Third, contributors emphasise the importance and effectiveness of embodied metaphors for their ability to provide safety and containment in the expression and resolution of the unspeakable.
- Fourth, the value of embodied relationality is largely discussed to show its role in the acknowledgement, witnessing, validation, and healing of the traumatised body.
- Fifth, several authors adopt a socio-political and historical perspective to discuss the traumatised body politic, systemic forces of traumatisation, the multifaceted and multidimensional aspects of trauma, and the need for culture-sensitive practices.
- Sixth, a number of contributions argue for the creation of community co-embodied spaces for the healing of trauma alongside more traditional individual approaches.

This volume doesn't claim to represent an exhaustive account of the innovative body of work exploring trauma and embodied healing from a dramatherapy, theatre and performance perspective. If anything, it sets the foundations for further exploration and research. Amongst its limitations, the dialogue between dramatherapy, theatre and performance studies is only emerging. The integration of theory and practice suggested in this volume can only enhance both fields of study and their capacity to effectively contribute to the complex area of trauma healing. The book also does not cover all categories of trauma. The reader will understand that such an undertaking was beyond its scope. It seems important however to extend to other presentations the insights and learnings contained in this volume. Lastly, there is a large number of embodied theatre traditions that undoubtedly could be explored for their therapeutic applications. The book only refers to a few. This fascinating investigation will hopefully continue beyond the content of these pages.

Before venturing further into the book, it feels necessary to flag up the following two points.

First, the reader will find different spellings of the word *dramatherapy* throughout the volume. This is because the discipline has developed and evolved differently in different parts of the world. It seemed important to respect these different traditions. The reader will find that what might look like a discrepancy is transcended by a common body of theoretical and practical knowledge.

Second, it is important to make the reader aware that, given the subject of this volume, some of its content may be perceived as disturbing or unsettling. The reader must be reassured that the material in the book was selected with the view of sensitively meeting its aims and of contributing to new knowledge. Having said this, I urge the reader to remain aware of the level of care that may be required to ensure a safe and rewarding reading.

Drew Leder (2020) reminds us that 'healing' shares the same etymological roots as 'whole' and describes a process of re-integration. As he writes, 'if there are healing strategies that focus on *separating* from the body, there are others that involve *embracing* the body, moving closer to it at times of challenge' (p.11). My hope is that this volume will contribute to healing strategies that acknowledge and value individual bodies located in worlds torn by trauma. It is also my hope that the reader will find in this book sources of knowledge and inspiration that embrace interdisciplinary perspectives.

References

Armstrong, C. R., Frydman, J. S., & Rowe, C. (2019). A Snapshot of Empirical Drama Therapy Research: Conducting a General Review of the Literature. *GMS Journal of Arts Therapies*, Vol. 1, 1–16.

Constien, T. & Junker, J. (2023). Analysis of the Body of Literature Based on a New Drama Therapy Literature Database. *The Arts in Psychotherapy*, Vol. 82. https://doi.org/10.1016/j.aip.2022.101989

de Witte, M., Orkibi, H., Zarate, R., Karkou, V., Sajnani, N., Malhotra, B., Ho, R. T. H., Kaimal, G., Baker, F. A., & Koch, S. C. (2021). From therapeutic factors to mechanisms of change in the creative arts therapies: A scoping review. *Frontiers in Psychology*. 12:678397. https://doi.org/10.3389/fpsyg.2021.678397

Feniger-Schaal, R. & Orkibi, H. (2020). Integrative systemic review of drama therapy intervention research. *Psychology of Aesthetics, Creativity, and the Arts*, 14(1), 68–80.

Frydman, J. S., Cook, A., Armstrong, C. R., Rowe, C., & Kern, C. (2022). The drama therapy core processes: A Delphi study establishing a North American perspective. *The Arts in Psychotherapy*, Vol. 80. https://doi.org/10.1016/j.aip.2022.101939

Johnson, D. R. & Sajnani, N. (2014). The role of drama therapy in trauma Treatment. In N. Sajnani & R. D. Johnson (Eds.), *Trauma-Informed drama therapy* (pp. 5–23). Charles C. Thomas Publisher.

Jones, P. (2005). *The arts therapies: A revolution in healthcare*. Brunner-Routledge.

Leder, D. (2020). The absent body (and beyond). *The Philosopher*, 108(3), 5–11.

Niedenthal, P. M. & Maringer, M. (2009). Embodied emotion considered. *Emotion Review*, 1(2), 122–128.

Nietzsche, F. (2005), *Thus spoke Zarathustra* (translated by G. Parkes). Oxford University Press.

Orkibi, H., Keisari, S., Sajnani, N. L., & de Witte, M. (2023). Effectiveness of drama-based therapies on mental health outcomes: A systematic review and meta-analysis of controlled studies. *Psychology of Aesthetics, Creativity, and the Arts*. https://dx.doi.org/10.1037/aca0000582

Shapiro, L. (2020). *The somatic therapy workbook*. Ulysses Press.

Voigt, K. (2019). The Great reason of the body: Friedrich Nietzsche, Joseph Beuys and the art of giving meaning to matter and earth. *Tate Papers*, no. 32. Retrieved from www.tate.org.uk/research/tate-papers/32/nietzsche-beuys-giving-meaning-matter-earth

Part I

Theoretical Perspectives

Chapter 1

The Imagined Body

Drama Therapy's Unique Contribution to Trauma Treatment

Craig Haen

It is now widely understood that trauma exposure impacts people multidimensionally, involving physiological, neurological, emotional, and cognitive domains. Traumatic events that are directly experienced almost always involve an overwhelming of one's agency and boundaries, with the body as the site of impact. Survivors' bodies serve as the archive of trauma's reverberations (Haen, 2022), storing embodied memories of what has happened and communicating the trauma narrative through symptoms, behaviors, and body language before words are accessible (Sutton, 2020). For this reason, there are a multitude of clinical approaches for treating trauma that engage the body: as a means of communicating and processing the emotional impact, as a source of self-regulatory practices to resolve hyperarousal of the nervous system, and as an experiential entity through which states of shutdown and freezing are evoked and reworked. Ironically, in this turn toward focusing on the body, practitioners have successfully argued against Cartesian mind-body dualism while also largely failing to consider the important mental function of imagination.

Mental imagery is an ever-present part of most humans' lives, with a flow of images constituting what we consider our stream of consciousness (Damasio, 2021). Our minds are continually shifting between focusing on the outside world and on the internal imaginative one (Carroll, 2020). Both voluntary and involuntary, imaginative processes undergird perception, problem-solving, decision making, empathy and self-expression, and can guide thoughts and behaviors (Blackwell, 2019; Chan, 2021). As Zabelina (2023) noted, intrusive mental imagery is also the characteristic symptom of people who have experienced trauma.

Several scholars have argued that increased attention be paid to imagination as a transtheoretical mechanism of change in psychotherapy generally (Chan, 2021), and in trauma treatment specifically (Haen, 2020; Malchiodi, 2020; Rubinstein & Lahad, 2022). However, an examination of foundational and recent texts on embodied trauma treatment approaches shows little explicit focus on use of imagination within dance/movement therapy (Dieterich-Hartwell & Melsom, 2022), sensorimotor psychotherapy (Ogden & Fisher,

DOI: 10.4324/9781003322375-3

2015), somatic experiencing (Levine, 2015), and polyvagal-informed therapies (Porges & Dana, 2018). Conversely, there has been scant consideration of embodiment within approaches that center the use of imagination, including guided imagery, imaginal exposure, imagery rescripting and rehearsal, and top-down treatment modalities based in cognitive-behavioral paradigms.

This chapter will attempt to bridge those gaps by considering the contributions of drama therapy to the treatment of psychological trauma, both for those who meet the diagnostic criteria of Post-Traumatic Stress Disorder (PTSD) and for the large patient population whose traumatic experiences have not been validated by that diagnosis. I will discuss ways that imagination is compromised by trauma and how re-accessing it within treatment is curative. However, I will argue that, unlike in sedentary approaches, the potential of trauma-specific drama therapy and other similar experiential therapies lies precisely in the pairing of imagination with embodiment. I will crystallize these ideas using the construct of the *imagined body*.

It is through the evocation of the imagined body that patient and therapist tap into emergent post-traumatic states of being which presage their development in the patient's life outside of the treatment space. I will draw on interdisciplinary theory and research, as well as case examples, to illustrate how drama therapy offers a clinical approach uniquely suited to working with traumatized people.

Imagination

Taylor (2013) defined imagination as the capacity to 'transcend time, place, and/or circumstance to think about what might have been, plan and anticipate the future, create fictional worlds, and consider alternatives to the actual experiences of our lives' (p. 3). Carroll (2020) noted three core processes from which all of the more nuanced and specialized forms of imagination derive: *simulation* (the creation of imaginative facsimiles of memory and experience), *mental time travel* (engagement with episodic memory of the past and projection into the future), and *perspective taking* (predicting others' thoughts and feelings through empathy and inference). Noting that mental imagery develops prior to language, Chan (2021) suggested that imagination may be 'a more primal medium through which all conceptual forms operate' (p. 68).

Rooted in the attachment relationship and developing out of childhood pretend play, imagination is gaining increased attention from developmental researchers for its links to skill acquisition in several domains, including executive functioning and emotion regulation (Haen, 2020; Harris, 2000). Historically, studies in the field of psychology have tended to focus on related constructs of creativity and innovation, rather than imagination (Thomson & Jacque, 2019). However, there has been a shift in recent years, marked by a greater number of empirical investigations from diverse fields, including cognitive neuroscience and evolutionary biology. Summarizing this research, Carroll (2020, p. 31) wrote:

> We can now say with confidence that the imagination is a neurological reality, that it is lodged in specific parts of the brain, that it consists of an identifiable set of components and processes, that these components and processes have adaptive functions, and that in fulfilling its functions imagination has been a major causal factor in making *Homo sapiens* the dominant species on earth.

Interest in imagination among neuroscientists has been spurred by the discovery of a network encompassing cortical midline regions of the brain that include the medial prefrontal cortex, posterior cingulate cortex, lateral parietal cortices, lateral temporal cortex, hippocampal formation, and precuneus (Chan, 2021). Named the default mode network (DMN) because it was originally thought to be the part that was active when the brain was doing little else, it has subsequently become known as the 'imagination network' due to its associations with daydreaming, rumination, mentalization, autobiographical recall, metaphorical thinking, theory of mind, empathy, cognitive flexibility, and creativity (Chan, 2021; Lanius et al., 2020). The DMN has been characterized as a hub that serves to integrate distributed representations from across the cortex (Villena-González & Cosmelli, 2020), making it 'the brain's most comprehensive network for the integration of information' (Carroll, 2020, p. 37).

One of the more striking features of the DMN is that it is equidistant from the central nodes of the sensory and motor networks. Lanius et al. (2020) noted the importance of this overlap, as distinct parts of the DMN's neuroanatomy have been associated with consciousness of thoughts and emotions, as well as with embodied sense of self. They reported that people with PTSD show reduced functional connectivity within the DMN compared to non-traumatized people, and suggested that this phenomenon correlates with the fuzzy self-experience often characteristic of trauma survivors. Deficiencies in sense of self are particularly apparent in somatically oriented descriptions such as, 'I feel dead inside' or 'I feel like my body doesn't belong to me.' Rubinstein and Lahad (2022) speculated that the experience of trauma may be related to these changes in the DMN. The neural connectivity of regions associated with both imagination and somatic processes suggests a concordance between body and imagination that can be harnessed in trauma treatment.

Traumatic Memory and Embodiment

Trauma is fundamentally rooted in memory: both experiencing repetitive, involuntary memories of intolerable past events, and difficulty recalling parts of those events in order to form a linear and coherent narrative. Intrusive memories usually present as brief flashes that provide a literal recall of aspects of the traumatic experience, although they also occasionally involve imagined elaborations. Compared to other psychiatric disorders in which patients struggle with disturbing thoughts and images, the memories of people with PTSD have been found to contain greater sensory components (Brewin & Vasterling, 2021). These elements are thought to be responsible for trauma memories being so difficult to integrate (Bryant, 2021).

Likewise, information processing models of PTSD propose that trauma memories contain visceral emotional, cognitive, and meaning-based aspects that are strongly wired within a fear network, so that the activation of one of these components triggers others (Bryant, 2021). This associative network is hypothesized to be the mechanism through which flashbacks are readily ignited by both external and internal stimuli. Lacking temporal anchoring, flashbacks involve an immersive reliving of the trauma without the double consciousness of remembering oneself in the past while also remaining rooted in the present (Hill, 2021).

People who have experienced trauma have been found to have similar challenges in imagining future events, especially positive ones (Brewin & Vasterling, 2021). Deficits in the ability to consider the future have ramifications for identity, agency, and problem-solving, as new actions and conversations are often preceded by first imagining them as possibilities. Imaginal preparedness is an important coping skill through which people can preview emotions that may accompany difficult circumstances, develop internal dialogues, and rehearse effective ways of responding (Lahad, 2019).

An additional, often-overlooked characteristic of trauma memories is that they frequently lack spatial coherence related to *scene construction*, which is the ability to accurately and vividly recall the environment in which the events took place (Brewin & Vasterling, 2021). Deficits in spatial processing lead to trauma memories that are often decontextualized and less open to modification and reworking. Attending to spatial elements and supporting trauma survivors in locating themselves within the landscape of their memories can reduce intrusive recall (Oulton et al., 2018), and help integrate the internal, embodied experience of trauma with the external and social contexts of these events (Goshen et al., 2019).

In addition to its impact on memory, trauma is also characterized by its negative effect on self-regulation. Affective dysregulation involves both hyper- (too much) and hypo- (too little) arousal as manifested in emotional flooding, flashbacks, panic, and nightmares on the one hand, and numbing, withdrawal, dissociation, and states of psychic deadness on the other. Each type corresponds to differences in consciousness that have notably distinct neural profiles, with hyperarousal likely involving right brain dominance and hypoarousal likely guided by the left brain (Hill, 2021). Best practice guidelines indicate that all trauma treatment approaches should be concerned with the management of these bodily-rooted states, with the goals of upregulating hypoaroused systems and downregulating hyperaroused ones in order to help patients move toward self-regulation (Ford et al., 2015). These guidelines also characterize effective treatment approaches as ones that increase mastery over both internal (somatic and affective) and external (environmental) triggers of trauma symptoms. Schore (2021, p. 51) concluded:

> The clinical organizing principle for working with any disturbance of affect regulation dictates that the psychobiologically attuned empathic therapist facilitates the patient reexperiencing overwhelming affects in incrementally titrated, increasing affectively tolerable doses in the context of a safe environment, so that overwhelmingly traumatic feelings can be regulated, come into consciousness, and be adaptively integrated into the patient's emotional life.

In order to engage in attunement at this level, therapists must have proficiency in their own bodies. Schore (2021) characterized empathy as a mature form of synchrony in which therapists' and patients' physiological, affective, and regulatory systems become linked. Synchrony may be particularly important in trauma treatment as it fosters safety and connection in the therapeutic relationship that counters the profound isolation that accompanies trauma and its aftermath. In addition to body-to-body coupling, empathy also involves imagination as therapists have to place themselves inside patients' often-unimaginable experiences as a primary means for understanding (Gerber, 2022).

Transforming Trauma

Recovery from trauma requires several understandings that are particularly difficult for survivors to integrate: (1) the knowledge that the present has been shaped by experiences of the past; (2) the belief that they deserve better treatment or circumstances than they received; (3) the trust that they did the best they could to respond to the trauma with the resources they had at the time; and (4) the sense that they can expect better for themselves in the future. These understandings are often blocked by shame, loneliness, and hypervigilance intended to guard against getting hurt again.

As Ecker and Vaz (2022) suggested, many evidence-based trauma treatments, particularly those rooted in cognitive-behavioral and exposure methods, target explicit cognitions and symptom suppression rather than working with deeply rooted traumatogenic beliefs. Top-down methods tend to label these trauma-based schemas as maladaptive or irrational rather than engaging with them directly. The result is that traumatized patients often express a desire to use coping skills to assist them in changing behavior outside of sessions. However, these techniques frequently fall flat in daily life when environmental reminders cue survivors' defense systems. Traumatized people, particularly those with histories of developmental and attachment trauma, often cannot utilize cognitive skills that require executive functioning when hyperaroused or emotionally dysregulated (Marks-Tarlow, 2021).

By contrast, transformational methods aim to modify the underlying, implicit beliefs that trigger symptoms. A framework for capturing the distinction between transformational approaches and more traditional ones is that of *memory reconsolidation*. Rooted in animal research, memory reconsolidation refers to a change process that capitalizes on neuroplasticity to modify aversive memories through their reactivation and pairing with novel or discrepant experiences in the present. The juxtaposition of frightening memories and disconfirming positive experiences marked by trust, connection, or vitality contests the semantic or schematic content of the memory, creating the conditions for it to be reprocessed and filed away properly (Goldman & Fredrick-Keniston, 2020). When a memory is reconsolidated, its intensity is reduced, the emotional valence can shift along the continuum from negative to positive, and new meanings can be associated with the experience (Stevens, 2018). This process can be thought of as one of 'unlearning' to associate the memory with fear.

Memory reconsolidation depends upon a 'genuine embracing and full, experiential inhabiting of the previously nonconscious core belief or schema underlying or generating the symptom' (Ecker & Vaz, 2022, p. 8). However, engaging directly with traumatic memories is threateningly painful for many survivors, so they protect themselves from further harm through avoidance. The imaginative structures of drama therapy allow for stepping into these memories and their associated core beliefs with the additional safety that the 'as if' state can provide. Some patients can do this work more directly, in a psychodramatic fashion (Giacomucci, 2023), while others need the cushioning and distance provided by metaphor and fictional content. Neuroscientific research supports that the imagination can be an effective vehicle for memory reconsolidation (Reddan et al., 2018).

Stepping into a role allows for activating trauma memories while reworking the experience with new aspects of agency, competency, empowerment, relative safety, connection, and potentially humor and joy. I first began to understand the power of this process over two decades ago while working with two profoundly traumatized boys whose mother had subjected them both to physical abuse and torture, including attempting to drown them in a hotel bathtub (McGarvey & Haen, 2005). The most damaging interpersonal violence involved tying the younger brother to a chair and cutting his face with shards of broken glass, rendering him disfigured. His older brother was coerced by their mother to participate in these assaults.

In working through their complex trauma during a psychiatric hospital admission, both boys were engaged in a re-enactment of scenes from the story of Peter Pan. This story, to which they were naturally drawn, held metaphoric resemblance to their abuse in the way that the child characters were tied up and forced to walk the plank to be drowned in the sea. In addition, the villain pirate threatened to cut them with his hand, which had been replaced by a sharp hook that he wielded as a weapon. The most transformative moment of their drama therapy session occurred when they decided to work together to tie up Captain Hook (who was played by me) with wrapping paper ribbon. In doing so, the boys ran in circles around Hook, getting tangled in the ribbon and laughing together in shared, unbridled joy. They shifted from their traumatized bodies (which had been constrained, damaged, controlled by their mother, and powerless to protect them) to their imagined bodies (which were free, alive, capable, and attuned to one another). Memory reconsolidation was apparent in a subsequent shift in their relationship from victim and perpetrator to allies in recovering from the trauma of their abuse. Previously, they would continually re-enact the abuse during their interactions by yelling hurtful things at each other, and expressing deeply embedded beliefs about themselves and each other rooted in one of them having borne the brunt of the abuse and the other having participated in it. After this session, they were better able to recognize and connect with the hurt parts in one another and often expressed a sense of collective strength that came from knowing they had survived together, bringing new meaning to their trauma experience.

The Imagined Body

Theatre is unique among the arts because it is, as Goldstein observed (2017, p. 28), the 'only art form in which audiences engage with real humans, creating relationships, actions, behaviors, and emotions meant to be read as truthful.' Watching events played out through dramatic action likely evokes the same neurological and emotional processes as responding to these same occurrences in real life. This mimetic effect gives theatre its unique potency for stimulating emotional engagement and catharsis. It makes intuitive sense, then, that approaches rooted in theatre would be used to channel imagination in service of healing; for, as Gilmore (2010) noted, improvisational acting is the closest adult equivalent to the state of modified consciousness that occurs during pretend play in young children.

Harris (2000) stipulated that children's pretend play is marked by the abandonment of typical rules about the world in favor of newly created ones based in imagination, while role play involves adopting the subjectivity of a character. In doing so, children 'are led to think about various transformations and capacities that would ordinarily be impossible' (p. 183). This expansion and transformation of self-experience was recently illuminated by a novel study involving wearable brain imaging technology. Greaves et al. (2022) found that when actors were in character, their response to hearing their own names shouted aloud was dampened in the left anterior prefrontal cortex. The researchers concluded that stepping into role involves suppression of one's sense of self.

While similar effects may happen through imagination alone, it is important to note that both acting and play come alive through *action*, as emotion is an embodied process. In fact, one of the first psychological theories of emotions, developed separately by William James and Carl Lange, located their origin within the body (Lang, 1994). They proposed that embodiment precedes emotion. For example, they suggested that we don't tremble in response to feeling scared, but instead tremble in response to a stimulus that in turn leads to feeling frightened. A modern neuroscientific update of the James-Lange theory is the theory of constructed emotions (Barrett, 2018). In this framework, emotions first arise at the level of affect, which is a bodily sensation that contains only two characteristics: arousal (high or low) and valence (positive or negative). The brain, which monitors bodily states through interoception, interprets this affect by applying past experiences and cultural contexts. It is this interpretation that is surmised to constitute the understanding of the sensation as emotion.

Other neuroscientists have presented more complex views, but many highlight the intertwined relationship between emotions and somatic states (e.g. Damasio, 2021). These theories bear resemblance to acting approaches in which performers are taught to first develop the physicality of their character, with the idea that emotional expression will follow. Indeed, positive correlations have been established between the elaborateness of children's pretend play and the use of their body within that play, including their capacities for somatic awareness, balance and touch (Roberts et al., 2017).

Imaginative practices allow for conceptualizing future possibilities, but the actualization of these possibilities in the real world can be too far of a leap for many trauma survivors without first having grounded that knowledge within the body. Transformative change often requires a confluence of both cognitive and embodied understanding. I propose that this nexus of embodiment and imagination contains what is potentially most effective about drama therapy's approach to trauma: the *imagined body*.

The imagined body can be defined as what happens when a person is able to transcend current realities by imagining new ways of being, feeling, and responding in concert with inhabiting the body either in new, healthier ways or in former ways that were disrupted by trauma. Taken together, imagining and embodying provide the kinds of disconfirming experiences that allow for moments of transcendence that, because they have been inhabited, can presage new realities and support memory reconsolidation. As drama therapists well know, the process of taking on a role allows for the development of parts of self that have yet to take root in a person's life, a rehearsal space for trying on future possibilities. Some trauma survivors might begin with embodiment by first engaging in movement, which then allows for imagining a new environment or narrative. For others, embodiment comes later as a concretization or elaboration of what was first imagined.

Key to the effectiveness of the imagined body is *absorption*, the impact of which has been understudied in psychotherapy. Kealy et al. (2019) defined absorption as the propensity to shift awareness from one's immediate surroundings to becoming fully immersed in imaginative and representational experiences. It manifests in a heightened attention to and involvement in artistic processes, fantasies, meditative practices, and emotions. Kealy et al. (2019) found that patients in group therapy who had higher levels of absorption were more likely to experience sessions as interesting and exciting early on, and that the degree to which they felt stimulated by the group predicted their improvement in psychiatric symptoms. This relationship between stimulation and treatment effectiveness did not hold true for group members with lower levels of absorption, leading the researchers to conclude that 'a capacity for imaginative and sensory immersion thus seems to facilitate the translation of enthusiasm for the group therapy experience into personal change' (p. 6).

On a brain level, there is a thin line between imagined and lived reality, both forming similar associations and neurological pathways. As Ecker and Vaz (2022) asserted, the more deeply patients can engage in role play and experiential work, the greater the potential for the work to have a meaningful impact that supports memory reconsolidation. When fully absorbed in the imagined body, survivors find they can integrate experiences and expand limiting self-definitions. Because trauma is shaped by experience, its remediation is best achieved through experience as well.

The Promise of the Imagined Body

Single-incident and mass trauma experiences, especially when they occur in adulthood, have a different impact and symptom profile from cumulative trauma that occurs during critical developmental periods of infancy, childhood, and adolescence (Hill, 2021). During single-event trauma, one experiences a rupture of previously held notions of self and others. In that instance, there is a clear demarcation between the pre- and post-trauma self. By contrast, complex trauma tends to shape one's personality, attachment style, and regulatory system, impeding the development of an embodied sense of safety, self-efficacy, or agency. Therefore, the imagined body can be thought of as allowing for two kinds of transformation in drama therapy: (1) restoring the body of the past that was lost during interpersonal or mass trauma; and (2) imagining the potential body of the future that transcends complex trauma. I will discuss each type of imagined body and provide case material to illustrate them, concluding with some thoughts about ramifications for clinical practice.

The Imagined Past Body

One hallmark of trauma is what Lifton (1988) termed *failed enactment*, the inability to respond to the traumatic event(s) in an effectively self-protective way. The somatic imprints of trauma often reside in the sense that one's body was constricted, weak, ineffectual, or a source of betrayal. By engaging clients in reprocessing their past trauma in an embodied way in which they re-inhabit the experience (whether as themselves or from the more distanced position of a character), drama therapists can work with them to experience their bodies in ways that are qualitatively different from back then. This process involves imagining other possibilities they couldn't envisage at the time because of shock or fear, which can allow for change in cases where evidence-based practices have been unsuccessful (Kaur et al., 2016).

My work with an adult named Cory[1] illustrates the use of the imagined past body in recovery from a frightening home invasion. Cory lived alone in an apartment in a major metropolitan city. As he stepped out of the shower one night, after returning home from the gym, he encountered an intruder who had entered through a window and had some of Cory's electronics in one hand and a gun in the other. Time slowed as the intruder pointed his weapon at Cory, freezing him in his tracks.

Cory entered treatment soon thereafter. He was psychologically healthy and, were it not for this event, would otherwise not have been in therapy. He was previously a confident and assertive person with a clear sense of self, but this incident had shaken him, leading to nightmares, anxiety about being alone, and questions about his self-efficacy. We worked in session on engaging his imaginative recall of the event, with Cory closing his eyes and describing what he remembered with as much sensory detail as he could tolerate, fleshing out each aspect of an encounter that lasted mere seconds but felt like an hour: the look on the intruder's face, his threat of violence, Cory's vulnerability at being covered only by a towel, and his inability to move. Most prominent in his mind was standing immobile as the gun was pointed at his chest. As he gradually immersed himself in the memory, we identified the actions he wished he could have taken at the time, which were thwarted by fear. These included expanding his body rather than cowering, making eye contact with the robber, and finding words.

After threatening Cory at gunpoint, the intruder escaped out the window, but inexplicably returned later that night after the police had left and attempted to break in again. This time, Cory's boyfriend had come over to stay with him. They were able to yell at the man and throw things at him as he climbed through the window. While these defensive actions were successful in getting the intruder to retreat, Cory's traumatic reactions were tied to the fear and immobilization from the first encounter when he was alone.

While holding the mental imagery and somatic sensations connected to the trauma event, we practiced slowly moving from the frozen, contracted posture his body had been forced to hold to a more expansive position with his shoulders drawn back and his gaze directed forward. He became grounded by tightening his fists in a defensive posture and centered by drawing conscious breaths. He moved through a repetitive oscillation between the traumatized body he had held and the stronger, imagined body he wished he could have inhabited – the one he typically existed in. We were working to incrementally embed the idea that moving out of helplessness and fear was within his control. Cory was able to then tolerate imaginally confronting the perpetrator by yelling clearly and forcefully for him to 'get the fuck out,' adding this to his sequence of movement.

Cory's work was augmented by two important practices. The first was that he began attending Krav Maga classes. This self-defense system, which has been a successful recovery tool for many trauma survivors with whom I have worked, involves grappling and repeatedly practicing getting put into holds and then fighting one's way out of them. In addition, I helped Cory to identify and internalize the strength he had shown, along with the support he had experienced, when he and his boyfriend successfully prevented a second intrusion into the apartment – thereby evading further danger.

In this work, Cory used the 'as if' space to pair his trauma experience with his well-developed sense of himself as capable and strong. By locating himself in the landscape of his traumatic memory and becoming fully absorbed in it, he was able to re-experience these events with greater continuity and spatial coherence that lent new meaning to the original event. Cory's work concluded after just a few sessions because he reported improvements in his anxiety, sleep, and ability to feel safe in his apartment. He reached out on the first anniversary of the break-in to say that these markers of successful treatment had persisted over time.

The Imagined Future Body

A prime difference between single-event trauma and complex trauma is the way in which sustained and repeated harm or polyvictimization can shape one's sense of identity. Living in chronic fear leads to alterations in the nervous system that prime a traumatized person for ongoing hypervigilance, redirecting mental resources toward threat detection. Complex trauma has noticeable impacts on the body as well, through *procedural learning* (Ogden & Fisher, 2015). When trauma is ongoing and inescapable – as is the case for a child who grows up in a chronically abusive household or violent neighborhood, or who faces repeated oppression from belonging to a racially marginalized group – people learn to survive using fight, flight, freeze, or appeasement. These responses become habitual, supported by adaptations to the carriage and posture of the body such as, for example, hunched shoulders, downcast eyes, tense fists, or efforts to make oneself small.

Procedural adaptations form a kind of *body armor*, to use a term introduced by Reich (1933/1980), that influences how individuals inhabit their bodies and move through the world. For these patients, the value of drama therapy lies in the imagined future body in which they learn to hold themselves in more expansive, empowered, and open ways through first trying on these physical changes in the 'as if' space of therapy. This kind of intervention holds promise not just for external changes but may alter body chemistry as well. In one study with trained actors, van Anders et al. (2015) found that wielding power in a role play contributed to the production of increased testosterone in females but not in males, suggesting that embodying status had particular impact for social groups that are less societally empowered.

A research-supported protocol for behavior change utilizes *mental contrasting* (Oettingen & Gollwitzer, 2019). This two-step process involves (1) imagining completing a future goal and experiencing the resultant positive feelings; and (2) identifying the obstacles in present reality to completing that goal – ultimately developing plans for how to overcome each obstacle, known as *implementation intentions*. Drama therapy can amplify the impact of mental contrasting by engaging the imagined future body.

For example, Justine, a 15-year-old patient, was contemplating setting limits with a peer at school whose overly physical way of joking with her was triggering this teen's past experiences of violence. Justine's early years were marked by physical and sexual abuse by her biological mother and several of her mother's boyfriends, which led to her being removed from her mother's care and placed with a relative out of state when she was an adolescent.

Through this experience, she learned to not make eye contact with others and had difficulty forming sentences, often becoming unable to access language in normatively challenging social situations, like talking to peers or speaking up in class. Being unable to respond effectively and instead shrinking would inevitably result in seeing herself as incapable, weak, and unworthy of connection – which led to profound loneliness and suicidality. Setting boundaries with her peer in an assertive way was difficult because her body's alarm system would falsely warn her that she was going to be attacked, like she had been in her childhood home. Previous cognitive interventions and attempts to help Justine respond differently to these situations had fallen apart once fear kicked in.

After a year of work on processing her past traumatic experiences and learning to regulate her emotions, we spent several months in session creating a character, first in imagination and then through embodiment. This incremental approach corresponded to Justine's increased tolerance of affect and agency. We started with miniature figures that allowed for distance and perspective, then gradually moved to her inhabiting this character, one she named Queeny. Queeny was a young monarch who had stepped into power after her father, the king, had been killed. Despite her youth, she was a decisive ruler who did not suffer fools. At first, Justine could only physicalize her from the neck up, speaking the character's words while her body remained sunken. We practiced her embodying Queeny more fully over time, eventually adding movement. This evolved into a co-created scene in which Queeny was challenged by various villagers who disagreed with her or tried to steal her power.

Moving from the metaphoric to the real, Justine initiated a discussion in one session about the dynamic with her peer at school, aware that this fellow student didn't present an actual threat to her safety – rather, her body was reacting as though in danger. I asked Justine to imagine what it would feel like to have successfully stood up to her peer – a level of assertion she had not yet accomplished – and to represent that feeling in a body sculpt. She then focused on two obstacles to meeting this goal: her fear of reprisal and her tendency to shut down during conflictual situations. Justine embodied these obstacles in a subsequent sculpt.

I facilitated an oscillation between the two poses as Justine was asked to think of a plan for overcoming her fear and possible shutting-down. Initially, she struggled with this task, but when asked what change she could make to the obstacle sculpt so that it more closely resembled the one of her achieving her goal, she was able to identify pulling her shoulders back. This adjustment straightened her body, redirected her gaze outward, and localized an embedded feeling of confidence she could access to counteract her fear-based shrinking and withdrawal. Justine remarked that she could find the Queeny within her as she worked on being more confident. She practiced tracking the false alarm activated by her trauma and then shifting her bodily positioning in order to remind herself that she was in the present.

Justine returned to session proud to report that not only did she successfully and peaceably confront her peer, but she was able to tolerate the interaction and see it through to a satisfying resolution by summoning strength in her shoulders several times during the conversation. This shift was the genesis of Justine's altered self-perception, which led to her defining herself as worthy of care and able to connect to others and form friendships. Self-assertion became not just a tool for establishing boundaries but also for positively influencing others, as she was eventually able to take on a leadership role in a school club – something that was previously unimaginable to her.

Conclusion

Just as the impact of trauma is complex and multi-dimensional, its treatment must be nuanced and holistic. Paradoxically, transformative treatment involves evoking and reprocessing the very memories that trauma survivors would most like to avoid. Experiential work with the body holds promise for settling the hyperaroused system or enlivening the hypoaroused one, while imagination offers buffering and safety that create the conditions for modifying the core beliefs that maintain and exacerbate symptoms. The *imagined body* is a nexus point where the principles informing exposure and cognitive-behavioral therapies and those underlying somatic approaches meet. The combination of imagination and embodiment has a synergistic effect that makes drama therapy and other similar experiential methods ideally suited to repairing the losses resulting from single-event trauma, as well as the more insidious developmental impacts of complex trauma.

Focusing on the imagined body gives drama therapists a lens for seeing what is most effective about the work, while situating our discipline within substantive evidence garnered from developmental psychology, animal research, neurobiology, and related fields. It also offers a window into thinking about how creative approaches may fill the gaps where existing evidence-based treatments fall short. Beyond individual behavior, the imagined future body might suggest new possibilities for one's family or social group, from the consideration of moral alternatives to an expanded sense of freedom that might lead to envisioning new sociopolitical structures (Chan, 2021; Gerber, 2022).

Social change is rooted in imagining one's oppressed body as defiant and unbound. We too might dream big, imagining a day in which we collaborate across disciplines and listen deeply to our patients and their intuitive sense of what is curative. Working in solidarity, mental health professionals might heal not only individual damaged bodies, but the collective body that has been wounded by hatred, division, self-interest, misuse of power, and resistance to accountability. All just outcomes begin with someone imagining 'what if….'

Note

1 Pseudonyms are used in clinical vignettes and all identifying details have been altered.

References

Barrett, L. F. (2018). *How emotions are made: The secret life of the brain*. Mariner.

Blackwell, S. E. (2019). Mental imagery: From basic research to clinical practice. *Journal of Psychotherapy Integration*, 29(3), 235–247. https://doi.org/10.1037/int0000108

Brewin, C. R. & Vasterling, J. J. (2021). Alterations in memory and other neurocognitive processes. In M. J. Friedman, P. P. Schnurr, & T. M. Keane (Eds.), *Handbook of PTSD: Science and practice* (3rd ed., pp. 117–134). Guilford.

Bryant, R. A. (2021). Psychological models of PTSD. In M. J. Friedman, P. P. Schnurr & T. M. Keane (Eds.), *Handbook of PTSD: Science and practice* (3rd ed., pp. 98–116). Guilford.

Carroll, J. (2020). Imagination, the brain's default mode network, and imaginative verbal artifacts. In J. Carroll, M. Clasen & E. Jonsson (Eds.), *Evolutionary perspectives on imaginative culture* (pp. 31–52). Springer. https://doi.org/10.1007/978-3-030-46190-4_2

Chan, A. (2021). *Reassembling models of reality: Theory and clinical practice*. Norton.

Damasio, A. (2021). *Feeling & knowing: Making minds conscious*. Pantheon.

Dieterich-Hartwell, R. & Melsom, A. M. (2022). *Dance/movement therapy for trauma survivors: Theoretical, clinical, and cultural perspectives*. Routledge.

Ecker, B. & Vaz, A. (2022). Memory reconsolidation and the crisis of mechanism in psychotherapy. *New Ideas in Psychology*, 66, Article 100945. https://doi.org/10.1016/j.newideapscyh.2022.100945

Ford, J. D., Grosso, D. J., Elhai, J. D., & Courtois, C. A. (2015). Treatment of adults with PTSD. In J. D. Ford, D. J. Grasso, J. D. Elhai, Jon, D., & C. A. Courtois, *Posttraumatic stress disorder: Scientific and professional dimensions* (pp. 299–366). https://doi.org/10.1016/B978-0-12-801288-8.00007-8

Gerber, N. (2022). *Imagination and arts-based practices for integration in research*. Routledge.

Giacomucci, S. (2023). *Trauma-informed principles in group therapy, psychodrama, and organizations: Action methods for leadership*. Routledge.

Gilmore, K. (2010). Pretend play and development in early childhood (with implications for the Oedipal phase). *Journal of the American Psychoanalytic Association*, 59(6), 1157–1181. https://doi.org/10.1177/0003065111427158

Goldman, R. & Fredrick-Keniston, A. (2020). Memory reconsolidation as a common change process: Moving toward an integrative model of psychotherapy. In R. D. Lane & L. Nadel (Eds.), *Neuroscience of enduring change: Implications for psychotherapy* (pp. 328–359). Oxford.

Goldstein, T. R. (2017). Live theatre as exception and test case for experiencing negative emotions in art. *Behavioral and Brain Sciences*, 40, Article e362. https://doi.org/10.1017/S0140525X17001704

Goshen, I., Huss, E., & Koch, S. C. (2019). Creating an embodied phenomenological typology for describing the qualitative experience of traumatic space from continued bombings. *Journal of Loss and Trauma*, 24(5–6), 460–472. https://doi.org/10.1080/15325024.2018.1507471

Greaves, D. A., Pinti, P., Din, S., Hickson, R., Diao, M., Lange, C., Khurana, P., Hunter, K., Tachtsidis, I., & Hamilton, A. F. C. (2022). Exploring theater neuroscience: Using wearable functional near-infrared spectroscopy to measure the sense of self and interpersonal coordination in professional actors. *Journal of Cognitive Neuroscience*, 34(12), 2215–2236. https://doi.org/10.1162/jocn_a_01912

Haen, C. (2020). The roles of metaphor and imagination in child trauma treatment. *Journal of Infant, Child, and Adolescent Psychotherapy*, 19(1), 42–45. https://doi.org/10.1080/15289168.2020.1717171

Haen, C. (2022). Foreword. In R. Dieterich-Hartwell & A. M. Melsom. *Dance/movement therapy for trauma survivors: Theoretical, clinical, and cultural perspectives* (pp. xiv–xvi). Routledge.

Harris, P. L. (2000). *The work of the imagination*. Blackwell Publishers.

Hill, D. (2021). Dysregulation and its impact on states of consciousness. In D. J. Siegel, A. N. Schore & L. Cozolino (Eds.), *Interpersonal neurobiology and clinical practice* (pp. 169–193). Norton.

Kaur, M., Murphy, D., & Smith, K. V. (2016). An adapted imaginal exposure approach to traditional methods used within trauma-focused cognitive behavioural therapy, trialled with a veteran population. *The cognitive Behaviour Therapist*, 9, Article e10. https://doi.org/10.1017/S1754470X16000052

Kealy, D., McCloskey, K. D., Cox, D. W., Ogrodniczuk, J. S., & Joyce, A. S. (2019). Getting absorbed in group therapy: Absorption and cohesion in integrative group treatment. *Counselling and Psychotherapy Research*, 19(3), 286–293. https://doi.org/10.1002/capr.12226

Lahad, M. (2019). The healing power of imagination: Playfulness in impossible situations. In Y. Ataria, A. Kravitz, & E. Pitcovski (Eds.), *Jean Améry: Beyond the mind's limits* (pp. 171–197). Palgrave Macmillan.

Lang, P. J. (1994). The varieties of emotional experience: A meditation on James-Lange theory. *Psychological Review*, 101(2), 211–221. https://doi.org/10.1037/0033-295X.101.2.211

Lanius, R. A., Terpou, B. A., & McKinnon, M. C. (2020). The sense of self in the aftermath of trauma: Lessons from the default mode network in posttraumatic stress disorder. *European Journal of Psychotraumatology*, 11(1), Article 1807703. https://doi.org/10.1080/20008198.2020.1807703

Levine, P. A. (2015). *Trauma and memory: Brain and body in a search for the living past*. North Atlantic Books.

Lifton, R. J. (1988). Understanding the traumatized self: Imagery, symbolization, and transformation. In J. P. Wilson, Z. Harel, & B. Kahana (Eds.), *Human adaptation to extreme stress: From the Holocaust to Vietnam* (pp. 7–31). Springer.

Malchiodi, C. A. (2020). *Trauma and expressive arts therapy: Brain, body, and imagination in the healing process*. Guilford.

Marks-Tarlow, T. (2021). Birds of a feather: The importance of interpersonal synchrony in psychotherapy. In D. J. Siegel, A. N. Schore, & L. Cozolino (Eds.), *Interpersonal neurobiology and clinical practice* (pp. 261–291). Norton.

McGarvey, T. P. & Haen, C. (2005). Intervention strategies for treating traumatized siblings on a pediatric inpatient unit. *American Journal of Orthopsychiatry*, 75(3), 395–408. https://doi.org/10.1037/0002-9432.75.3.395

Oettingen, G. & Gollwitzer, P. M. (2019). From feeling good to doing good. In J. Gruber (Ed.), *The Oxford handbook of positive emotion and psychopathology* (pp. 596–611). Oxford.

Ogden, P. & Fisher, J. (2015). *Sensorimotor psychotherapy: Interventions for trauma and attachment*. Norton.

Oulton, J. M., Strange, D., Nixon, R. D. V., & Takarangi, M. K. T. (2018). Imagining trauma: Memory amplification and the role of elaborative cognitions. *Journal of Behavior Therapy and Experimental Psychiatry*, 60, 78–86. https://doi.org/10.1016/j.jbtep.2018.04.003

Porges, S. W. & Dana, D. (2018). *Clinical applications of the polyvagal theory: The emergence of polyvagal-informed therapies*. Norton.

Reddan, M. C., Wager, T. D., & Schiller, D. (2018). Attenuating neural threat expression with imagination. *Neuron*, 100(4), 994–1005. https://doi.org/10.1016/j.neuron.2018.10.047

Reich, W. (1980). *Character analysis* (3rd ed., V. R. Carfagno, Trans.). Farrar, Straus and Giroux. (Original work published 1933.)

Roberts, T., Stagnitti, K., Brown, T., & Bhopti, A. (2017). Relationship between sensory processing and pretend play in typically developing children. *The American Journal of Occupational Therapy*, 72(1), Article 7201195050. https://doi.org/10.5014/ajot.2018.027623

Rubinstein, D. & Lahad, M. (2022). Fantastic reality: The role of imagination, playfulness and creativity in healing trauma. *Traumatology*. Advance online publication. https://doi.org/10.1037/trm0000376

Schore, A. N. (2021). The interpersonal neurobiology of therapeutic mutual regressions in reenactments of early attachment trauma. In D. J. Siegel, A. N. Schore, & L. Cozolino (Eds.), *Interpersonal neurobiology and clinical practice* (pp. 27–58). Norton.

Stevens, F. L. (2018). Affect regulation and affect reconsolidation as organizing principles in psychotherapy. *Journal of Psychotherapy Integration*, 29(3), 277–290. https://doi.org/10.1037/int0000130

Sutton, S. (2020). *Psychoanalysis, neuroscience and the stories of our lives: The relational roots of mental health*. Routledge.

Taylor, M. (2013). Transcending time, place, and/or circumstance: An introduction. In M. Taylor (Ed.), *The Oxford handbook of the development of imagination* (pp. 3–10). Oxford University Press.

Thomson, P. & Jacque, S. V. (2019). *Creativity, trauma, and resilience*. Lexington Books.

van Anders, S. M., Steiger, J., & Goldey, K. L. (2015). Effects of gendered behavior on testosterone in women and men. *PNAS*, 112(45), 13805–13810. https://doi.org/10.1073/pnas.1509591112

Villena-González, M. & Cosmelli, D. (2020). Imagination and mind wandering: Two sides of the same coin? A brain dynamics perspective. In D. D. Preiss, D. Cosmelli, & J. C. Kaufman (Eds.), *Creativity and the wandering mind: Spontaneous and controlled cognition* (pp. 93–120). Academic Press.

Zabelina, D. L. (2023). Imagination. In A. B. Bakker, F. Gander, W. Ruch, & L. Tay (Eds.), *Handbook of positive psychology assessment*. Hogrefe.

Chapter 2

The Emotional Body

A Somatic and Trauma-Informed Practice for Cultivating Expressive Capabilities for the Actor and the Individual

Laura Facciponti Bond

Introduction

Actor is defined not just as one who acts in a play, movie, or television show, but also as *one who behaves as if acting a part* (Merriam-Webster, 2023). Whether one is acting professionally or in devised theatre projects, improvisational fictionalized skits, scenes, or stories, the *actor* performs roles and could be experiencing many of drama's disciplinary challenges and potential for mental instability inherent within the practice. Yet, acting is used for personal and cultural transformational catharsis, communication of new ideas, and the opportunity to unite communities. The challenge here is how to provide the benefits of the art form, while preserving and protecting the individual providing its craft: *the actor*.

Actors have been particularly overlooked and are often not prepared for potential impacts of the emotional and psychological challenges required of acting. Taking on the life of a fictionalized character for long periods of time adds to the psychological hazards of the discipline (Brandfonbrener, 1992). Since theatre's story structure relies on conflict, many actors are portraying characters who are highly distraught victims, villains, or those struggling with great loss. Therefore, actors can live and relive intense emotional episodes for hours every day. For these reasons, explain the authors of the Australian Actors' Wellbeing Study, 'performers are more at risk than others for anxiety, depression, substance abuse, poor emotion regulation, sleep disruption, crises of confidence, identity blurring, and suicide' (Maxwell et al., 2015).

Getting into character is not simply 'putting on' or 'taking off' a role. Some common practices for connecting with a character are the use of emotional substitutions or tapping into personal histories to evoke the emotions required of a role. When using these methods, many actors have reported difficulties switching off the emotional, psychological, and physical engagements of their roles, leaving them struggling to return back to their previous state (Robb & Venning, 2016). When a deeply distressing or disturbing life experience is triggered and relived repeatedly, some can experience anxiety disorders, panic attacks, trauma, and significant decrease in their immune systems (Medina, 2008).

DOI: 10.4324/9781003322375-4

Some acting methods engage the use of imagination or the 'what if' concept, where an actor imagines how they might feel if they were a character in a specific situation. As the brain does not always distinguish between imaginative and real events, actors can remain within these emotional states if effective methods for de-roling or letting go of imaginative circumstances are not used (Kemp, 2012). Professional actors have reported experiencing dissociative processes that alter self-perception and blur boundaries between 'me' and 'not me' when they create characters (Thompson & Jacque, 2012). Similar concerns were also raised in recent studies where researchers found that actors experienced additional levels of destabilization when inhabiting difficult psychological territory, lost sight of the boundary between self and character (Robb & Clemence, 2017), and desired a clearer understanding of emotion and specific methods for how to access and exit emotion states (Stroud, 2022).

Research has highlighted the emotional and psychological toll on actors in the discipline when healthy methods are not implemented. Unfortunately, the belief that actors need to struggle and suffer for their art is still perpetuated by many within the discipline. In his report summarizing a fellowship dedicated to studying holistic healthcare of actors, Dr. Mark Seton explained that theatre educators' responses demonstrate 'starkly the reluctance to change and the stigma attached to considering psychological and emotional well-being in contexts of performing arts training' (Seton, 2009).

Meanwhile, drama and the use of *acting a part* is expanding well beyond the formalized and historical spaces of stage and screen. For example, dramatherapy utilizes drama, role playing, and essentially acting as 'an embodied practice that is active and experiential' and is used 'as a means for individuals to tell their stories, set goals and solve problems, express feelings, or achieve catharsis' (North American Drama Therapy Association, 2023). Neuroscience informs us that acting exercises and role playing in any situation can have an impact on an individual's wellbeing (Kemp, 2012). All acting or role playing circumstances require as much consideration for assisting the individual in healthy ways to take on and then de-role from, or release the emotions, actions, and imaginary circumstances required of their roles, so they return to a centered, calm, and clear sense of their true selves.

Traumatized individuals may have additional challenges with acting exercises or role playing unless they learn clear and accurate means to access and fully embody emotional states. Bessel van der Kolk (2014) explains that traumatized individuals

> can't figure out for themselves what they're really feeling about any given situation or what makes them feel better or worse. This is the result of numbing, which keeps them from anticipating and responding to the ordinary demands of their bodies in quiet, mindful ways.

Van der Kolk states that traumatized individuals can learn to tolerate their sensations, befriend their inner experiences, and cultivate new action patterns. He recommends using activities like focused attention on breathing, learning to notice feeling to help foster emotional regulation, and beginning to develop body awareness. Van Der Kolk contends that to recover from trauma, individuals need to become familiar with and befriend the sensations of their bodies. In order to move beyond their trauma, they first need to become aware of their sensations to help their bodies interact with the world around them. Physical self-awareness is the first step in releasing the trauma of the past (van der Kolk, 2014).

Fortunately, drama and theatre practitioners worldwide are becoming more proactive in seeking trauma-informed practices. According to the National Center for Trauma-Informed Care (NCTIC), a trauma-informed practice seeks to realize the widespread impact of trauma, recognize its signs and symptoms, integrate knowledge about it within their practice, and actively avoid re-traumatization (National Center for Trauma-Informed Care, 2021). The trauma-informed care principles and mindfulness practices supported by NCTIC are central to many of the teaching guidelines for the Emotional Body® method (Emotional Body, 2017). Its evidence-based emotional effector patterns and foundations as a somatic and embodied process have become a sought-after trauma-informed practice for helping individuals develop physical emotion regulation and expanding expressive capabilities. Training in the Emotional Body method has many somatic therapeutic benefits, including assisting individuals in addressing the physical disconnections, disembodiment, and numbness often associated with various aspects of trauma.

In this chapter, I will demonstrate how the Emotional Body method can serve as a somatic and trauma-informed practice for cultivating expressive capabilities for the actor and the individual. The chapter reveals how the method assists individuals in raising and refining their interior somatic perception skills, as well as their exterior proprioceptive and movement abilities during lessons in basic human expression and communication. Pedagogical theories and practitioner methods are described in detail to reveal how learners develop skills in somatic emotion regulation, affect labeling, and emotional granularity. Examples of how learners discover inherent emotion patterns that exist within their own behavior, while also learning how to create new feelings and expressive patterns of choice, are also provided. The therapeutic benefits of the Emotional Body method for the individual and the practitioner are explained throughout.

Discovering the Emotional Effector Patterns

The Emotional Body method's origins began with researchers asking whether it was possible to identify and differentiate between physiological measurements of emotional states within the human body. Professor Susana Bloch and her collaborators, theatre director Pedro Orthous and neurophysiologist Guy Santibañez-H, planted powerful seeds beginning with this research question in the early 1970s. They then extended their research question by asking whether these physiological occurrences could be willfully replicated by a practitioner as a means of emotion regulation. The team did discover measurements of emotional states – they called these emotional effector patterns – and began initial developments in a method for its instruction and practice called the BOS method, using the first letters of their last names to form the acronym (Bloch, 2002).

The original BOS research team concluded that specific emotions were linked to patterns of breathing, facial expression, degrees of muscular tension, and postural attitudes. They termed this form of somatic emotional measurement 'effector patterns' and equated its use to classic emotion standards close to those determined by Darwin (Bloch et al., 1987), as well as recognizing its connections to the James-Lange theory (Bloch, 2002). The BOS method allows people to induce an emotion state by the voluntary reproduction of specific respiratory-postural-facial patterns (Bloch et al., 1987).

The research team identified and analyzed six basic emotions[1]. Basic or pure emotions, according to classic emotion theory, are objective physiological fingerprints of emotion that would be considered common among most human beings (Barrett, 2017). These basic emotions can be voluntarily evoked by activating the corresponding effector pattern, which is composed of: (1) a breathing pattern, characterized by amplitude and frequency modulation; (2) a muscular activation characterized by a set of contracting and/or relaxing groups of muscles, defined in a particular posture; (3) a facial expression characterized by the activation of different facial muscle patterns (Bloch et al., 1987). Emotional Effector Patterns (EEP) became the practice term for this foundational emotion measurement and modulation method.

The EEP were a significant discovery for actor training and for physical emotion regulation methods. In future decades, the EEP became known in multiple disciplines. As Rick Kemp explains, 'consciously chosen muscular activity can generate the affective states of different emotions. These are no less or more "real" than those generated through mental exercises such as "emotion memory"' (Kemp, 2012, p.18). Emotional intensity and control are modulated in EEP training using somatic elements to regulate muscle engagement levels. No personal histories or imaginative circumstances are used in this method. Additionally, the BOS team introduced a physical Step Out procedure that includes a Neutral Breath pattern that incorporates slow deep cycled breathing along with calibrated arm and hand movements, and finishes with a full body shake out and vocalized release to help discharge emotional induction (Bloch et al., 1987). After developing proficiency in the EEP, a person can evoke complex emotions by mixing somatic elements of the effector patterns, much like primary colors mix to produce new colors.

Developing the Emotional Body Method

In my early career as a university instructor of Theatre in the 1990s, I was aware of many unhealthy practices inherent within the acting profession and was determined not to teach young performers psychologically and emotionally damaging practices. I had the opportunity to experience the EEP when Professor Bloch presented a workshop at a conference for the Association for Theatre in Higher Education in the US in the late 1990s. I was convinced of the EEP's potential for theatre, interdisciplinary studies, and somatic and embodied therapeutic purposes. With few certified practitioners in the world at the time, I spent years traveling to master the EEP, researching their relevance to human expression, and their application to physical emotion regulation and the performance profession.

After attending a 2003 workshop in New York where Susana Bloch was a guest teacher, I began a dialogue with her about the possibility of coming to Chile to study with her and other colleagues who were using the EEP in therapeutic and somatic practices as well as theatre. In 2005, I spent a sabbatical in Santiago where Professor Bloch and several of her colleagues designed a special teacher training for me. During this time Susana granted me her highest recommendation for teaching the EEP and a master certification in her individual method for teaching the EEP that she called Alba Emoting. I was encouraged to advance the teaching of the EEP by studying and incorporating more interdisciplinary somatic and vocal methods. Upon my return to the United States in 2006, I began offering regular classes on the method. Determined to share the method worldwide, I regularly trained new teachers and brought the first workshops in the method to Great Britain and Canada. Since that time, interest in the EEP has broadened to other professions.

After more than 15 years of conscious practice research, development, and training in additional interdisciplinary methods, it became clear that the Emotional Body® method of teaching the EEP had become its own method, and was dramatically different in pedagogy, style, and delivery than the BOS and Alba methods (Bond, 2017). I made significant advancements on the EEP teaching by strengthening its instructional approach using additional evidence-based methods and somatic education theories. While co-teaching seminars annually with Feldenkrais Awareness Through Movement® practitioners from 2007 to the present, I integrated somatic education theory into the EEP instruction, including research on anatomy and its relationship to human expression within recent neuroscience and psychology fields. Additionally, I included vocal patterns within the Emotional Body method, an element missing in the original EEP. I published a comprehensive book on the method, *The Emotional Body: A Method for Physical Self-Regulation*, and developed clear guidelines for levels of study and teacher training to ensure consistent practice of the Emotional Body method of instruction worldwide.

Emotional Body courses are attended by individuals from various professions, many of whom are from the therapeutic and somatic fields, seeking to add this method to their practice. The development of clear study and teacher training guidelines has assisted many of these individuals in pursuing competent training in the method, while informing the public on the careful and thoughtful process the method has taken in its development and training. The paragraphs that follow will assume that any instructor or therapist using the Emotional Body method in their practice has followed the published Emotional Body teacher training guidelines for its use and practice. Although Emotional Body trained ranks range from Practioner to Leader Instructor, for semantic purposes in making this chapter succinct in its writing, I will refer to an Emotional Body trained teacher or therapist as the *practitioner*, and the person they are teaching, coaching, or guiding as the *learner*.

A Somatic and Embodied Therapeutic Modality for Emotion Regulation

The central curriculum of the Emotional Body method is the lessons on the EEP, beginning with a process of raising the learner's somatic awareness while developing skills in emotion regulation and resiliency. The lessons then progress to exercises on how to embody and release the EEP and obtain a neutral or restored and calm state. The series of lessons described in the following paragraphs are provided in the order they are often used within a full intensive training program. However, an experienced practitioner can use any of the exercises described throughout this chapter out of this sequence to serve a specific purpose within their practice.

When learning the EEP, an individual can obtain skills in emotional self-regulation and resilience by developing abilities to recognize stress signals in the body, call upon 'physically hard' muscular stances or emotionally challenging states at will, and then learn to release them when not needed. During Emotional Body lessons, students learn methods for achieving physical relaxation, attaining a sense of neutrality, increasing beneficial emotional states, and ways to apply them to activities within their life and profession. According to the American Psychological Association (APA), resilience has been defined as the process and outcome of successfully adapting to difficult or challenging life experiences, especially through mental, emotional, and behavioral flexibility and adjustment to external and internal demands (American Psychology Association, 2022). Resilience can include larger cultural contexts and is a complex process that can present itself in differing degrees of abilities across multiple domains of life. This includes the workplace, educational settings, personal life, and relationships. Resilience skills can be developed within such practices as: recognizing stress in the body, building physical hardness, strengthening the relaxation response, and increasing positive emotions (Riopel, 2019). Therefore, awareness development attained through somatic sensing, physical emotion regulation, and the ability to embody physically hard and soft emotions is assisting in the development of skills in resilience through learning the Emotional Body method.

According to Kain and Terrell (2018), if resiliency skills were not acquired during early childhood or impaired due to traumatic experiences, many of them can be learned by adults who develop somatic sensing capabilities or raise their awareness interoceptively. Interoception is a process of noticing our internal state, evaluating combined sensations and perceptions of physical processes to assess our interior environment and determine what it is telling us about our feelings, state of being, and identity. We use these somatic observations to make many important life evaluations about our actions, sense of safety, assessments of wellbeing, and sense of belonging (Kain & Terrell, 2018). Practitioners are aware of the somatic therapeutic benefits these lessons can have in assisting the learner in developing and reporting on their somatic sensing capabilities throughout training.

When teaching the Emotional Body method, practitioners serve in the dual role as instructors and co-regulators, managing a delicate somatic dialogue with the learner. This requires a continuous mutual adjustment of actions and intentions, an ability to recognize when something or someone triggers us, and how to communicate and act in such a way that encourages our empathic response (Kain & Terrell, 2018). During Emotional Body lessons, the practitioner provides slow, gentle guidance to learners using precise vocal instructions. The learner begins lessons lying down so their body is engaged in the least amount of physical activity, allowing for the greatest degree of inner perception of physical, emotional, and mental sensations, guided by an instructional principle – 'do less, to find more.' The learner explores interior sensations of breathing patterns and small muscle movements designed to raise interoceptive capabilities. Learners are reminded to take each instruction with a sense of slow, gradual, and controlled physical curiosity and use an interior lens to sense and perceive how they feel throughout each step.

Learners are first invited to examine their own habitual state as a means of personal data collection concerning habitual breath, muscle, thought, and emotion patterns. At this point of personal inquiry, they are collecting valuable information concerning subtle habitual patterns. Later, reflections and discussions with a practitioner may reveal discoveries about lingering low-level emotions, emotional traits, and habitual muscular patterns which may have been present within what they had believed to be their 'resting' or 'neutral state.'

Evaluating and Creating New Patterns

Throughout the course, a learner will continue to evaluate their personal patterns, potentially making valuable discoveries concerning patterns that consistently appear. Practitioners describe these as *emotional entanglements*, when an individual wishes to express a pure emotional state like a 'take me seriously' expression of *anger*, but can't seem to express it without it being accompanied with tears, fearful eyes, a trembling lip, or a smirking smile. The same person who finds that their anger is often accompanied with tears may also discover that their expressions of joy and laughter often companion with crying, even their sensuality with others is coupled with sighs and slightly watery eyes. Susana Bloch would often describe in her teaching how an emotional entanglement is like a plant that wants to grow straight, strong, and independent, but is impeded by another vining plant that has taken a hold of it, affecting all of its movements and expressions. Identifying entanglements can be a personally revolutionary discovery with mixed reactions of desires for their immediate dismissal, and storied reasons for how and why they were formed.

Discovering consistent entanglement patterns of one emotion like *sadness* can also reveal information about the person's long-standing emotional traits. A trait is considered a long-term characteristic revealed through a person's behavior, feelings, and actions (Brown, 2021). Practitioners recognize that traits take a lifetime to develop. Emotional entanglements therefore require respectful and careful handling. It *is* possible to clear entanglements but it does take considerable time and patience in a series of gradual lessons designed with the intention of gently unentangling this vining emotion pattern from its host(s).

Soon after habitual patterns are explored, learners are introduced to a neutralizing pattern, titled 'zero' as a reminder to return to a zero level of emotional engagement. Zero serves as a home base used throughout the course for restorative practice, and as a resting point that is considered emotion-less. Learners do not receive verbal indicators of 'neutral' or 'zero' during its first introduction to avoid leading their experience or directing sensations through suggestion. The students experience what it is like to move between zero and their own personal pattern or 'resting state' to make discoveries between the differences. Learners are then asked to share a word or phrase that best describes how they felt within the new pattern. Their words are always honored as being perfect and right for their experiences. Discussions and questions follow concerning these and the process continues. Contemporary neuroscience has helped us realize that lessons like these assist in developing a better sense of who we are as we develop clearer connections with our bodies (Damasio, 1999).

Eventually the EEP are introduced to bring the learner into and out of small variances of felt sensations that can be described as subtle emotional shifts or states. In the original BOS method, each EEP was repeated and gradually prolonged to allow the learner to experience activation and identify a particular emotion (Bloch et al., 1987). This later developed into the term of creating an emotional induction, which can come and go at any time during EEP learning and practice. During these lessons, learners are encouraged to develop a sense of internal physical curiosity and somatic discovery. Practitioners refrain from referring to any of the basic emotion patterns as either positive or negative. Recognizing that pure emotional states are designed to assist human life in its thriving and surviving, it is only when these emotions bring us into a dysregulated state or no longer serve our health, wellbeing, or ability to thrive within our world or society that an alternative emotion is recommended for the occasion. After this introductory lesson, learners are invited to share an emotion word or phrase to describe their felt sense of what the EEP evoked for them.

In the Emotional Body method, each EEP is titled with a number and letter: 1a, 1b, 2a, 2b, 3a, and 3b[2]. A numeric-alpha title removes all possible leading language concerning the experience and assists in making connections between interoception and affect labeling development. Affect labeling development, or more specifically its use within Affect Regulation (AR), has become well known for its effectiveness in emotion regulation and as a companion within various therapies. Affect is considered a more encompassing term that includes a person's emotions, feelings, motivations, impulses, and moods. Many practitioners tend to use the terms affect and emotion interchangeably (Berking & Whitley, 2014). As learners make connections between somatic sensations and emotional vocabulary, they develop skills in affect labeling. They become more proficient in emotional granularity, which is the ability to accurately recognize and label emotions. Individuals with highly developed skills in emotional granularity have shown to improve emotion regulation skills and enhance psychosocial wellbeing (Brown, 2021).

Between each shift out of a new EEP, learners return to zero and are coached to sense EEP in the muscles or breath. This is a form of pendulation, gently moving in and out of internal sensations. Pendulation is used in many different types of somatic therapy practices (van der Kolk, 2014). The form of pendulation in the Emotional Body method is taught without the use of memory associations or imagery. Pendulation lessons can help the learner explore the somatic properties of moving from a low-level emotion to a mid and high one, and then back down again to zero. Learners can also pendulate between two different EEP patterns and slowly explore the somatic properties and sensations of moving from one emotional state to another, while feeling how the two emotions mix in the middle of the pendulating exercise. Practitioners call this a 'polarizing exercise,' as learners explore two different emotional poles and what lies between them. For example, we may start in a pattern that the learner describes as evoking a sense of *fear* and direct them to gradually add elements of a pattern that the learner may describe as inducting a state of *happiness*. While they invite the somatic elements of *happiness*, they may learn about all the mixed states that occur when various somatic aspects of these two basic patterns merge. In a later exercise, these mixed states may then be turned into fully embodied choices of new patterns for expressive explorations. Within this polarizing exercise, learners can also check their bodies for residual tensions from the *fear* explorations, learn about how their bodies hang on to emotional states, and what it takes to fully clear these emotional experiences by using zero and other restorative practices.

Learners can make discoveries about where, when, and how much affect may be lingering in their bodies after they experience an EEP in a condition commonly called emotional residue or emotional hangover. The BOS team described this as a tonic state of emotion that is maintained over time and not specifically caused by a direct stimulus (Bloch et al., 1987). Learners are invited to review their somatic sensing for emotional residue and reconsider the use of additional restorative practices to achieve a deeper embodied and holistic sense of neutrality. Such skill development is extremely valuable for all individuals as they learn more about their emotional habits and abilities to self-regulate. It is particularly important for those managing the effects of trauma as they learn methods to calm their nervous systems and achieve an embodied sense of safety (van der Kolk, 2014).

Applications of the Method

As Emotional Body lessons progress, learners gradually rise from the floor and explore the EEP with physical positions from seated to standing, walking, and interactive activities. Learners begin to recognize how these patterns relate to day-to-day experiences. These lessons involve more muscle engagement and activity. The potential is increased for greater intensity of the EEP due to many factors. More breath intensity is required to support additional activity and exteroceptive engagement causes higher rates of activation of the nervous system and limbic emotional responses. Kain and Terrell (2018) explain that exteroception helps individuals perceive and make sense of the external environment by pulling information from a variety of sources: (1) the attention-oriented senses of sight, hearing, taste, smell, touch; (2) their relationship to their vestibular or balance-centered system; and (3) the proprioceptive system, which provides information on how the parts of their selves are in relationship to each other, their rate of movement, and feelings. It is important for practitioners to recognize that a person's methods and processing of their external environment can be altered by past trauma or temporary stress physiology. Therefore, lessons during this stage are designed as short and controlled physical visits in and out of each EEP, and are always followed by instructions for returning to zero with additional restorative practices as needed.

Emotional dysregulation or trauma histories may be revealed during exercises on the EEP facial and postural patterns. Individual blocks and physical struggles to access certain emotions as well as emotional entanglements, may come up for some individuals as they attempt to embody the muscular aspects of these patterns in the face and posture. According to Dr. Stephen Porges (2011), some traumatized individuals present features of gaze aversion, flat facial affect, or a posture that is poised to fight or flee. Porges recommends that when recognizing these signs, it is important to engage using calming postures and vocal tones to assist them in downregulating to a sense of calm and safety. In addition to vocal modulations during their instructions, practitioners remind learners to apply the zero pattern, which has a smooth elongated exhale. This brings about a calming effect in the body and introduces an opposite emotional direction from the learner's default position of fear, sadness, or anger. Considering its potential for somatic and embodied therapeutic purposes, the learner is then invited to cultivate new embodied patterns towards developing personal agency for the various emotional states of joy, tenderness, courage, pride, or sensuality.

Management of emotional levels of intensity are introduced as the learner feels the ability to progress to this stage of increased physical engagement. They are provided with ways to sense and understand how to control higher levels of induction without causing states of dysregulation or becoming unsettled. Emotional intensity is modulated in three levels: minimal, moderate, and maximal (Bloch, 2002), while also reinforcing the choice of reversing back to zero – all while receiving reminders that the learner is in control of their experience and levels of intensity. At this stage in the course, these conscious and controlled shifts in and out of emotional states and self-regulated degrees of emotional intensity assist learners with becoming more comfortable with the sensations and emotions they may not typically allow themselves to feel outside of a controlled exercise or learning environment. They reinforce the learner's physical and emotion regulation abilities and assist them in developing adaptive qualities for emotional resilience. Additionally, learners can establish a better sense of their internal locus of control and personal agency.

Application lessons are the final stages in an introductory Emotional Body training. This consists in using the EEP in various activities so that learners can recognize how the patterns exist within everyday interactions and their relevance to professional disciplines including the craft of acting. At this point, learners are given a collection of exercises designed for this purpose that involve applying the EEP to physical blocking or movement activities, speaking text or telling stories, singing, improvisation, presenting short scenes, or engaging in brief dialogues with others. Within this process, when learners consciously apply the EEP to these actions they acquire an understanding of how to fully embody the activity. Simultaneously, they need to maintain the emotion's pure state of expression. This synthesis of the EEP with activities will raise their awareness of how emotional mixes can unknowingly enter their practice and assists the learner in refining their abilities in affect regulation.

Powerful insights are gained about how the cognitive aspects of the brain can draw the learner's attention away from purely somatic practices when verbal language and imagery are applied in exercises. Controlled somatic pattern exercises are essential steps toward assisting the individual with integrating the patterns into life activities. A common life example of this adaptation might be equal to a person who has just learned to ride a bicycle. They have practiced for quite some time, applying all their attention-oriented senses as well as vestibular and proprioceptive abilities to the act of riding a bike through space. Then, as the person determines that they have achieved this ability to ride a bike well, they combine it with more experiences and interactions with others. They listen to music or podcasts while riding, use hand signals in traffic, wave and talk to others as they pass by or dodge unexpected obstacles. They combine these brand-new somatic skills with cognitive brain activities like language, imagery, and emotions. Within an Emotional Body course, the learners are guided through this process with practitioners who assist them in their primary focus on the patterns first. In addition, practitioners add new elements to the learner's environment. The intention is to gradually engage them in multi-tasking interdisciplinary somatic tasks to ensure they can eventually reach a fully integrated stage of the EEP's potential.

Eventually, mixed states are introduced by combining the EEP into what Bloch called 'emotional mixes' (Bloch, 2002, p.63). Referring to the metaphor of the painter's palette and the EEP as primary colors, Bloch explained that any other emotion felt beyond the EEP would be a subjective mixture of the EEP into a secondary 'mixed emotion,' and represent most of the emotions experienced within adult human behavior. An example of an emotional mix would be combining specific aspects of 1a and 1b to create pride. Learning how to identify and create mixed emotions would provide individuals with the opportunity to create their own embodied experiences within their lives and professions, and expand their emotional expressions and the ability to consciously create new patterns.

Full integration is achieved once a learner can construct and deconstruct the EEP and reach a point where mixed emotional states are easily accessed and identified. At this point, they are encouraged to freely express, perform, and practice deconstructing events and activities much like transcribing a dance or language into basic EEP. An individual who has achieved full integration of the method can fluidly move from constructing and using pure EEP patterns to creating conscious mixes or simply expressing and being aware of emotional states that present within their expressions. These skills are particularly useful for the craft, practice, and the personal health and well-being of the actor.

Therapeutic Potential for the Method

The applications and benefits for the Emotional Body method as a somatic and embodied educational and therapeutic tool are multidimensional and encompass various aspects and levels within the training process. Considering the benefits described throughout this chapter and gained by observing students during their developmental stages of exploring and embodying the EEP, practitioners collect valuable information about when and how emotions linger in the learner's body. These observations can inform the practitioner about the learner's emotion regulation abilities for the following three aspects:

1 receiving and physically following verbal descriptions for pattern practice;
2 their emotional stimulus response and release tolerance levels; and

3 recognizing where a student's personal sense of safety lies within the pattern exploration while the lessons are still within a low level of interoceptive exploration and physical engagement.

Practitioners observe learners following verbal descriptions of each of the EEP during initial lessons, and if, for example, the learner mixes in other EEP elements by habit, a practitioner gains information of the learner's potential for entangled emotional patterns. A learner's emotional stimulus response and release tolerance levels could be best described by acknowledging each individual's area known as their 'window of tolerance,' which is their optimal area within which a person can respond to a stimulus without becoming overly aroused or unsettled to the point of becoming dysregulated (Siegel, 1999). The third aspect concerning the learner's sense of safety is vital and the cornerstone of every Emotional Body course. To this end, practitioners are advised to keep instructions for intensity levels extremely low during initial lessons to establish an environment where the learner can explore EEP patterns within their personal window of tolerance. This avoids bringing the learner to higher levels of activation too soon, where they might instinctively engage protective rigid behaviors or experience dysregulated chaotic states that could cause them to become unsettled or feel unsafe (Siegel, 2020). However, some learners might push the emotional intensity of pattern application out of enthusiasm yet potentially taking them beyond their tolerance window at the same time. In another scenario, a learner may automatically begin to engage protective blocks and barriers from the pattern instructed, and find that they have unintentionally mixed in a second emotional pattern not currently in practice.

These various reactions provide feedback while also offering information about a learner's neuroception and their ability to self-regulate. Porges (2004) coined the term neuroception to describe how the vagus nerve, a long wandering nerve that runs from the brain to the base of the spine and is connected to all the internal organs and the autonomic nervous system, informs the entire body through neural circuits using sensory input, and distinguishes whether situations or people are safe, dangerous, or life-threatening. Neuroception takes place in the primitive part of the brain and allows the body to instinctively, and outside of conscious awareness, trigger defensive behaviors of fight, flight, or freeze. In such cases, a learner may suddenly enter a place where they may have difficulty clearing to zero or neutrality and become dysregulated, unsettled, or further traumatized. Practitioners collect and compare this type of information about learners through observations and adjust their instructions for those who might need extra guidance to keep them within a tighter window of activation. Practitioners use regular gentle reminders to guide the learners back to neutrality, keep their practice of the patterns in low intensities during the beginning stages of exploration, and remind learners they can return to neutral on their own at any time and listen to the rest of the lesson rather than push their tolerance levels too far. Keeping trauma-informed practices in mind as the EEP are introduced, along with the use of consent-based invitational language and respect for individual learning space and pace, Emotional Body practitioners establish a learning environment where individuals can feel greater personal control within their experience and tolerance levels.

Conclusion

The Emotional Body method has been established through years of development investigating how the EEP can assist individuals with accessing and releasing emotions through purely physical means. Dramatherapy, theatre, and therapeutic practitioners have the opportunity to apply this evidence-based and trauma-informed embodied modality for emotion regulation and healthy restorative practices to their discipline. Although practitioners and hundreds of learners have reported on the method's benefits and effectiveness for emotion regulation, it was further validated in a recent research project on the EEP conducted with professional actors by Emotional Body instructors (Buchli & Stroud, 2022). The grant-funded project aimed to determine if the EEP could provide a safe, practical, and effective methodology to: (1) identify or detach actors from the character; (2) monitor and regulate personal vulnerability; and (3) minimize post-performance stress. The project's final data revealed that research participants reported that the EEP improved their affect labeling abilities, provided a shared common language for communicating and understanding emotion, gave them a specific method for entering and exiting an emotion, enabled them with an ability to regulate levels of emotional expression and experience, and provided better personal agency within the demands and diversities of acting environments.

Whether the Emotional Body method is used to help train actors or practitioners to be better prepared for the entertainment or therapeutic disciplines, learning this method for emotional expression and regulation can be beneficial in the following ways. The method assists individuals in obtaining the ability to clearly observe and identify emotion in self and others, by developing highly nuanced skills in somatic sensing and aligning them with interoceptive and exteroceptive observations of the specific EEP patterns. By learning how the EEP's basic emotion patterns eventually mix into more complex states that can be constructed or deconstructed by using the EEP as the basic elements, individuals acquire a clearer understanding of emotion and cultivate the ability to construct new emotional patterns of expression in their lives. Recognizing that all emotions stem from the six primary expressions and mix into new states that can be categorized back to their original base emotions, individuals develop keen abilities in affect labeling and more nuanced skills in sensing and describing what they are feeling, expressing, and seeing in others. With the method's purely physical approach that is not reliant on the use of imaginative or psychological stimuli, individuals achieve a practical method for entering and exiting an emotional state and regulating its intensity level at will and with less risk of experiencing emotional residue or psychologically disturbing adverse effects. Finally, the Emotional Body method consistently supports and repeatedly provides individuals with healthy self-care and restorative practices designed to soothe the nervous system and invite a sense of calm and peace within the body.

The Emotional Body method is used within many different professions where there is an interest in physical emotion regulation, somatic sensing development, and restorative practices. After nearly two decades of research and somatic educational development of the Emotional Body method, we have successfully improved the pedagogy and delivery of the EEP, so that its somatic and embodied therapeutic purposes and interdisciplinary applications have become more plausible.

Notes

1 In an article titled 'Effector Patterns of Basic Emotions: A Psychophysiological Method for Training Actors' the BOS research team in 1987 labeled the six emotional effector patterns as: Happiness-laughter, Sadness-crying, Fear-anxiety, Anger-aggression, Sex-eroticism, and Tenderness. Over the years names for the patterns would fluctuate largely due to the subjective nature of affect labeling.

2 I labeled the emotional effector patterns during the development of the Emotional Body method to remove subjective bias in the teaching and learning process of the patterns. Since Susana Bloch often referred to the Neutral Breath pattern as returning to a zero state, I first labeled Neutral as zero. I then identified the six emotion patterns as three cognate pairs based on the breathing patterns. There were two patterns each of (1) nose breathing; (2) mouth breathing; and (3) nose/mouth combined. Each cognate pair also brings a person from what many might refer to as a positive (a) emotional state and negative (b) emotional state. This is how the labeling 0, 1a, 1b, 2a, 2b, 3a, 3b was created.

References

American Psychology Association (2022). *Resilience*. Retrieved from www.apa.org/topics/resilience

Barrett, L. F. (2017). *How emotions are made: The secret life of the brain*. Houghton Mifflin Harcourt.

Berking, M. & Whitley, B. (2014). *Affect regulation training: A practitioner's manual*. Springer Science & Business Media.

Bloch, S. (2002). *The alba of emotions: Managing emotions through breathing*. Grijalbo.

Bloch, S., Orthous, P., & Santibanez-H, G. (1987). Effector patterns of basic emotions: A psychophysiological method for training actors. *Journal of Social and Biological Structures*, 10, 1–19.

Bond, L. (2017). *The emotional body: A method for physical self-regulation*. Pure Expressions.

Brandfonbrener, A. (1992). The forgotten patients. *Medical Problems of Performing Artists*, 7 (4), 101–102.

Brown, B. (2021). *Atlas of the heart: mapping meaningful connection and the language of human experience*. Random House.

Buchli, I. & Stroud, T. (2022). *Rethinking emotion in contemporary theatre* [Conference Presentation]. University of Winnipeg, Manitoba, Canada.

Damasio, A. (1999). *The feeling of what happens: Body and emotion in the making of consciousness*. Harcourt.

Emotional Body (2017). *Emotional Body Instructional Understandings and Instructor Level Guidelines*. Retrieved from https://emotionalbody.co/instructors/

Kain, K. L. & Terrell, S. (2018). *Nurturing resilience: helping clients move forward from developmental trauma*. North Atlantic Books.

Kemp, R. (2012). *Embodied acting: What neuroscience tells us about performance*. Routledge.

Maxwell, I. A., Cariston, M., & Szabo, A. M. (2015). *The australian actors' wellbeing study: A preliminary report*. Retrieved from www.senseconnexion.com/wp-content/uploads/2015/08/The-Australian-Actors-Wellbeing-Study.pdf

Medina, J. (2008). *Brain Rules: 12 principles for surviving and thriving at work, home, and school*. Ear Press.

Merriam-Webster (2023, January 18). *Actor*. Retrieved from www.merriam-webster.com/dictionary/actor

National Center for Trauma-Informed Care (2021). *What is trauma-informed care?* Retrieved from www.traumainformedcare.chcs.org/what-is-trauma-informed-care

North American Drama Therapy Association (2023, January 10). *What is drama therapy?* Retrieved from www.nadta.org/what-is-drama-therapy

Porges, S. W. (2004). Neuroception: A subconscious system for detecting threat and safety. *Zero to Three: Bulletin of the National Center for Clinical Infant Programs*, 24(5), 19–24.

Porges, S. W. (2011). *The polyvagal theory: Neurophysiological foundations of emotions, attachment communication, and self-regulation*. W.W. Norton & Company.

Riopel, L. (2019). Resilience Examples: What Key Skills Make You Resilient? Retrieved from https://positivepsychology.com/resilience-skills/

Robb, A. E. & Clemence, D. (2017). Exploring psychological wellbeing in acting training: An Australian interview study. *Theatre, Dance and Performance Training*, 8(3), 297–316.

Robb, A. E. & Venning, A. (2016). Exploring psychological wellbeing in a sample of Australian actors. *Australian Psychologist*, 53(1), 77–86. https://psycnet.apa.org/record/2016-30419-001

Seton, M. (2009). *The Gilbert Spottiswood Churchill Fellowship to Study Holistic Healthcare of Actors in Training and in the Workplace* [Report]. The Winston Churchill Memorial Trust of Australia. Retrieved from https://senseconnexion.com/ChurchillReport_ActorsHealthcareUK.pdf

Siegel, D. J. (1999). *The developing mind. Toward a neurobiology of interpersonal experience*. Guilford.

Siegel, D. J. (2020). *The developing mind: How relationships and the brain interact to shape who we are* (3rd ed.). Guilford.

Stroud, T. (2022, June 14). *Challenging the taboo of emotion in theatre practice* [Conference Presentation]. Canadian Association of Theatre Research Conference, University of Lethbridge, Alberta, Canada. Retrieved from https://catracrt.ca/conference-catr-2022/

Thompson, P. & Jacque, V. S. (2012). Holding a mirror up to nature: Psychological vulnerability in actors. *Psychology of Aesthetics, Creativity and the Arts*, 6(4), 366–367.

van der Kolk, B. (2014). *The body keeps the score: Brain, mind and body in the healing of trauma*. Penguin Books.

Chapter 3

Playful and Poetic Embodiment for Indirect Processing of Trauma Using Masks

A Drama Therapy Framework Inspired by Lecoq's Physical Theatre Pedagogy

Shiu Hei Larry Ng

Introduction

This chapter aims to bring together Jacques Lecoq's physical theatre pedagogy, drama therapy and trauma healing, and to show how the first one can be a bridge between the other two. Lecoq's physical and kinaesthetic approach to theatre pedagogy based on a progressive sequence of systematically structured improvisational explorations has much to inspire, especially in relation to trauma healing. I will outline why and how masks can be useful in drama therapy from the perspective of Lecoq's dynamic poetics of physical theatre, which is different from the common understanding of mask as a projective tool. I will also argue how drama therapy can contribute to trauma healing by offering 'indirect forms of traumatic memory/experience processing' (Ford, 2017, p.240), which are somatic, metaphorically experiential, and holistic.

The two key teachings of Lecoq (1921–1999) on mime and mask, as well as the five stages of his pedagogical and exploratory sequence with masks, will be of particular importance in this task. Drawing from my experiences as a drama therapist working with clients affected by developmental trauma and/or social trauma in Hong Kong, with also a formal training in Lecoq's pedagogy, I will suggest a framework that (almost) reverses the original stages of masks in Lecoq's pedagogy to best care for traumatized clients. I will start this chapter by introducing Lecoq's pedagogy, and then present the therapeutic framework that will focus on the first four stages.

Lecoq's Pedagogy on Mime and Mask for a Trauma-Specific Drama Therapy

Lecoq's physical theatre pedagogy trains the actor-creator through movement, mime and mask, and their interrelationships. Besides being a revolutionary approach to theatre, it is more fundamentally a way to understand our relationship to the world, as well as how we learn and create.

DOI: 10.4324/9781003322375-5

The point of departure for Lecoq is that 'everything moves' (Lecoq, 2002, p.187). We are moved and we move as a body in space. Lecoq emphasizes that we are moved by the space while we also move the space. We are not just moved by the surrounding world causally and then react mechanically to it as consequence, we are also moved in a mimetic manner, leaving a dynamic impression that, played out in the body, becomes an inspiration to move creatively. This two-fold process of identification and transposition (Lecoq, 2002) is the source of our creative acts. Echoing Aristotle's philosophy and Marcel Jousse's anthropology of gesture (Jousse, 2016), Lecoq considers humans as miming beings, and miming as our basic way to learn and create.

Mime represents a more advanced level of movement through which a person moves in a more articulated manner by identifying with the dynamic structures of other beings in their surroundings, and by transposing their movements into further embodied constructions based on the original dynamic structure. As a creation method, this is called 'mimodynamics' (Lecoq, 2002, p.48). This also refers to how a person's sensorimotor literacy develops, and where higher cognitive functions, including language, are grounded. That is why Lecoq built his pedagogy of movement on miming movement, which essentially translates our dynamic relationship to the world.

Based on such a dynamic structure, movements are metaphors, physical and embodied, of both outer and inner phenomena, including emotions, thoughts, and desires, where outside and internal world mutually transform one another. For Lecoq, getting access to this dynamic – which he names 'the essence of life' (Lecoq, 2002, p.47) – is the key that connects self, others, and the world. It constitutes the foundation of metaphor, which he calls 'the universal poetic awareness' (my translation of *le fond poétique commun*, originally in Lecoq, 2002, p.47). Thus, his teaching can be considered as a pedagogy of playful and poetic embodiment.

Lecoq's teaching of mime echoes the phenomenology of corporeality of Merleau-Ponty (2012) and the analysis of Lakoff and Johnson (2003) about the fundamental role of metaphor in human cognition and action, and its sensorimotor base. Lecoq's pedagogy reflects the paradigm shift in cognitive science towards embodied cognition, as some theatre scholars have pointed out (Kemp, 2016; Murphy, 2019), and that grounds the possibility for indirect processing. Indirect processing refers to the way in which traumatic experiences and memories are processed through metaphorical and artistic means, as opposed to verbal means in more traditional forms of trauma therapy (Forbes et al., 2020; Kiyimba et al., 2022). It appears important to understand the possibility and mechanism of indirect processing in trauma healing, and to show how drama therapy can have a unique contribution to make to the field. My experience has convinced me that the teaching of Jacques Lecoq can significantly contribute to that undertaking.

Another key component in Lecoq's pedagogy is mask. Lecoq's view on mask was largely inspired by his collaboration with Amleto Sartori (1915–1962), a sculptor and key figure in the modern revival of masks in European theatre. For Lecoq and Sartori, masks are effective on stage because of their sculptural and dynamic structures characterized by their spatial qualities (Estévez, 2015). As a mask is an unfinished structure to be completed and animated by the actor's body moving it and moved by it, it invites or urges actors to 'push the space' (as Lecoq and teachers in his pedagogy often say) through gestures and movements. Therefore, an effective mask moves the actor not from a psychological internal state but rather through physical impulses that echo its shape, or more precisely the inherent dynamics of that shape. Such physical impulses are the base for any imaginative associations that develop in the actor's mind about the mask and that are mediated by the mask. In other words, masks here are not primarily considered as projective tools, as it is usually the case in drama therapy (Jones, 2007).

For Lecoq, the spatial dynamics of the mask enables students to transcend personal history into something more universal. This is also why Lecoq used many types of masks from different traditional origins, intentionally neglecting the cultural associations by focusing on the spatial-dynamic features of the masks. For Lecoq, masks approached from their codified traditions are at risk of losing their vitality and possibilities. Therefore, students under Lecoq's pedagogy are guided to see masks as spatial-dynamic objects and to understand their features and dynamic structure before playing them. This process is akin to the phenomenological *epoché* (or bracketing) whereby existing cultural references or social codes are set aside (Zahavi, 2017).

To summarize, movement, mime, and mask form a three-level developmental continuum in Lecoq's pedagogy, based on his fundamental insight about dynamics as the base of everything and the source of poetic creation. Lecoq's philosophy of poetic dynamic and his corresponding pedagogy provide an opportunity for an exploration of the therapeutic power of masks, and its application to trauma healing.

Lecoq's pedagogy can be taken as a reference for a new approach to how masks can be used in drama therapy, especially because it theoretically and practically illustrates (1) how drama and theatre are grounded in sensorimotor processes and emerge from playful embodiment; (2) how metaphors originate in movements that connect with the natural and social world, the psychological and the transpersonal; (3) how one can become an actor-creator who can actively claim their own experience through play and develop creative autonomy; (4) how different types of masks can have different transformative effects based on their specific dynamics; and (5) how improvisations with masks contribute to change and personal transformation.

I now briefly introduce Lecoq's typology of masks and its corresponding pedagogical sequence, and then present a way of applying it for trauma healing in (almost) reversed order.

Lecoq's original mask sequence consists of five types of masks in the following order: Neutral Mask, Larval Mask, Expressive Mask, Commedia dell'arte Half-Mask, and Red Nose (Lecoq, 2006; Wright, 2002). This is a sequence from equilibrium to increased disequilibrium, ordered according to the size of masks from the largest to the smallest. It firstly brings students to a zero point, or universal ground, where they are free from personal and socio-cultural interferences, and then gradually introduces them to different unbalanced states reflecting different types of dynamic structures and touching on different parts of our humanity.

From my experience working in groups with clients with developmental trauma and social trauma, I found that starting with the Commedia dell'arte Half-Mask and then reversing the pedagogical sequence works better therapeutically for those whose conditions and needs are largely different from those of students in a theatre school. The revised therapeutic sequence that I suggest can be presented as follows:

1 Commedia dell'arte Half-Masks are fun and bold. They liberate the clients' spontaneity, life drives, desires, survival wisdom, playfulness, humor, and psychological flexibility.
2 Expressive Masks enable the client to get in touch with strong but suppressed emotions, usually about relationships, mortality, and individual-group tension.
3 Larval Masks enable play, curiosity, and innocent responsiveness to (re)activate the subtle sensitivity and fresh vitality of the inner child.
4 The Neutral Mask leads to a state of calm readiness and openness that brings the most containing, harmonizing, and integrative power, as well as a kind of transpersonal dimension.
5 The Red Nose is used in the final stage for clients to individuate their transformation creatively and ascertain their uniqueness in body and mind.

This framework is particularly helpful in working with clients suffering from trauma-related conditions as the process in this sequence reflects different facets of trauma healing:

1 reactivating aliveness, increasing resilience, flexibility, and tolerance through the Commedia dell'arte Half-Mask;
2 processing complicated and entangled emotions, as well as mourning and core sadness through the Expressive Mask;
3 reconnecting to the pre-traumatized core of vitality and growth through the Larval Mask;
4 consolidating a mindful mind-body state for integration and self-regulation through the Neutral Mask;
5 facilitating personal integration and recognition of one's own uniqueness through the Red Nose.

From this, we can glimpse a possibility for the indirect processing of traumatic experience through mask work embedded in Lecoq's movement-mime-mask sequence. The way in which masks are viewed as incomplete dynamic structures can only be addressed by taking into consideration the whole sequence. Consequently, to enter the work with masks and for them to become effective, preparation through movement and mime is necessary. In the remainder of this chapter, I discuss in detail the first four stages of the reversed pedagogical sequence. Due to limited space, I will not discuss the Red Nose as it mainly remains optional in my practice.

Stage 1: Commedia dell'arte Half-Mask

Starting with half-masks has several practical advantages in a therapeutic context. Firstly, for less experienced clients, covering only half of the face feels less scary than the whole face. Because half-masks do not have complete features, it is the player who gives them life. Once the client takes off the half-mask, it will lose its power. By contrast, for masks with a complete face, it may be easier to imagine that they still have life even when not worn. Secondly, half-masks encourage the use of energetic sound and big movements through which the physical expressivity and presence of clients can be fully engaged. Thirdly, in the original Lecoq sequence, Commedia dell'arte Half-Masks are more straightforward and playful to use.

The Commedia dell'arte Half-Masks represent the stock characters in this theatre genre, usually classified into four groups, namely the Old Men, the Lovers, the Servants, and the Capitano (Fava, 2007). Each of them is considered to be the bearer of a specific condition of permanent survival. The differentiation of these characters also forms a model of hierarchical social structure. It is worth noting that not all these characters are masked (the lovers and the female servants are usually unmasked), and that the stock characters constitute different variations within each group, named, for instance, Pantalone, il Dottore, Tartaglia, Arlecchino, Brighella, Pulcinella, Zanni, or il Capitano.

These half-masks have a dual quality of being comic and cruel, and of playfully and primitively expressing life force and the dark side of living. We can observe this in their sharp geometrical and dynamic features in space, which can be seen as an exaggeration of human features. The duality that they express is also between the straightforward manifestation of desire towards fulfillment and enjoyment, without any sense of shame and guilt, and the inevitable brutality of existence that brings suffering and injustice to all mortals. The characters, represented by the masks, live between these two realities with an active and resilient flexibility of survival from which all kinds of oblique strategies for life engagement can be devised. A straightforward, strong, and resilient 'yes!' to life and destiny can be discovered, despite their sound complexities.

Trauma can result in difficulties engaging with life and in a loss of aliveness (Levine, 2010; van der Kolk et al., 2007). It is crucial for traumatized clients to regain a sense of safety in their own bodies and to overcome a fear of involvement with life itself (van der Hart et al., 1993), including giving and taking pleasure, and confronting their helplessness and shame (van der Kolk et al., 2007; Maté, 2022). Working with the Commedia dell'arte Half-Masks can be particularly effective in the first stages of trauma treatment for these problems, for the following reasons:

1 These masks can release the primitive or wild playfulness of the client and naturally create a playful group atmosphere. This is important for trauma healing because, as Ogden (2015, p.847) writes, 'clients are often challenged when it comes to a full-bodied capacity to enjoy life and to play'. She describes how play helps develop 'a flexible nervous system that can adapt quickly to all kinds of stimulation and a wide range of life events' (p.855). Porges (2021) also describes play as a neural exercise, suggesting that 'the roots of play are linked to the evolution of a neural mechanism that enables mammals to shift between mobilized fight-flight and calm, socially engaging states' (p.97). In earlier writing, he also illustrated how play can be seen as 'a therapeutic model in which autonomic state is disrupted and then stabilized through the recruitment of social engagement system' (Porges, 2018, p.62). Porges clearly contributes to the neurological understanding of how play supports greater resilience and the regulation of physiological states.
2 These masks, with their dynamic sculptural and spatial characteristics, can help clients reconnect with their primitive, instinctive life force, vitality, and desire through play and physicality. By reconnecting to such primitive energy in playing with the mask, and then bringing the character into action within the structure of a Commedia scene, the residual energy frozen in the nervous system's survival mechanism can be discharged within a safe containing structure. The masks allow for this energy to be safely released but also contained, while the action allows for it to be channeled and completed (Levine, 2010). It is a crucial processing for both somatic activation and stabilization through imaginative embodiment for traumatized clients, prior to engaging in the other stages of healing.
3 The stock characters in Commedia dell'arte are doomed to encounter a series of failure. They must deal with misfortune and the consequences of their mistakes. Protected by these masks, clients can become more playfully tolerant and resilient towards failure. This playful acceptance paves the way for loosening up the commonly shared pattern of self-blame for traumatized clients.
4 Commedia Half-Masks can help clients play with the shadow (in a Jungian sense), including social taboos, with energy and fun. The shadow (Jung, 1959) refers to what is suppressed and hidden under our personal or social mask, including primitive desires, cruelty in social interaction, power struggle, as well as our foolishness as mortals. Being aggressive, cunning, or greedy can be embraced playfully without seeing them simply as evilness. This can especially help clients to loosen up rigid patterns related to shame

and guilt, which are commonly internalized in traumatized clients' bodies (Maté, 2022).

5 These masks provide protection to play with the dynamics between oppressor and oppressed, usually mediated by plots of subversion. This is useful in trauma work because such dynamics and roles are usually 'automatically internalized and psychologically re-arrange one's internal sense of self' (Hudgins & Durost, 2022, p.59). The masks provide clients with contained opportunities to de-sensitize and explore themes of oppression and power, make these more tolerable (and playable), and liberate from internalized role structures.

For this very first stage using Commedia dell'arte masks, explorative improvisations with the masks are kept brief. This moving in and out of play is similar to titration and pendulation (Levine, 2010) to enable reconnection with the body's sensations and rechanneling energy through embodied action. At this stage, clients do not explore personal material explicitly but fully enjoy the playful, aesthetically distant, and decentered experience through which the body, emotions, and imagination can engage.

Stage 2: Expressive Mask

Expressive Mask and Larval Mask (in Stage 3), which both cover the whole face, enable clients to engage with more personal trauma material gradually and indirectly through associations. Although the Expressive Masks have full facial features, they still require a body to move and complete them. There are originally eight Sartori's Expressive Masks often used by Lecoq. Compared to the Larval Masks, they are 'more elaborate with finer details. They need only small movements to come alive' (Lecoq, 2006, p.106). As Lecoq keeps suggesting, 'they must be able to transform, to be sad, happy, excited, without ultimately becoming fixed in the expression of a single moment' (Lecoq, 2002, p.57). This is possible because these masks are primarily not portraits of singular facial expressions, but structures consisting of multi-directional or even conflicting dynamics.

The word 'expressive' can be misleading. These masks are not directly or intentionally expressive. They are expressive in multiple indirect ways as they do not directly speak. Because of this, the masks can effectively show overwhelmingly speechless moments in life, when 'words are no longer necessary or not necessary yet' (Lecoq, 2006, p.106). They are powerful in their subtlety and silence, responding to moments and situations in which not even a single word or gesture can possibly be expressed. Their gestural expressions can be indirect or interrupted, staying small, halfway, tight, or ambivalent, if not totally paralyzed. In my opinion, a more suitable term might be 'suppressive masks', because of their avoidance of expressing explicit emotions, although these still can leak out subtly and unintentionally. By contrast, both Commedia dell'arte Half-Masks and Larval Masks are straightforwardly expressive.

Consequently, this type of mask is therapeutically useful to explore suppressed feelings and overwhelming moments such as separation, catastrophe, or unbearable fate. The structural lines of these masks can be seen as traces of distortion and deformation from the sufferings caused by external or internal forces beyond the individual's control, or existential wounds from life history (see Figure 3.1).

Compared to the previous stage that focused on reconnecting to and grounding in a primitive vitality, this stage is concerned with fragmented meanings and unsettled emotions. The experience of feeling overwhelmed is an

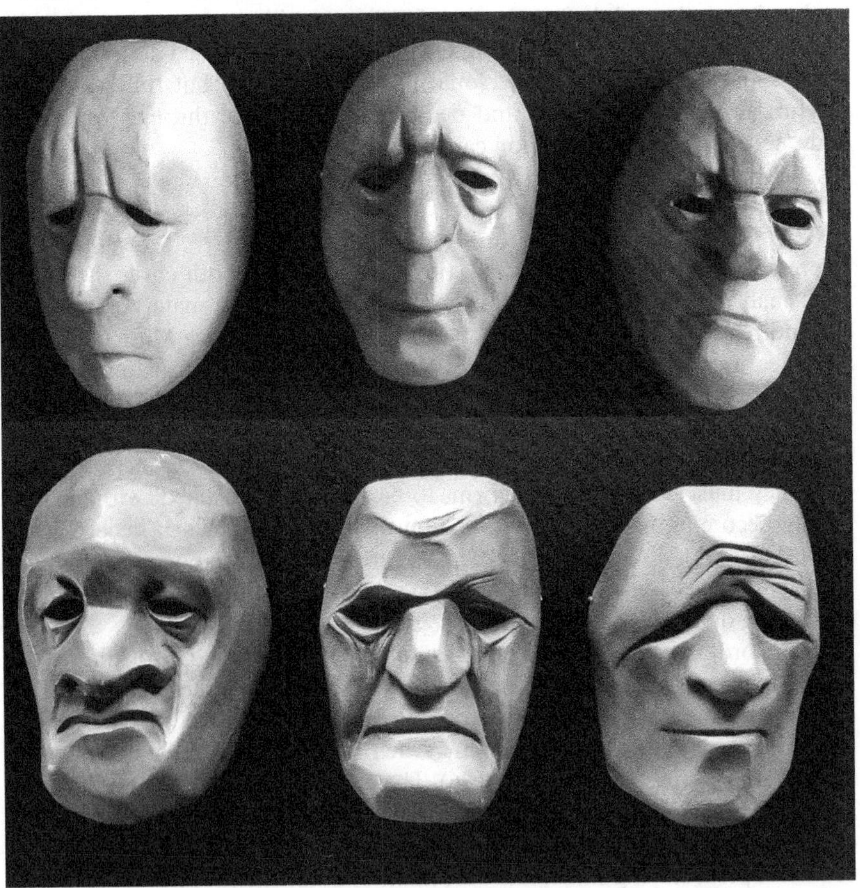

Figure 3.1 Expressive Masks designed and made by Matteo Destro, trained by Jacques Lecoq and Donato Sartori

essential component of trauma. The entanglement of manifold emotions emerging from it constitutes a 'complex' (Wilson, 2004). This was initially described by Jung (1919, p.66) as 'the total number of presentations relating to a definite experience that is charged with emotions'. Expressive Masks have great potential to get in touch with clients' traumatic experiences indirectly and to slowly disentangle them. In this second stage, putting the masks or the masked actors in fictional scenes that are carefully selected provides a structure for these chaotic and entangled experiences that are emotionally charged. Through these structures, emotions and the related non-verbal materials therein can be rechanneled.

Trauma experts recognize that the reframing of traumatic memories for new meaning to emerge is key in the healing process, alongside somatic stabilization (Herman, 1992; Ogden, 2006). Yet, as van der Kolk (2014) points out, many practitioners also discover that merely a reconstruction of the trauma experience into a coherent narrative is often not enough, implying that something is missing in terms of non-verbal material distant from cognitive and conceptual awareness, although still articulated instead of just being chaotic.

Authors in the field of trauma generally agree that the intrusive reliving in trauma belongs to a separated second memory system that is pre-verbal and very often fragmented (Brewin, 2014; Herman, 1992; van der Kolk, 1994; Levine, 2015), and hence cannot be processed directly via verbal means. Besides the primitive emotions for survival, there are also higher emotional states, such as grief, shame, guilt, or despair, that are associated with unprocessed memories.

Phenomenologically speaking, the Expressive Masks function like a 'magnet' attracting the fragmented images and disorganized impulses of those memories, as well as the emotional energies attached to them, so that they can come together under an aesthetic holding, similar to a process of crystallization. The images created through working with Expressive Masks enable the recollection of fragmented materials floating in implicit memories alienated from the conscious ego and autobiographical memory (van der Kolk, 1994; Levine, 2015). This is a key part of indirect experiential processing which will also be illustrated in the next stage with the Larval Masks.

The indirect processing that happens at this stage can also be associated with mourning. Authors have highlighted the importance of mourning in trauma treatment, especially for developmental trauma (Bowlby, 1980; Herman, 1992). Remembrance and mourning constitute the second stage in the three-stage recovery model proposed by Herman (1992). She describes how mourning is a subtle and complicated process whose facilitation requires skills. To mourn and to complete the mourning process, the suppressed and buried emotions must be recognized, released, and contained. The core sadness is then to be worked through with care and compassion, followed by acceptance.

An essential aspect of the mourning stage is its transpersonal and spiritual dimension. Some key trauma practitioners have argued that any effective and comprehensive treatment cannot avoid the question and the role of spirituality in trauma healing (Kalsched, 2013; Park et al., 2016). From these authors' perspective, moving towards the transpersonal and spiritual horizon is crucial for the completion of mourning.

I have identified three stages in the use of Expressive Masks that can facilitate the mourning process and the journey from the existential to the transpersonal. I have named these stages: poetic play, ritual play, and mythological play. They can be described as follows:

1 Poetic play describes scenes with masked characters depicting intense moments in daily life with existential themes. This stage is called 'poetic' play because the fictional scenes are stylized, so that those intense moments are presented in theatrically poetic forms that, therapeutically, provide emotional protection. The poetic form helps highlight what is precious at the core of loss and sadness, as well as our existential finitude, which is a key step in mourning.
2 Ritual play with mask consists in the transformation of the strong and deep emotions from the poetic play. A horizon between the existential and the transpersonal emerges as ritual is an interface between the individual mortal and experiences that extend beyond the personal. Such shift of horizon is key for transforming the core grief and sadness during mourning.
3 Mythological play with mask provides greater distance and an overview perspective of the world that allow clients to fully embody a transpersonal viewpoint to see life as a whole, in which the individual is only a part. The shift away from the individual's perspective provides a holistic space of containment for the mourning process.

To summarize, the Expressive Masks function like a magnet for the emotionally charged yet unprocessed fragments of traumatic memories. The poetically and aesthetically constructed dramatic scenes with masked characters give coherence and articulation to this material, which is then further transformed through a transition from the existential to the transpersonal as part of a mourning process.

Stage 3: Larval Mask

Larval Masks, also called Naive Masks (Wright, 2017), have a simple, rough, and bold shape, which has a momentum to go off-balance, making the wearer feel like they will fall. Despite being non-figurative and sometimes having no eyes, they still retain the features of a face. These masks can be recognized for their simplicity and purity, with clear dynamic features in their shape. In Lecoq pedagogy, this type of mask helps develop sensitivity and re-discover our

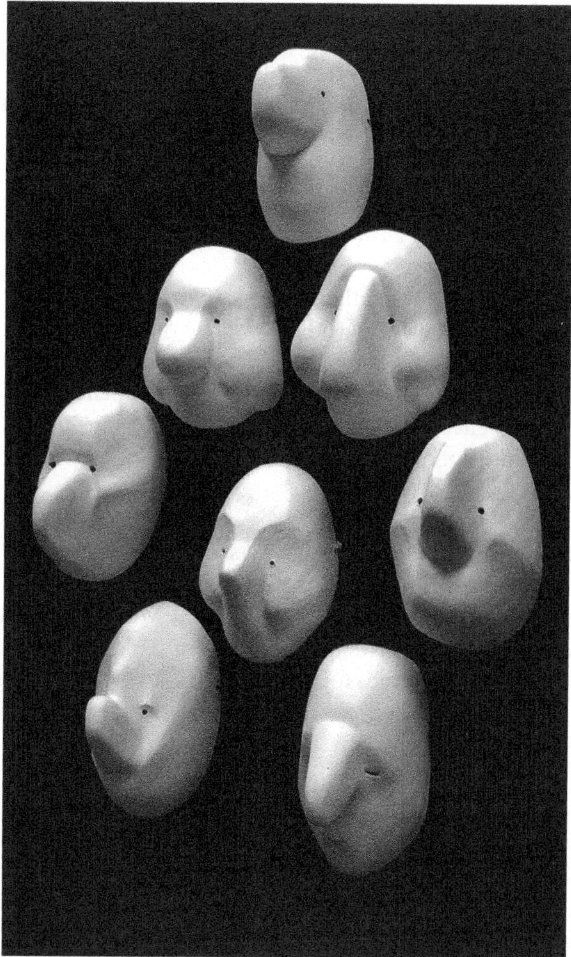

Figure 3.2 Larval Masks designed and made by Matteo Destro
© Matteo Destro

impulsive reaction to the environment prior to the interference of fear (see Figure 3.2).

Therapeutically, these masks can be beneficial because of the way in which they create a simple and safe space whereby one can feel free to explore the world with a sense of curiosity and playfulness deprived of fear. A space in which the clients' inner world can reconnect to the outer world and others, as it was before the traumatic event. These masks can therefore provide a corrective experience for developmental repair to reconnect with pre-traumatized parts.

There is an intimate and deep relationship between Larval Masks and trauma work as they can symbolize the inner child that was developmentally traumatized. Kalsched (2013) emphasizes that a main consequence of trauma is that our innocence, which is also the core of our creative vitality and growth, is paradoxically hidden and imprisoned by an archetypal self-care system aimed at protecting it. Furthermore, Kalsched (2017, p.474) suggests that:

> Only when the wounded, orphaned, and innocent part of the personality is allowed to suffer experience again – this time with the promise of new outcome – can true healing of trauma occur.

Larval Masks can represent an effective way to do this. A first step consists in simple play that enables the corrective experience of re-awakening or returning to a pre-traumatized playful and curious core. In simple play, clients return to a childlike state where they are invited to explore the environment and objects. Because of the innocence of the masks, spontaneous play and free exploration will emerge. Two additional stages can follow that simple play:

1 Cruel play enables the internalized perpetrators or oppressors from developmental or collective trauma to be released, externalized, and contained in an embodied manner, so that clients become conscious of them. In cruel play, the child character represented by Larval Mask is put into a series of intense encounters with unfriendly, indifferent, cold, or even abusive adult characters that are unmasked, forming a matrix of cruel adult-child dynamics from the collective unconscious. This processing works not only for the masked player, but also for the unmasked players. Cruel play provides a contained space for a safe (re-)experiencing of the suffering of the wounded part (metaphorically embodied and protected with the masked character), which according to Kalsched (2017) quoted above, is part of the trauma healing process.
2 Nurturing play consists in developing the inner nurturing capacities of the client. The clients are invited to use the Larval Masks as an image of a child character to imagine corrective nurturing experiences between child and caregivers, to explore, embody, and experiment with ideal and good enough parenting, and to help develop an internal capacity for self-care from these parenting images. This nurturing play leads to the imaginative embodiment of a new outcome that is experientially real for the previously wounded part (Kalsched, 2017).

From my experience, Larval Masks are not only useful for working with developmental trauma, as they are not only childlike but also innocent in essence. It can be argued that every relational traumatic experience, including social trauma, alienates an innocent part of the personality that feels victimized and helpless. As Kalsched (2017) pointed out, it is that part that needs to be released and nurtured for a thoroughgoing transformation. The Larval Masks can function as a metaphor of the innocent victim for us to reach and take care of. As such, this stage is a core part of the indirect processing of trauma.

Stage 4: Neutral Mask

The term 'Neutral Mask' can be misleading. Some might imagine that the word 'neutral' means zero and think about a state of dead calmness. But if we look at the Neutral Mask designed by Amleto Sartori, it is obvious that 'it has nothing in common with white masks used in carnival processions or demonstrations [as] those are dead masks, at the opposite pole from neutrality' (Lecoq, 2002, p.36). In short, the Neutral Mask is a mask of readiness, availability, and openness, that places the actor 'in a state of discovery, of freedom to receive, of perfect balance and economy of movement' (Lecoq, 2002, p.36). Its wide open eyes and comfortable open mouth imply a state of full opening towards the space, ready to enter that space and to create a dynamic balance with its surroundings. It is a mask of being one with everything and of harmony (see Figure 3.3).

To enter this mask, a combination of the Feldenkrais Method® and guided imagination for embodiment are used to help clients approach this state of openness, readiness, and harmony. Neutral Mask in this stage is used as a mask of integration, another key aspect of trauma healing. The core work in this stage also has three sub-stages:

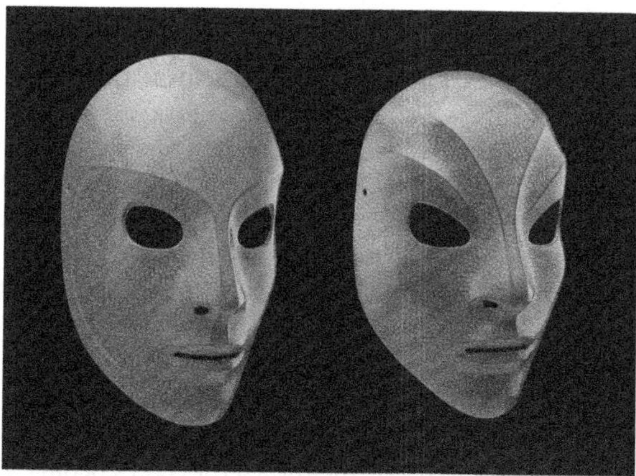

Figure 3.3 Neutral Masks (male on the left and female on the right) designed and made by Amleto Sartori from natural leather 1968

1 The first step consists in guiding clients to contemplatively review their previous experiences and learnings with the different types of masks, under the state of calm openness of the Neutral Mask. They review the ways in which the chosen masks have activated different inner parts in their healing journey. This constitutes a mindful process of integration, searching for an ultimately containing and coordinating state that regulates these different energies activated and re-channeled by the different masks to reach a dynamic and lively harmony.
2 Supported by the integration of these inner resources gathered through the different masks, clients are also invited to stay in this embodied contemplative state of the Neutral Mask to further review their personal life journey. This constitutes a step of moving back towards the personal after the journey into metaphor of the previous stages. The choice is given to the client as to how they would like to reassess the integration of their autobiographical narrative.
3 Clients are then invited to imagine new possibilities for their lives and their future, which is also emphasized as the final stage of trauma treatment (Herman, 1992; Ogden, 2006). Clients are supported to integrate their personal life materials reviewed in the previous stages with renewed possibilities for their future in a montage of body movements under the guidance of the Neutral Mask. Therein, images of the past and the future are anchored in the present to form a dynamic, aesthetic, non-linear totality, or 'temporal integration' (Siegel, 2012) in which 'we differentiate our longings for certainty, permanence and immortality from – and link them with – the reality of life's uncertainty, transience, and mortality' (p.286).

Following Lecoq's dynamic principle, these three sub-stages are not static. They resemble a moving meditation with the help of the Neutral Mask as a guiding image. For clients with trauma, the Neutral Mask holds important learnings as it helps keep them present and open to life, with increased capacity for self-regulation and integration. The openness and readiness of the Neutral Mask also prepare clients to engage in their real life with a renewed dynamic balance between the self and the surrounding world.

After this stage of the Neutral Mask, there can be several possible options, depending on the context. One option is to bring the journey to a close. Another one is to revisit previous stages for another cycle in the case of long-term work. A third option is to go into clown work and Red Nose for a deeper, more personalized consolidation and integration.

Table 3.1 provides a summary of the reversed Lecoq's pedagogical sequence of using different types of masks for trauma healing.

The therapeutic journey making use of mime and mask inspired by Lecoq's pedagogy has an arch shape, culminating at Stage 3. From Stage 1 to Stage 3, it is a journey from our corporeal life to our emotional self and the innermost core of creativity and growth. From Stage 3 to Stage 5, it is a process of rebirth,

Table 3.1 Framework of reversed pedagogical sequence of using masks for indirect processing of trauma in therapeutic settings

	Stage 1	*Stage 2*	*Stage 3*	*Stage 4*	*Stage 5*
Type of Mask	Commedia Half-Mask	Expressive Mask	Larval Mask	Neutral Mask	Red Nose
Client's inner resources	primitive life-force, desire, vitality	sentiments from love/value	the innocence, the soul, or the growing core of vitality	the containing and coordinating function	creativity through and for personal uniqueness
Therapeutic Possibilities	discharging and flowing of survival energy that was previously frozen	mourning and re-channeling of emotional energies that were previously suppressed	reconnecting with the source of human potentials, nurturing and re-activating human development	integration, self-regulation and harmonization	individuation or actualization of uniqueness
Sub-stages	–	1 poetic play 2 ritual play 3 mythological play	1 simple play 2 cruel play 3 nurturing play	1 integration of therapy journey 2 autobiographical integration 3 temporal integration	–

from an innocent and vulnerable core to an extensive consciousness and universal humanity of a creative individual. The process is progressive and can only move between stages when the client is ready.

Concluding Remarks

In this chapter, I have presented a therapeutic framework based on two interrelated core teachings in Lecoq's pedagogy. The first one refers to mimodynamics, the fundamental miming embodiment of human beings, which is the source of metaphorical cognition and imagination, and grounds the universal dynamism of his pedagogy. The second one is about masks as incomplete dynamic structures at the interface between embodiment and imagination. The therapeutic framework I have discussed is characterized by a progressive sequence making use of five different types of masks, in (almost) reversed order of the Lecoq's pedagogical sequence, modified for clients who have suffered trauma. It has shown how masks provide a strong container and are catalysts for healing and transformation.

At the core of this sequence is indirect experiential processing which first crystallizes and then transforms the fragmented traumatic materials. This phenomenon shows that pre-verbal, non-autobiographical images are not necessarily chaotic or fragmented but can have their own order when mediated by mask play and art forms. It illustrates how verbal processing is not the only way to process the fragmented materials of trauma, as suggested by other trauma therapies. I have shown, in this chapter, how working with masks provides effective strategies for the expression of non-verbal material as forms of indirect processing for trauma healing.

A limitation of this chapter is that it is mainly based on my practical clinical experience. It is an attempt to contribute to an initial stage of conceptualization for key concepts in the fields of physical theatre and trauma for future researchers and other practitioners to take as a point of reference. More empirical research is therefore needed for systematic testing and refinement or modification of the framework presented in this chapter. Besides, the model calls for further research in the following two areas. Firstly, more in-depth and systematic investigation is required with regards to the basic thesis of embodied, sensorimotor-based, and metaphorical cognition put forward by Lecoq, as well as the phenomenon of preverbal articulation and crystallization of images mediated by masks for indirect processing. This is especially relevant to trauma healing because the traumatic symptomatology is largely built upon the phenomenological and experiential distinction between episodic and perceptual memory (Brewin, 2014), or between explicit and implicit memory systems (van der Kolk, 1994), while more comprehensive understanding of indirect processing can help clarify the interaction between these memory systems and the possible mediation mechanisms in such interaction. Secondly, although Lecoq proposed that the spatial dynamics of the mask transcends personal history and cultural differences, and touches upon something more universal and fundamental, this requires further examination as to whether this is empirically valid especially in the context of multiculturalism, and whether such perspective limits our awareness of cultural diversity, or on the contrary assists intercultural communication.

Trauma can be experienced as invasive, and traumatic symptoms are akin to ghosts attached to or wandering within the self of the client. In contrast, masks are incomplete dynamic structures that can guide body movement and sensorimotor-based and embodied imagination to create contained spaces in which these ghosts can gather, play, and transform into something digestible for the psyche of the client. Metaphorically speaking, as in a masquerade carnival, the ghosts of trauma are invited as guests for temporary incarnation through play and a series of embodied metamorphosis until a higher harmony is achieved.

References

Bowlby, J. (1980). *Attachment and loss: loss, sadness and depression* (Vol. 3). Basic Books.

Brewin, C. (2014). Episodic memory, perceptual memory, and their interaction: foundations for a theory of posttraumatic stress disorder. *Psychological Bulletin*, 140(1), pp. 69–97.

Estévez, C. (2015). Mask performance for a contemporary Commedia dell'Arte. In J. Chaffe & O. Crick (Eds.), *The Routledge companion to Commedia dell'Arte* (pp. 130–138). Routledge.

Fava, A. (2007). *The comic mask in the Commedia Dell'Arte: Actor training, improvisation, and the poetics of survival*. Northwestern University Press.

Forbes, D., Bisson, J. I., Monson, C. M., & Berliner, L. (2020). *Effective Treatments for PTSD* (3rd ed.). The Guilford Press.

Ford, J. D. (2017). Emotional regulation and skill-based interventions. In S. N. Gold (Ed.), *APA Handbook of Trauma Psychology Vol. 2* (pp. 227–252). American Psychological Association.

Herman, J. (1992). *Trauma and recovery: The aftermath of violence—from domestic abuse to political terror*. Basic Books.

Hudgins, K. & Durost, S. W. (Eds.) (2022). *Experiential therapy from trauma to post-traumatic growth: Therapeutic spiral modal psychodrama*. Springer.

Jones, P. (2007). *Drama as therapy: theory, practice and research Vol.1*. Routledge.

Jousse, M. (2016). *In search of coherence: Introducing Marcel Jousse's anthropology of mimism*. Pickwick Publications.

Jung, C. G. (1919). *Studies in word association* (M. Eder, Trans.). Moffat, Yard & Company.

Jung, C. G. (1959). The shadow. In G. Adler & R. F. C. Hull (Eds.), *Collected works of C.G. Jung, Volume 9 (Part 2): Aion: Researches into the phenomenology of the self* (pp. 8–10). Princeton University Press.

Kalsched, D. (2013). *Trauma and the soul: A psycho-spiritual approach to human development and its interruption*. Routledge.

Kalsched, D. (2017). Trauma, innocence and the core complex of dissociation. *Journal of Analytical Psychology*, 62(4), 474–500.

Kemp. R. (2016). Lecoq, emotion and embodied cognition. In M. Evans & R. Kemp. (Eds.), *The Routledge companion to Jacques Lecoq* (pp. 199–207). Routledge.
Kiyimba, N., Buxton, C., Shuttleworth, J., & Pathe, E. (2022). *Discourses of psychological trauma*. Palgrave Macmillan.
Lakoff, G. & Johnson, M. (2003). *Metaphors we live by*. University of Chicago Press.
Lecoq, J. (2002). *The moving body*. Bloomsbury Methuen Drama.
Lecoq, J. (2006). *Theatre of movement and gesture*. Routledge.
Levine, P. (2010). *In an unspoken voice: How the body releases trauma and restores goodness*. North Atlantic Books.
Levine, P. (2015). *Trauma and memory: Brain and body in a search of living past: A practical guide for understanding and working with traumatic memory*. North Atlantic Books.
Maté, G. (2022). *The myth of normal: Trauma, illness & healing in a toxic culture*. Penguin Random House LLC.
Merleau-Ponty, M. (2012). *Phenomenology of perception*. Routledge.
Murphy, M. (2019). *Enacting Lecoq: Movement in theatre, cognition, and life*. Palgrave Macmillan.
Ogden, P. (2006). *Trauma and body: A sensorimotor approach to psychotherapy*. W. W. Norton & Company.
Ogden, P. (2015). *Sensorimotor psychotherapy: Interventions for trauma and attachment*. W. W. Norton & Company.
Park, C. L., Currier, J. M., Harris, J. I., & Slattery, J. M. (2016). *Trauma, meaning and spirituality: Translating research into clinical practice*. American Psychological Association.
Porges, S. W. (2018). Polyvagal theory: A primer. In S. W. Porges & D. Dana (Eds.), *Clinical applications of the polyvagal theory: The emergence of polyvagal-informed therapies* (pp. 50–72). W. W. Norton & Company.
Porges, S. W. (2021). *Polyvagal safety: Attachment, communication, self-regulation*. W. W. Norton & Company.
Siegel, D. (2012). *The Developing mind: How relationships and the brain interact to shape who we are*. The Guilford Press.
van der Hart, O., Steele, K., Boon, S., & Brown, P. (1993). The treatment of traumatic memories: Synthesis, realization, and integration. *Dissociation*, *6*, 162–180.
van der Kolk, B. A. (1994). The body keeps the score: Memory and the evolving psychobiology of posttraumatic stress. *Harvard Review of Psychiatry*, 1(5), 253–265.
van der Kolk, B. A. (2014). *The body keeps the score*. Penguin.
van der Kolk, B. A., MacFarlane, A. C., & Weisaeth, L. (Eds.) (2007). *Traumatic stress: The effects of overwhelming experience on mind, body, and society*. The Guilford Press.
Wilson, J. P. (2004). The abyss experience and the trauma complex: A Jungian perspective of posttraumatic stress disorder and dissociation. *Journal of Trauma & Dissociation*, 5(3), 43–68.
Wright, J. (2002). The masks of Jacques Lecoq. In F. Chamberlain & R. Yarrow (Eds.), *Jacques Lecoq and the British theatre* (pp. 71–84). Routledge.
Wright, J. (2017). *Playing the mask: Acting without bullshit*. Nick Hern Books.
Zahavi, D. (2017). *Husserl's legacy: Phenomenology, metaphysics, and transcendental philosophy*. Oxford University Press.

Chapter 4

Engaging the Body From a Distance

Online Dramatherapy with Traumatised Children

Christiana Iordanou

Introduction

Recent developments in neuroscientific research focus on the interrelationship between body and mind (Panksepp, 2007; Porges, 2009). Specifically, research shows that when trauma occurs, it is not processed verbally but rather stored in the body. Psychological treatment should therefore first and foremost target the body itself (van der Kolk, 2015). Childhood trauma can have deleterious consequences for a child's development. To facilitate healing, several therapeutic approaches which utilise the body in the process of treatment have been developed, one of which being dramatherapy (Sajnani et al., 2019). Traditionally, these methods are used in in-person therapeutic settings where children engage in play and/or other embodied activities in the same physical space as the therapist. Given that the lockdowns imposed by Covid-19[1] enforced an immediate shift to online therapy, dramatherapists were forced to adjust their practice to digital spaces and come up with ways to apply these methods from a distance to support traumatised children. As online dramatherapy is already used widely in therapeutic provision (Emunah & Butler, 2020), this chapter aims to discuss how it can engage the body in the treatment of traumatised children. The main goal of this chapter is to show that embodied work with traumatised children is feasible virtually as long as dramatherapists are open to the idea that online therapy is not inferior to face-to-face work but merely different. Accordingly, my aim is to provide an outline of what online dramatherapy with traumatised children may involve and how embodied practices can be incorporated in online work. I will first outline the consequences of childhood trauma to help the reader appreciate the magnitude of the problem and hence the need for effective online interventions.

Childhood Trauma and Its Consequences

Childhood trauma encompasses a host of traumatic events such as domestic, physical, and sexual abuse (van Westrhenen & Fritz, 2014). According to Terr (1991), there are two types of childhood trauma: (1) Type I includes single

DOI: 10.4324/9781003322375-6

traumatic incidents which are sudden and unexpected (e.g. physical disasters, terrorist attacks, or a single episode of abuse); (2) Type II involves prolonged and repeated incidents, such as repetitive sexual/physical abuse, domestic/community violence, war, etc. Terr's typology has been enriched by extensive research on developmental trauma, such as ongoing abusive experiences throughout childhood, which disrupt the formation of a healthy attachment bond and the child's ability to express and regulate emotions (D'Andrea et al., 2012; van der Kolk, 2009).

The data on trauma related to childhood is alarming. Overall, older children are more likely to have lived through more traumatic events than younger ones leading to harmful mental health consequences (Grasso et al., 2013). Adolescents are more susceptible to new traumatic experiences compared to younger children, and girls are more in danger compared to boys due to higher rates of sexual assault which affect them three to four times more than their male counterparts. In fact, adolescent girls represent the child population with the highest risk for traumatic experiences (Saunders & Adams, 2014). The Covid-19 pandemic added to the trauma experienced by children. During this time, there was an observed increase in several types of child abuse, including domestic and online abuse and child sexual exploitation (Romanou & Belton, 2020).

Childhood trauma has detrimental consequences for a child's development. As trauma is stored in the body, it can result in long-lasting psychological and/or health effects (Malchiodi, 2015; Sesar et al., 2022). When trauma occurs early in life, it can lead to developmental trauma disorder (DTD) which is a syndrome that extends the posttraumatic stress disorder diagnosis (PTSD) and involves several symptoms of emotional, somatic, cognitive, behavioural, and self/relational dysregulation (Spinazzola et al., 2021). If it is prolonged, such as in the case of persistent abuse and/or when children are the victims of multiple traumas, attachment and emotional development can be disrupted, with effects that can last for decades and be passed from one generation to the next (Greene et al., 2020; Perry, 2008; Thoma et al., 2021). Childhood trauma may also be related to symptoms of depression and/or dissociation because the neural pathways which connect self-awareness to the perception of one's body have broken down (Lim et al., 2020). It can further cause disruption between implicit and explicit memory, which can lead to disconnection between the context of the traumatic event and the emotions surrounding it (Malchiodi, 2003). Clearly, these findings indicate that the treatment of childhood trauma is crucial.

Childhood Trauma and the Body

Empirical work suggests that trauma is stored in the body and that the memory of traumatic events manifests in somatic experiences (van der Kolk, 2015). From an evolutionary perspective, trauma triggers a fight, flight, or freeze reaction in the brain, meaning that people respond by fighting back, running away, or freezing to the spot (Tyler, 2012). This is supported by research which shows trauma-related neuroimaging processes in the brain (Serlin & Zhou, 2022). When trauma occurs, it manifests in the body at a subconscious level and is then processed by the amygdala (Rothschild, 2000). The amygdala allows individuals to detect danger and stores the trauma in the form of sensory experiences (Homann, 2010). If people have sensory reminders similar to the traumatic event, they may interpret the current event as dangerous and react with emotional activation analogous to that related to the traumatic event. Due to this emotional activation, trauma affects the body's stress response and disrupts the brain's ability to deal with it effectively (Ursano et al., 2009). Further neuroscientific research shows that when trauma occurs, the right hemisphere of the brain, which involves nonverbal communication, takes the lead while the left hemisphere, which is responsible for linguistic communication, is sluggish, leading to inability to express oneself verbally (van der Kolk, 1996). As a result, traumatised individuals may be unable to verbalise their experience and may require nonverbal methods to express their feelings, thoughts, and emotions. Collectively, these findings suggest that interventions which target sensory memory and include embodied practices may be more appropriate than language to facilitate healing (Laird & Mulvihill, 2022).

Many of the embodied therapeutic approaches discussed in the literature on trauma treatment are theoretically grounded in attachment theory. According to this, infants need to form a positive attachment relationship with a trusted parental figure to regulate their emotions (Schore & Schore, 2008). A responsive caregiver will attend to an infant's needs by attuning to their facial expressions, gestures, and movements. Through these bodily and nonverbal cues, the child learns to form a healthy attachment. If, however, the caregiver does not respond to the child's needs, the child's development may be impaired and their ability to form healthy attachment bonds in the future may be severely compromised. Since children develop a sense of self through their body (Hanna, 1970), these embodied experiences also affect their social experiences (Price & Shildrick, 1999; Weiss, 1999). This suggests that the body plays a significant role in social interaction. As these nonverbal communication cues reside in the right part of the brain, children with trauma history may struggle to express themselves verbally and may require nonverbal means such as movement, rhythm, and attunement to understand and process their trauma (Schore & Schore, 2008; Serlin & Zhou, 2022). Thus 'bottom up' therapeutic approaches which start from the body and move up to the brain may be more successful in the healing process than verbal interventions (Ogden et al., 2006). Such approaches involve practices that help children gain body awareness by first paying attention to physical sensations. Children can then process the nonverbal experience cognitively and understand their trauma responses by observing what is happening in their body.

Working Through Childhood Trauma From an Embodied Perspective

Dramatherapy utilises embodied interventions to deal with childhood trauma. According to Jones (2007, p.113), 'embodiment in dramatherapy involves the way the self is realized by and through the body. The body is often described as the primary means by which communication occurs between self and other'. As we primarily learn through our bodies, children who have experienced trauma, particularly physical trauma, require physical play to feel safe again in their body (Jennings, 2015). Play in several of its forms – i.e. sensory play, projective play, role-play – is children's way of expressing their trauma, often leading to emotional release (Ogawa, 2004). It has a prominent role in children's development and is related to aspects of cognitive development such as perspective taking, self-awareness, coping, and self-regulation (Bolton et al., 2021). It helps children deal with traumatic events while building their confidence and self-mastery, which are important for those who have felt frightened and belittled. Play comes naturally to children and helps them make sense of their experiences by keeping a safe distance from the event and working through it (Jones, 2015). It further enables children who feel 'small' and scared to experiment with several roles and find new ways to understand the situation they are in. This approach helps them create a new narrative which allows them to recognise what happened, challenge it, and finally detach from it (Newman, 2017).

One of the earliest embodied forms of play with infants in dramatherapy is Neuro-Dramatic Play (NDP) which involves sensory, rhythmic, and dramatic play, and supports the formation of healthy attachments (Jennings, 2011). This type of play usually happens six months before to six months after birth but can be returned to with traumatised children to achieve healing. The different forms of developmental play can be described as follows. Sensory play such as playing with slime or blowing bubbles helps children experiment with their senses. Messy play such as finger paints and sand play allows children to express the mess of their experience and start creating some order. Rhythmic play, which entails dancing, clapping, singing, and drumming, helps children rediscover their rhythm. Dramatic play essentially involves role-play and enables children to explore their experience symbolically. These activities help children develop a sense of self and, by working with their body, learn to feel safe in it again (Jennings, 2015).

One way for embodied play to be utilised in dramatherapy for the treatment of childhood trauma is through Jennings's Embodiment-Projection-Role (EPR) paradigm (2015) which follows the progression of dramatic play from birth up to the seventh year of life. In this model, embodiment involves the first 13 months of life during which infants explore the world through their body and senses. Neuro-Dramatic Play happens during this stage. Projection extends between 13 months and 3 years, during which children play with toys and art media. Role takes place between three and seven years. Here children can enact roles and stories. It is imperative that children are offered the opportunity to enact roles which are outside of their own reality, as paradoxically, they are more likely to understand their own experience better if they adopt a distanced role (Jennings, 1998). This can be achieved by engaging with roles which involve single feelings, such as 'the angry person' or 'the sad person', using masks or animal characters to create a story, or working with characters that emerged during projective play.

Overall, NDP and EPR involve embodied activities which enable children to make use of their imagination and symbolism to heal trauma. By using these methods, dramatherapists can create a dramatic reality which allows children to explore their experience safely (Pendzik, 2006). Dramatic reality is the space between reality and fantasy, where one's imagination takes form. In dramatic reality, traumatised children can explore a victimised hero's feelings with the knowledge that they are not actually the character, and hence work through and overcome the role's difficulties. In face-to-face dramatherapy, this is achieved through projective and embodied play which enable children to connect with their own body and experiment with being physically close with the therapist in the safety of the therapy room. In this process children face their traumatised parts and accept them in the here and now. Here, children can engage with roles from stories and fairy tales and process the traumatic event from a safe distance (Jennings, 1994). In dramatherapy, this distance is called aesthetic distance. In the context of trauma, aesthetic distance is the space between over-distance, which involves cognitively detaching from the traumatic event, and under-distance, which involves reexperiencing the event and being flooded by emotions (Landy, 1983; Scheff, 1981). Aesthetic distance creates a balance between these two states: the child can revisit a past event securely without being too close to it (under-distanced) or entirely withdrawn from it (over-distanced). The aesthetic distance created in dramatherapy allows children to be both an observer and a participant in a situation and hence understand it and work through it effectively. As an example, when a child engages in role-play, they can participate in the character's journey while also observing the character's progress and realisation of the desired outcome.

Using embodied practices in dramatherapy not only helps children distance themselves emotionally from the distressing event but also minimises the anxiety related to verbally recalling it (Haen, 2015). This is particularly beneficial in child sexual abuse cases where the body has been violated, and children have difficulty narrating the incident (Bannister, 2003; Iordanou, 2019). It further enables children to put fragmented memories regarding the traumatic experience into a chronological context and process them effectively (Sesar et al., 2022).

Transition From Physical to Online Spaces

Due to the social restrictions imposed during the pandemic, there was an immediate shift to online therapy, which became the primary means of providing psychotherapeutic treatment, leading many dramatherapists to adjust their work to digital spaces (Feniger-Schaal et al., 2022). This shift from a three-dimensional to a two-dimensional reality had serious implications, particularly for dramatherapy provision which is grounded in creativity, action, and embodied practices (Schubert, 2022). Some scholars argue that in an online space the body expresses itself differently and misses the opportunity to engage in the present moment with another person with whom it coexists (Dementyeva, 2020). This is because, in online spaces, the felt sense – the somatic experience of oneself and the other in the moment – may be lost (Gendlin, 1981). In fact, as body postures, distance, rhythm, and movements may be distorted in an online environment, one can argue that online therapeutic work may be disembodied (García et al., 2022).

As aesthetic distance is an integral part of dramatherapeutic work, a pertinent question is whether it can be recreated online to facilitate children's healing from trauma. When working online, one needs to carefully consider the transitional space created from the real-life distance of physical environments to the child's personal space (Schubert, 2022). In face-to-face dramatherapy, this is primarily achieved through ritual which creates a transitional time to and from the session. This transitional time may be lacking in online spaces. Additionally, engaging our senses and full body may not be possible online, suggesting that working from a distance may in fact hinder embodied work (Krasanakis 2021; Regula, 2020).

Although these challenges of online dramatherapy are real and valid, recent research findings suggest that engaging the body from a distance is feasible if therapists accept that the online setting is not lacking compared to an in-person setting but is merely different (Atsmon et al., 2022). Technological communication can indeed be embodied as it happens in the context of habitual sensorimotor engagement with one's environment (García et al., 2022). Thus, dramatherapeutic work through the screen does not have to replace face-to-face work but provides a different approach for traumatised children to experiment with embodied practices (Schubert, 2022). Moreover, as traumatised children may be afraid of physical proximity, the distance created by digital mediums may offer them the space they need to experiment safely with their body. They may feel more secure when entering the session from their room, not only due to the physical distance between themselves and the therapist but also the security experienced in their own space (Regula, 2020; Wood et al., 2020). Besides, one should not forget that younger individuals are generally more familiar with technologies which are part of their lives and thus may feel more at ease engaging in online work. Lastly, for any action to take place online, children must give consent (e.g. children should be asked if they are willing to share their drawing on camera) (Schubert, 2022). Although this is not exclusive to online working, the issue of consent is nevertheless a powerful healing process for traumatised children as trauma is accompanied by a sense of loss of control (Ogawa, 2004).

Engaging the Body From a Distance: Online Dramatherapy With Traumatised Children

Accordingly, dramatherapists can apply their creativity and adjust their toolkit in online settings with the knowledge that their work is not intended to supplement face-to-face therapy but rather create a new avenue of communication and healing. In this section, I will outline a series of activities that can be used online to facilitate this work with traumatised children.

In online dramatherapy the virtual space replaces the therapist's practice and constitutes a new therapy room which is partly digital and partly physical (Schubert, 2022). Inevitably, the coexistence of bodies is missing. However, the camera can act as the eye of an imaginary audience: traumatised children can see their body postures and movements on the screen and gain body awareness which in a face-to-face session would be achieved through the eyes of the therapist (Atsmon & Pendzik, 2020). As with face-to-face therapy, the priority when working with traumatised children online is to ascertain that each child feels safe during the session. Given that healing depends on the formation of a trusting relationship between therapist and child, building rapport with children should also be prioritised. When engaging with children online, the developmental stage of each child should be considered carefully (Bolton et al., 2021). As setting up the scene allows children to know what to expect, the physical space should be prepared beforehand so that it is in clear view from the camera (Ogden & Goldstein, 2020). This can reduce stress related to the unknown and is imperative because trauma is related to unpredictability and uncertainty (Brothers, 2007). From the beginning of the session, the therapist should inform children about the process: letting them know that they will be meeting in a virtual space in which they can talk about whatever they desire, explore their concerns in whatever manner they wish, and have control of their screen and mouse (Bolton et al., 2021). This latter action is remedial as trauma is characterised by powerlessness (Ogawa, 2004). Starting from manipulating the computer, children can then engage in embodied activities in the room (Ogden & Goldstein, 2020).

In their work with traumatised children dramatherapists can adopt the three-phase model included in the guidelines of the International Society for the Study of Traumatic Stress (Foa et al., 2009). They can start the session with some form of stabilisation which involves grounding and that can be achieved through imagery. As an example, through the image of a tree, children can be guided to imagine that they have roots in the earth, which allows them to feel the earth's energy radiating through their legs. They may also be guided to feel that their body is as strong and firm as a tree trunk and experiment with being both flexible and forceful (Serlin & Zhou, 2022).

After the grounding phase, children can be invited to explore emotions in their body through movements. They can move around quickly or slowly, graciously, or clumsily, or reach their hands up to express hope (Stavrou, 2020). In this process, it is important to consider the transition from one movement to the next as conscious movement allows one to identify the stored trauma in the body (Hartley, 2004). One way to accomplish this is by using polarities. Polarities such as 'open and close' or 'up and down' involve archetypal movements and resemble early developmental movements of infants (Serlin, 1993). Here, children can experiment with movements of direct and indirect flow while visualising images such as flowing water. Considering the child's space or lack of it and the manner they relate to it can promote further movement and create new ways to share one's story (Engelhard & Furlager, 2021). As the session unfolds, the therapist can invite children to move closer or away from the screen and find the appropriate distance for themselves. They can move in the room freely, choose their pace, and gain body awareness. This helps them set boundaries and instils a sense of security which is lost with trauma (Ogawa, 2004). Throughout this procedure, the therapist needs to ascertain that the child can return to an inner safe space of stability if the movements become too intense (Serlin & Zhou, 2022). Further embodied activities such as mindfulness, meditation, and progressive muscle relaxation can be performed here to reduce trauma-related stress (Pitre et al., 2016; van der Kolk, 2015). These can also be used in the initial stages of the session to facilitate stabilisation.

The last stage involves reflection and a return to the self in the here and now (Serlin & Zhou, 2022). This helps children evaluate the insights that came about through the movement exercises.

Throughout a session, children can experiment with further embodied practices which promote closeness and exposure (Engelhard & Furlager, 2021). They can throw soft toys on the screen, press buttons on the computer, turn the camera and microphone on and off, show the therapist different parts of their body, move to other locations, change the position they are in, etc. Imagination and creativity can be limitless. As Engelhard and Furlager suggest (2021, p.79):

> passing an imaginary ball between therapist and client, or pulling on an imaginary rope while paying attention to the intensity and speed happening on the other side of the screen, as well as 'offering hands' while nudging the back of the hands to the boundaries of the zoom frame, are all examples which invite exercises of make-believe experiences, into which the client pours the content of his/her inner world.

As it has already been stated, one of the consequences of childhood trauma involves distorted attachment bonds between the child and important others (Spinazzola et al., 2021). Working through impaired attachment online can be achieved through methods such as doubling and mirroring. These methods are developmental processes characteristic of the child–caregiver relationship and help build a strong therapeutic alliance (Bannister, 2003; Iordanou, 2019). Recent research evidence on the role mirror neurons play in the development of empathy shows that mirroring one another's movements through a screen is effective (Buk, 2009). By working with these methods, children can experiment with movement, rhythm, and attunement, which are characteristic of the non-verbal communication taking place between infant and caregiver early in the child's development, and facilitate the formation of healthy attachments (Schore & Schore, 2008).

Additionally, dramatherapists can incorporate projective play in their online work with traumatised children. Projective play can involve interaction with puppets and toys, creating stories, and exploring characters and relationships to help contain the terrifying feelings related to trauma (Bannister, 2003; Sesar et al., 2022). Although it is not primarily an embodied technique, it offers children the opportunity to project their emotions and thoughts to the items on the screen and hence 'exercise control over their world rather than being overwhelmed with epic size experiences' (Jennings, 1999, p.6). One type of projective play which can happen online involves virtual sand trays. Sand tray is a trauma-informed sensory intervention which nurtures children's attachment needs and enables them to communicate their experience through metaphors and symbols (Lyles & Homeyer, 2015). It offers the opportunity to re-enact events creatively and facilitates the expression of thoughts and emotions (Duffey & Somody, 2011). There are various online platforms which offer virtual sand trays (Fried, 2020) that include a virtual sandbox and other props which, in their physical form, can be found in numerous therapy practices (Bolton et al., 2021). Here, children are encouraged to interact with several characters and create stories and scenes they wish to work on. Once the scene has been created, the sand tray can be saved virtually to remind children of their work. The story making related to the sand tray can then inspire themes for further embodied play which can be enacted during the session.

Drawing is another playful projective activity which can be used with traumatised children and form the basis of embodied play. Drawing allows children to express their thoughts and emotions regarding the traumatic event (Driessnack, 2005; Iordanou et al., 2021). When they draw, children create a narrative of the experience and understand it better in a stress-free manner. Talking about the drawing helps them process the painful memories and heal from trauma (Laird & Mulvihill, 2022; Malchiodi, 2003). The drawing can further be used for embodied work through creating a story based on its content, role-playing it or drawing a character who can come to the child's aid and then creating a story/role-play about this character's adventures.

Improvisation and role-play can also be achieved virtually allowing for playful embodied experiences to take place (Quigley, 2020). Here, children can make use of their imagination. They can be a warrior, a dwarf, a giant, or a superhero. By using their imagination, they can recreate their story and feel stronger to overcome their sense of powerlessness (Ogawa, 2004). Through role-play, children can come closer to their traumatic experience while keeping an emotional distance from it. In this process, a strong bond is created in the space between the therapist and the child, which helps the latter learn to build healthy attachment relationships while decreasing the possibility of re-traumatisation (Bannister, 2003). One way to engage children in this type of play is by initiating the activity and asking them to join in. In her clinical work, Quigley (2020) observed that clients found it easier to engage in embodied activities virtually if she initiated the movement and gently invited them to join her. This approach can potentially strengthen the therapeutic relationship and the child's ability to connect.

Finally, to help children fully work through the trauma, the session should end with reflection (Foa et al., 2009) to process the embodied work cognitively and connect it to their experience. If role-play is pursued, de-roling should be an integral part of the session. De-roling helps children leave behind the role they played and return to themselves again and creates a balance between the activities taking place in the virtual environment and going back to life outside of it (Gualeni et al., 2017). Encouraging children to de-role or leave the space where the session took place helps defuse the energy related to the therapeutic process in a healthy manner and allows them to return to their everyday life feeling safe and secure (Quigley, 2020).

Concluding Remarks

Dramatherapeutic work with traumatised children involves utilising embodied techniques and creating a dramatic reality in which children can process their trauma symbolically. This work traditionally takes place physically. The Covid-19 pandemic forced many dramatherapists to move their work online, causing concerns regarding the feasibility of engaging in sensory and bodily practices from a distance. Research shows that this shift has been possible and that working therapeutically online is not worse or better than in-person work but, rather, different. As long as dramatherapists can provide children with a sense of control and security which are paramount in the treatment of trauma, healing can still be facilitated from a distance. Providing children with a trusting and consistent therapeutic environment can actually 'defrost frozen feelings' relevant to the trauma (Ogawa, 2004, p.21). If the therapeutic relationship is nurtured in online spaces, treatment can still be successful. One of the characteristics of dramatherapists is their ability to adjust to adversity in a creative manner, and creativity can still take place in online spaces to engage the body in therapeutic work.

To be able to work with traumatised children in a virtual space, key steps should be considered and put in place. Firstly, dramatherapists should ensure that a trusting therapeutic relationship is built between themselves and the child. Each session should start with grounding so that children are ready to engage in therapeutic work. Secondly, children should be encouraged to engage in different types of play which allow them to work through their trauma symbolically and metaphorically. Lastly, reflection and/or de-roling should take place so that children leave the session feeling safe and secure.

I hope to have shown in this chapter that the applications of embodied practices traditionally used in face-to-face therapy can be utilised effectively online to help address the effects of trauma in children. As this type of work is relatively new, extensive research is needed to ascertain the reliability and validity of dramatherapeutic interventions in the treatment of childhood trauma in digital spaces. Training is also required, especially for those therapists who are newer to technologies. Suffice to say that when working online with children, issues of privacy, confidentiality, and safeguarding should be prioritised. The possibilities the digital world offers for interaction and clinical work with children are limitless. It is my hope that this chapter will form the basis for further exploration of ways to facilitate the healing journey of traumatised children.

Note

1 In the UK, the first lockdown period started on 23 March 2020 until 13 May 2020, when people from one household were allowed to meet one person from another household outside while keeping a two-metre distance. The second lockdown was imposed from 5 November 2020, for four weeks. A third lockdown followed starting from 5 January 2021 and gradually ending from 8 March 2021.

References

Atsmon, A. & Pendzik, S. (2020). The clinical use of digital resources in drama therapy: An explorative study of well-established practitioners. *The Drama Therapy Review*, 6(1), 7–26.

Atsmon, A., Katz, T., & Pendzik, S. (2022). 'Migrated onto the Screen': The impact of the COVID-19 pandemic on the clinical practice of drama therapy. *The Arts in Psychotherapy*, 79, 101913. https://doi.org/10.1016/j.aip.2022.101913

Bannister, A. (2003). The effects of creative therapies with children who have been sexually abused. *Dramatherapy*, 25(1), 3–9. https://doi.org/10.1080/02630672.2003.9689619

Bolton, C. A., Thompson, H., Spring, J. A., & Frick, M. H. (2021). Innovative play-based strategies for teletherapy. *Journal of Creativity in Mental Health*. Advance online publication. https://doi.org/10.1080/15401383.2021.2011814

Brothers, D. (2007). *Towards a psychology of uncertainty: Trauma-centred psychoanalysis*. Routledge.

Buk, A. (2009). The mirror neuron system and embodied simulation: Clinical implications for art therapists working with trauma survivors. *The Arts in Psychotherapy*, 36(2), 61–74. https://doi.org/10.1016/j.aip.2009.01.008

D'Andrea, W., Ford, J., Stolbach, B., Spinazzola, J., & van der Kolk, B. A. (2012). Understanding interpersonal trauma in children: Why we need a developmentally appropriate trauma diagnosis. *American Journal of Orthopsychiatry*, *82*(2), 187–200. https://doi.org/10.1111/j.1939-0025.2012.01154.x

Dementyeva, L. (2020). Reflection of developmental trauma in lockdown situations. *Analytical Psychology: Theory and Practice. Scientific Practical Jungian Journal*, 1, 93–98.

Driessnack, M. (2005). Children's drawings as facilitators of communication: A meta-analysis. *Journal of Pediatric Nursing*, 20, 414–423. https://doi.org.10.1016/j.pedn.2005.03.011

Duffey, T. & Somody, C. (2011). The role of relational-cultural theory in mental health counseling. *Journal of Mental Health Counseling*, 33(3), 223–242. https://doi.org/10.17744/mehc.33.3.c10410226u275647

Emunah, R. & Butler, J. (2020). The current state of the field of drama therapy. In D. Johnson & R. Emunah (Eds.), *Current approaches in drama therapy* (pp. 22–36). Charles C. Thomas.

Engelhard, E. S. & Furlager, A. Y. (2021). Remaining held: Dance/movement therapy with children during lockdown. *Body, Movement and Dance in Psychotherapy*, 16, 73–86. https://doi.org/10.1080/17432979.2020.1850525

Feniger-Schaal, R., Orkibi, H., Keisari, S., Sajnani, N. L., & Butler, J. D. (2022). Shifting to tele-creative arts therapies during the COVID-19 pandemic: An international study on helpful and challenging factors. *The Arts in psychotherapy*, 78, 101898. https://doi.org/10.1016/j.aip.2022.101898

Foa, E. B., Keane, T. A., Friedman, M. J., & Cohen, J. A. (Eds.) (2009). *Effective treatments for PTSD: Practice guidelines from the International Society for Traumatic Stress Studies*. Guilford Press.

Fried, K. (2020). *Online sand tray by Dr. Karen Fried*. Oaklander Training. www.onlinesandtray.com/

García, E., Di Paolo, E. A., & De Jaegher, H. (2022). Embodiment in online psychotherapy: A qualitative study. *Psychology and psychotherapy*, 95(1), 191–211. https://doi.org/10.1111/papt.12359

Gendlin, E. T. (1981). *Focusing*. Bantam.

Grasso, D. J., Saunders, B. E., Williams, L. M., Hanson, R., Smith, D. W., & Fitzgerald, M. M. (2013). Patterns of multiple victimization among maltreated children in Navy families. *Journal of Traumatic Stress*, 26(5), 597–604. https://doi.org/10.1002/jts.21853

Greene, C. A., Haisley, L., Wallace, C., & Ford, J. D. (2020). Intergenerational effects of childhood maltreatment: A systematic review of the parenting practices of adult survivors of childhood abuse, neglect, and violence. *Clinical Psychology Review*, 80, 101891. https://doi.org/10.1016/j.cpr.2020.101891

Gualeni, S., Vella, D., & Harrington, J. (2017). De-roling from experiences and identities in virtual worlds. *Journal of Virtual Worlds Research*, 10, 1–18. https://doi.org/10.4101/jvwr.v10i2.7268

Haen, C. (2015). Vanquishing monsters: Group drama therapy for treating trauma. In C. A. Malchiodi (Ed.), *Creative arts and play therapy. Creative interventions with traumatized children* (pp. 235–257). The Guilford Press.

Hanna, T. (1970). *Bodies in revolt: A primer in somatic thinking*. Freeperson Press.

Hartley, L. (2004). *Somatic psychology: Body, mind and meaning*. Whurr.

Homann, K. B. (2010). Embodied concepts of neurobiology in dance/movement therapy practice. *American Journal of Dance Therapy*, 32, 80–99. https://doi.org/10.1007/s10465-010-9099-6

Iordanou, C. (2019). 'The space between': Role play as a tool in the treatment of child sexual abuse. *Dramatherapy*, 40(3), 134–141. https://doi.org/10.1177%2F0263067219899044

Iordanou, C., Allen, M., & Warmelink, L. (2021). Drawing in eyewitness testimony: What is the content of children's drawings and how does it differ from their verbal reports? *Empirical Studies of the Arts*, 40, 245–258. https://doi.org/10.1177/02762374211047971

Jennings, S. (1994). 'Prologue', in S. Jennings, A. Cattanach, S. Mitchell, A. Chesner, & B. Meldrum (Eds.), *The Handbook of dramatherapy* (pp.1–11), Routledge.

Jennings, S. (1998). *Introduction to dramatherapy*. Jessica Kingsley.

Jennings, S. (1999). *Introduction to developmental play therapy*. Jessica Kingsley.

Jennings, S. (2011). *Healthy attachments and neuro-dramatic-play*. Jessica Kingsley.

Jennings, S. (2015). Trauma: The body, the play, and the drama. *BCPC Children and Young People, and Families Journal*, 40–45. Retrieved from www.bacp.co.uk/bacp-journals/bacp-children-young-people-and-families-journal/september-2015/trauma-the-body-the-play-and-the-drama/

Jones, P. (2007). *Drama therapy: Theory, practice and research* (2nd ed.). Routledge.

Jones, P. (2015). Trauma and dramatherapy: Dreams, play and the social construction of culture, *South African Theatre Journal*, 28(1), 4–16. https://doi.org/10.1080/10137548.2015.1011897

Krasanakis, S. (2021). Questions that emerge from practising drama therapy in the untouchable, odourless play space of the internet. *Drama Therapy Review*, 7(2), (287–292). https://doi.org/10.1386/dtr_00079_7

Laird, L. & Mulvihill, N. (2022). Assessing the extent to which art therapy can be used with victims of childhood sexual abuse: A thematic analysis of published studies. *Journal of Child Sexual Abuse*, 31(1), 105–126. https://doi.org/10.1080/10538712.2021.1918308

Landy, R. J. (1983). The use of distancing in drama therapy. *The Arts in Psychotherapy*, *10*(3), 175–185. https://doi.org/10.1016/0197-4556(83)90006-0

Lim, B. H., Hodges, M. A., & Lilly, M. M. (2020). The differential effects of insecure attachment on post-traumatic stress: A systematic review of extant findings and explanatory mechanisms. *Trauma Violence & Abuse*, 21(5), 1044–1060. https://doi.org/10.1177/1524838018815136

Lyles, M. & Homeyer, L. E. (2015). The use of sandtray therapy with adoptive families. *Adoption Quarterly*, *18*(1), 67–80. https://doi.org/10.1080/10926755.2014.945704

Malchiodi, C. A. (2003). *Handbook of art therapy*. The Guilford Press.

Malchiodi, C. A. (2015). *Creative interventions with traumatized children*. The Guilford Press.

Newman, T. (2017). Creating the role: How dramatherapy can assist in re/creating an identity with recovering addicts. *Dramatherapy*, 38(2–3), 106–123. http://doi.org/10.1080/02630672.2017.1340492

Ogawa, Y. (2004). Childhood trauma and play therapy intervention for traumatized children. *Journal of Professional Counseling: Practice, Theory & Research*, 32(1), 19–29. http://doi.org/10.1080/15566382.2004.12033798

Ogden, P. & Goldstein, B. (2020). Sensorimotor psychotherapy from a distance: Engaging the body, creating presence, and building relationship in videoconferencing. In H. Weinberg & A. Rolnick (Eds.), *Theory and practice of online therapy: Internet-delivered interventions for individuals, families, groups, and organizations* (pp. 47–63). Routledge.

Ogden, P., Pain, C., & Fisher, J. (2006). A sensorimotor approach to the treatment of trauma and dissociation. *Psychiatric Clinics of North America*, 29(1), 263–279. https://doi.org/10.1016/j.psc.2005.10.012

Panksepp, J. (2007). The power of the word may reside in the power of affect. *Integrative Psychological and Behavioral Science*, 42(1), 47–55.

Pendzik, S. (2006). On dramatic reality and its therapeutic function in drama therapy. *The Arts in Psychotherapy*, 33, 271–280.

Perry, B. D. (2008). Foreword. In C. A. Malchiodi (Ed.), *Creative interventions with traumatized children*. The Guilford Press.

Pitre, R., Mayor, C., & Johnson, D. R. (2016). Developmental transformations short-form as a stress reduction method for children. *Drama Therapy Review*, 2, 167–181. http://dx.doi.org/10.1386/dtr.2.2.167_1

Porges, S. W. (2009). Reciprocal influences between body and brain in the perception and expression of affect: A polyvagal perspective. In D. Fosha, D. Siegel, & M. Solomon (Eds.), *The healing power of emotion: Affective neuroscience, development, and clinical practice* (pp. 27–54). W. W. Norton.

Price, J. & Shildrick, M. (1999). *Feminist theory and the body*. Routledge.

Quigley, C. A. (2020). ProReal®: The 'good enough' online alternative to face-to-face Dramatherapy. *Dramatherapy*, 41(2), 90–99. https://doi.org/10.1177/02630672211020886

Regula, J. (2020). Developmental transformations over video chat: An exploration of presence in the therapeutic relationship. *Drama Therapy Review*, 6(1), 67–83.

Romanou, E. & Belton, E. (2020). *Isolated and struggling: social isolation and the risk of child maltreatment, in lockdown and beyond*. NSPCC. Retrieved from https://learning.nspcc.org.uk/research-resources/2020/social-isolation-risk-child-abuse-during-and-after-coronavirus-pandemic#:~:text=There%20are%20indications%20that%20the%20conditions%20caused%20by%20the%20coronavirus,exploitation%20and%20child%20sexual%20exploitation

Rothschild, B. (2000). *The body remembers: The psychophysiology of trauma and trauma treatment*. Norton.

Sajnani, N., Mayor, C., Burch, D., Feldman, D., Davis, C., Kelly, J., Landis, H., & McAdam, L. (2019). Collaborative discourse analysis on the use of drama therapy to treat trauma in schools. *Drama Therapy Review*, *5*(1), 27–47. https://doi.org/10.1386/dtr.5.1.27_1

Saunders, B. E. & Adams, Z. W. (2014). Epidemiology of traumatic experiences in childhood. *Child and Adolescent Psychiatric Clinics of North America*, *23*(2), 167–184. https://doi.org/10.1016/j.chc.2013.12.003

Scheff, T. (1981). The distancing of emotion in psychotherapy. *Psychotherapy: Theory, Research and Practice*, 18(1), 46–53. https://doi.org/10.1037/h0085960

Schore, J. R. & Schore, A. N. (2008). Modern attachment theory: The central role of affect regulation in development and treatment. *Clinical Social Work*, 36, 9–20.

Schubert, M. (2022). Seeking dramatic reality in the digital world. *Dramatherapy Review*, 8(2), 235–248.

Serlin, I. (1993). Root images of healing in dance therapy. *American Dance Therapy Journal*, 15(2), 65–75.

Serlin, I. A. & Zhou, G. (2022). Dance movement therapy in the time of COVID-19. *Creative Arts in Education and Therapy (CAET)*, 32–41. Retrieved from https://caet.inspirees.com/caetojsjournals/index.php/caet/article/view/390

Sesar, K., Dodaj, A., Sesar, D., Smoljan, I., & Mikulic, M. (2022). The creative arts therapies with children and adolescents with traumatic experiences. *Central European Journal of Paediatrics*, 18. https://doi.org/10.5457/p2005-114.319

Spinazzola, J., van der Kolk, B., & Ford, J. D. (2021). Developmental trauma disorder: A legacy of attachment trauma in victimized children. *Journal of Trauma Stress*, 34, 711–720. https://doi.org/10.1002/jts.22697

Stavrou, D. (2020). The medium is the message: The transformation of drama therapy practice during COVID-19. *Dramatherapy Review*, 6(Suppl. 2), 181–185.

Terr, L. C. (1991). Childhood traumas: An outline and overview. *American Journal of Psychiatry*, 148(1), 10–20.

Thoma, M. V., Bernays, F., Eising, C. M., Maercker, A., & Rohner, S. L. (2021). Child maltreatment, lifetime trauma, and mental health in Swiss older survivors of enforced child welfare practices: Investigating the mediating role of self-esteem and self-compassion. *Child Abuse & Neglect*, 113, 104925. https://doi.org/10.1016/j.chiabu.2020.104925

Tyler, A. T. (2012) The limbic model of systemic trauma, *Journal of Social Work Practice*, 26, 1, 125–138. https://doi.org/ 10.1080/02650533.2011.602474

Ursano, R. J., Zhang, L., Li, H., Johnson, L., Carlton, J., Fullerton, C. S., & Benedek, D. M. (2009). PTSD and traumatic stress: From gene to community and bench to bedside. *Brain Research, 1293*, 2–12. https://doi.org/10.1016/j.brainres.2009.03.030

van der Kolk, B. A. (1996). The complexity of adaptation to trauma: Self-regulation, stimulus discrimination, and characterological development. In B. A. van der Kolk, A. C. McFarlane, & L. Weisaeth (Eds.), *Traumatic stress: The effects of overwhelming experience on mind, body and society*, (pp. 182–213). The Guilford Press.

van der Kolk, B. A. (2009). Entwicklungstrauma-Störung: Auf dem Weg zu einer sinnvollen Diagnostik für chronisch traumatisierte Kinder [Developmental trauma disorder: towards a rational diagnosis for chronically traumatized children]. *Praxis der Kinderpsychologie und Kinderpsychiatrie*, 58(8), 572–586. https://doi.org/10.13109/prkk.2009.58.8.572

van der Kolk, B. A. (2015). *The body keeps the score: Brain, mind, and body in the healing of trauma*. Viking.

van Westrhenen, N. & Fritz, E. (2014). Creative arts therapy as treatment for child trauma: An overview. *The Arts in Psychotherapy*, *41*(5), 527–534. https://doi.org/10.1016/j.aip.2014.10.004

Weiss, G. (1999). *Body images: Embodiment as intercorporeality*. Routledge.

Wood, L., White, S., Gervais, D., Owen, M., Moore, S., Boylan, Z., Cosby, O., Ansted, J., Capitman, J., & Ciempa, T. (2020). Challenges and strategies delivering group drama therapy via telemental health: Action research using inductive thematic analysis. *Drama Therapy Review*, 6(2), 149–165.

Chapter 5

Therapy of Gesture

Integrating Psychophysical Approaches from Theatre and Therapy in the Healing of Trauma

J. F. Jacques

Introduction

My intention in this chapter is to outline an integrative psychophysical approach to trauma healing that is grounded in the art form of theatre, more specifically in the teaching of the Russian actor and director Michael Chekhov (1891–1955). My aim is to suggest an original embodied practice that integrates findings in neuroscience, embodied cognition, and emotion; learnings from approaches in theatre that have emphasised the connection between physicality and the internal emotional life; and some of the advances made by embodied forms of therapy in the treatment of trauma, most notably Somatic Experiencing and Sensorimotor Psychotherapy. I have named this approach the *therapy of gesture*.

Psychophysicality will be described in this chapter as amounting to the bi-directionality between the human mind and human body. Human gestures, that I define as being the different configurations adopted by the body in space either through will or constraint, constitute the nodal points of bi-directionality and therefore the vehicle for the understanding, expression, and resolution of traumatic experiences. I will attempt to explain how this approach provides additional resources to enable and support the embodied healing of trauma, as well as considering its applications and limitations. My hope is that this chapter will provide an example of how the artistic can meet the therapeutic to address the needs of the traumatised body.

Embodied Mind and Mindful Body

In his novel *La Main* (*The Hand*) (1968), the Belgian writer Georges Simenon (1903–1989) describes how the sensation of a hand translates a realisation of unbearable and disavowed desires that cannot possibly be acted on, but also how a simple audacious gesture ('*l'audace du geste*') could feel like a deliverance. In other words, whilst the awareness of the hand brings clarity to a turbulence of conflicting emotions, the possibility of a gesture holds the potential for the emergence of new emotional states. What Simenon's novel illustrates is the clear links between embodied experiences, emotions, and cognition.

DOI: 10.4324/9781003322375-7

His contemporary, the French phenomenological philosopher Maurice Merleau-Ponty (1908–1961) described how we primarily experience the world and others through our bodies and that, as such, our perceptions are direct expressions of our embodied lived experiences. As Merleau-Ponty wrote, 'the perceiving mind is an incarnated mind' (Merleau-Ponty, 1964, p.3). Furthermore, consciousness is first and foremost embedded in the body. The experiences accumulated by the body contribute to the emergence of a consciousness that very largely predates reflective and symbolic representations. 'All consciousness', writes Merleau-Ponty, 'is perceptual consciousness' (Merleau-Ponty, 2009, p.459). As perception is embodied, so is consciousness. Embodied consciousness therefore describes how the direct perceptual, sensory, and motor experiences of the body shape our internal working models, our capacity to orientate in the world, and our relationships to others. Recent research has shown how the bodily roots of consciousness go back as far as *in utero* experiences, therefore reflecting the profound co-embodied relationality that prefigures its emergence (Ciaunica et al., 2021).

The significance of the body in the construction and organisation of experience as outlined by Merleau-Ponty led to the emergence of the concept of the embodied mind (Varela et al., 2016). This translates the way in which the body is not a satellite of central neurological processes in the brain but rather the nexus of cognition itself. This overturns the cartesian argument of a *cogito* – describing the cognitive capacities of individuals to think about and reflect on themselves – detached from the body and the senses. If Descartes (1596–1650) put forward that thinking was the ontological marker of being, recent advances in cognitive science have suggested that we are and have a body before being able to think about it. Descartes's principle can therefore be recast as *sum corpus, ergo cogito et sentio* – I am a body, therefore I think and feel.

In its most simplistic form, the embodied mind describes a structural connection between internal mental processing, physiological constituents, and the ecological system. It expresses the way in which the mind – which includes a set of mental operations including reasoning, distinguishing, recognising, categorising, conceptualising, and meaning-making – is located in a body that, in interaction with an environment, shapes its constitution. Cognition is therefore embodied, involving perception and action, as opposed to what was suggested by earlier models in cognitive science that reduce the mind to a set of mental and symbolic representations autonomously organised into configurations of meaning in a way that is asomatic and amodal (Foglia & Wilson, 2013; Fincher-Kiefer, 2019).

Embodied cognition asserts that cognitive processes and conceptual knowledge are grounded in and mapped within the sensory-motor system (Gallese & Lakoff, 2005; Glenberg, 2015). As Gallese & Lakoff write (2005), 'the sensory-motor system not only provides structure to conceptual content, but also characterises the semantic content of concepts in terms of the way that we function with our bodies in the world' (p.456). In other words, the understanding and schematic knowledge that we have or hold about ourselves, others, and the world are directly based on sensory-motor activity and embodied interactions. Consequently, observe Foglia and Wilson (2013, p.319), 'the body intrinsically constraints, regulates, and shapes the nature of mental activity'.

Furthermore, research not only indicates that the body is directly involved in cognitive processing, but that mental representations stored in memory continue to be supported by embodied responses that in turn constrain mental activity (Foglia & Wilson, 2013). The hypothesis is that a body action or gesture, for example, carried out or experienced in a given context will have cognitive and psychological correlates that will continue to be enacted through similar embodied patterns in different environments. This suggests that an embodied approach to cognition reflects a bi-directionality between mental and bodily processes (Draguhn & Sauer, 2023).

Similarly, research in neuroscience has shown the embodied basis of emotions. Emotions, like cognition, are grounded in modality-specific systems (Winkielman et al., 2008). Although they differ in nature and function, they might not be as separate as we might imagine as they appear to share a common neural substrate, and to contribute to an integrated and interactive model of the embodied mind. Equally, the separation of cognition and emotions as belonging to different structures of the brain has been criticised for presenting a simplistic and erroneous image that overlooks more complex phenomena (Feldman Barrett, 2017). As Okon-Singer et al. write (2015, p.8), 'emotional and cognitive regions dynamically influence one another via a complex web of recurrent, often indirect anatomical connections in ways that jointly contribute to adaptive behaviour'.

The neurophysiology of emotions and the role of perceptual and peripheral mechanisms in their creation has been particularly studied by Damasio (2000). Damasio and Carvalho (2013) introduce a distinction between feelings and emotions that translates both physiological states. According to them, if both feelings and emotions are mental constructs, they are 'triggered by the perception or recall' (Damasio & Carvalho, 2013, p.144) of different body stimuli. Feelings reflect experiences of the internal interoceptive system (i.e. the perceptions and sensations of what is happening inside the body), whereas emotions reflect experiences of the external exteroceptive system (i.e. the information provided by the five senses). They both constitute an axis of body states that triggers what Damasio and Carvalho call 'action programmes' (p.145) that constitute adjustments within a system to ensure homeostatic regulation. They argue that medical disorders can be traced back to the physiology of emotions and feelings.

Research has indicated that the bi-directionality that is constitutive of embodied cognition is also a characteristic of embodied emotion. Niedenthal and Maringer (2009) show how a given experience, such as for instance witnessing a hawk pouncing on a chick, will trigger feelings and emotions grounded in perceptions and sensations (for instance fear) that will be encoded and stored in the physiology of the body. The recall of the event, or similar experiences that can be associated with it, will not only reactivate the feeling but also its physiology leading to a 'multimodal reenactment' (p.123). This suggests how body states and emotional states mutually inform one another.

If the mind is embodied, the body can also be mindful of its own processes. This is quite an essential element of what it means to have and be a body as it provides the awareness of the sensory-motor and perceptual knowledge and the information held by it. Being mindful means attending to and attuning into the signals that the body constantly sends and that may remain concealed from the emotional-cognitive brain. The mindful body translates a process of becoming one as mind and body through an awareness of sickness and pain but also through a propensity for healing (Scheper-Hughes & Lock, 1987). In other words, it describes ways in which one becomes accustomed to the language of the body, and to its different modulations, inflections, and variations in sensations, perceptions, and gestures. As in Simenon's novel mentioned earlier, the mindful body informs our most intimate and deep turbulences whilst also providing the means for release and the possibility of liberation.

Psychophysical Approaches in Theatre

The integration of recent advances in cognitive science and neuroscience within the theory and practice of theatre and performance is fairly new (Kemp & McConachie, 2019). However, one could argue that theatre intuitively discovered what cognitive science took much longer to uncover. Jacques Lecoq (1921–1999) wrote that 'the body does know things that the head doesn't know yet' (Lecoq, 1997, p.22), a statement that prefigures a lot of what cognitive science would confirm, even though in much simplified terms. As Kemp (2019) observes, 'this principle of Lecoq's correlates with the foundational concept of embodied cognition, that sensorial and motor experiences form the neural foundations for mental concepts' (p.180). Physical gestures are for Lecoq located at the interface between the external world, sensations, and emotions. A gesture does not refer to a certain part of the body in isolation from others but encompasses its whole moving physicality and physiology. Lecoq describes gesture as the primary mode of communication that reflects conscious and unconscious knowledge, or voluntary and involuntary intention. The work of the actor consists in becoming aware of gestures in order to be able to use them deliberately. 'Little by little', writes Lecoq (2006, p.6), 'these gestures acquire clarity', and will reveal something about the internal life of those to whom they belong. Lecoq was greatly influenced by the French anthropologist Marcel Jousse (1886–1961), author of *The Anthropology of Gesture* (2018), initially published between 1974 and 1978. It is worth considering some of Jousse's ideas on gesture before pursuing the discussion of psychophysical approaches in theatre.

Jousse famously wrote that 'man thinks with the whole of his body' (2018, p.30). For Jousse, human gesture is the most fundamental mechanism of the body through which it is mimetically constituted but also expresses itself. Jousse defines gesture as 'the living energy that drives the global whole' that is the human body (2018, p.50). It is a tool to understand and access the deepest abysses of the mind. He observes that since not all gestures are conscious, gaining awareness also requires gestures. In other words, gestures constitute, for Jousse, the road to the unconscious and translates the psychophysicality of the human body and its history. Jousse also identified three fundamental physiological mechanisms. One of them is bilateralism that he designates 'the symmetrical structure of the human body which, he believed, shapes all forms of human expression, mental and physical' (Tardan-Masquelier, 1993, p.19). Jousse describes bilateralism as the expression of 'the spontaneous law of human equilibrium' (2018, p.213) between above and below, right and left, and in front and behind. Bilateralism can be observed in all human acts or behaviours such as in walking, which represents a constant sway from left to right and vice versa. Swaying, which characterises bilateralism, is for Jousse the natural and universal way for human beings to express themselves, and that expression is constituted of gestures. Jousse observes that any situations that force the human body out of its natural balanced structure can only severely affect the psychological functioning of human beings, and the way in which they interact with the world around them.

Jousse, like Lecoq, suggests an embodied pedagogical approach (Nixon, 2019) that is also shared by the Russian actor and director Michael Chekhov, founder of a psychophysical technique of acting. The remainder of this section will focus on some important elements of his teaching to keep exploring the interplay between body and mind from a theatre perspective. For Chekhov, the body is the most important and natural tool of the actor. Chekhov does not believe in a psychology that can be accessed from within but rather from without. Acting is first and foremost about sensations that inform and reveal psychological depth and feelings. Sensations are awakened by paying close attention to the actions and movements of the body, which are commonly termed by Chekhov 'gestures'. The psychological content of a gesture is more specifically revealed by its quality, directionality, and tempo. This is what constitute a psychological gesture that is a window into the emotional life of a character[1]. As Chekhov writes, psychological gesture means 'the gesture together with the feelings connected with it' (1991, p.60). The connection between body and inner life that defines psychological gesture means that a particular movement can help elicit feelings, wishes, needs, or desires, but also that the internal psychology of the body reveals itself physically through gestures. There exists therefore a psychophysical loop between physicality and feeling as they end up mutually informing one another, in the same way as the bi-directionality previously mentioned. As Sinéad Rushe (2019, pp.68–69) writes:

> Just as emotional content cannot be separated from its physical embodiment, the inner life must continually adjust to the actions, gestures and positions of the physical body. We no longer know where one thing starts in the chain reaction; both are continuously influencing and adapting to each other.

I now look a bit more closely at three other singular aspects of Chekhov's method: the ideal centre, the quality and directionality of movements.

The Ideal Centre

The ideal centre describes a source of vitality within the body. It represents a core and original point of energy that permeates the whole body and from which life naturally flows and expresses itself. At a most fundamental level, connecting with the ideal centre enables us to experience 'the concrete reality of ourselves and our body' (Rushe, 2019, p.38). It characterises a process of attunement leading to discoveries but also a serious acceptance of who we are in our own physicality. It constitutes the most fundamental step to ground the creative and imaginative work that will follow. As such, to connect with the source becomes a way to familiarise ourselves with the knowledge of the body and of its natural impulses that precede all movements (Chekhov, 2014). Furthermore, Chekhov describes the ideal centre as 'a source of inner activity and power' within the body (Chekhov, 2014, p.7). This power reacquaints us with the fact that we are a body before having a body. We are and remain subjects despite what the body might have endured. The ideal centre encourages us to reclaim the body for what it is as opposed to what it has become, and to uncover its concealed strengths and potential. It puts us in a state of presence and receptivity that 'awakens the realization that we have resources at our disposal, if we choose to tap into them' (Rushe, 2019, p.39). This sense of presence might make us aware of possible resistances that may be indicative of deeper conflicts. But the sense of receptivity that the ideal centre invites allows us to receive these without judgements or criticisms. It puts the body into an active state of empathic and deep 'embodied listening' (Rushe, 2019, p.58) to reveal its most fundamental impulses, needs, and desires, and to realign its physical expression with its emotional content. Receiving in that sense means allowing ourselves to become aware of the impressions that our body makes on us as well as those that are being made on it. As the body gradually feels able to receive, it also radiates from the inside out as if 'sending out rays' into the space around it (Chekhov, 2014, p.12). The practice of radiating can be seen as the opposite of receiving although they appear interdependent in their relationship, as in the natural action of breathing in and out. Radiating helps cultivate a sense of openness within ourselves and towards others through external expression. It could be argued that the ideal centre through its natural movements towards the inside and the outside, receiving and sending out, modulates the capacity of the body to self-regulate in relation to the environment.

Quality of Movements

Another aspect of Chekhov's teaching concerns the 'psychological qualities' of the movements and gestures of the body (Chekhov, 1991, p.48). Chekhov's approach can be described as psychophysical because of the way in which the morphology of the body constantly relates to the content of its inner life. In that sense, all the exercises suggested by Chekhov are not intended to be purely physical but rather to 'penetrate all of the parts of the body with fine psychological vibrations' (Chekhov, 1991, p.43). The quality of a movement refers to the particular way in which it is executed and to the sensations and feelings that will be activated as a result. As Rushe writes (2019, p.126), 'if action is the verb or *what* I am doing, [...] quality is the adverb or *how* I am doing my action'. Amongst these qualities is the feeling of form that describes the body's relationship to space and the way in which it is shaped by it as much as shaping it. The feeling of form consists in bringing awareness to the body as a 'living form in space' (Rushe, 2019, p.65). It refers to a process of kinaesthetic or proprioceptive awareness that, alongside interoceptive and exteroceptive experiences as discussed by Damasio and Carvalho (2013), awakens emotions and feelings. Equally, as the actions of the body and the internal emotional life inform one another as we have seen, feelings are also endowed with forms and shapes. They have spatial qualities that compose the body like the special arrangement of notes compose a piece of music. Feeling the form of the body reveals the emotional intricacies of its internal landscape. The number of qualities can be infinite although Chekhov identifies four main ones that tend to correspond to the four elements of nature. Without having the space to review them all here, we can nevertheless observe that all have psychological correlates that only gain visibility and meaning through curiosity for the singular ways in which movements are executed. Amongst the other qualities, Chekhov mentions, for instance, the following adverbs: 'calmly, fiercely, thoughtfully, angrily, hastily, staccato, legato, painfully, decidedly, slyly, wilfully, rigidly, softly, soothingly' (Chekhov, 1991, p.38).

Directionality of Movements

Finally, the structure of the body, its gestures and movements also have directional qualities. A simple observation of people rapidly shows how they hold themselves and how they tend to inhabit their space. Their bodies might be showing different types of directionality, either forward, backward, upward, downward, right, left, or a combination of those (Rushe, 2019). Each of these polarities illustrate the bilateralism of the human body, as described above (Jousse, 2018). If they might not compromise the overall balance of the body, they nevertheless illustrate a physical proneness with a psychological content, also reflecting and activating sensations and feelings, as was the case for the qualities of movement previously discussed. In addition, the directionality of the body does not only connect psychological states to spatiality but also to temporality. The adoption by the body, or its awareness, of different directional postures may 'activate a specific moment' (Rushe, 2019, p.148), image, or memory that may trigger feelings. The body therefore holds in its own physicality the unfolding of time, from the past to the present and the future.

Psychophysical Approaches in Trauma-Focused Therapy

Marcel Jousse was a student of Pierre Janet (1859–1947), the French psychologist and neurologist contemporary of Freud, who was one of the first physicians to suggest that psychic trauma is an essential causation factor for mental health disorders (Bülher & Heim, 2001). There doesn't appear to be any detailed study exploring how the theories of Janet might have been foundational in Jousse's thinking, but we can reasonably believe that the psychophysicality of the human gesture, as suggested by Jousse, is a development of Janet's ideas, especially on psychological automatism (Janet, 1998).

Janet described how human behaviour is made up of automatisms, or repeated patterns, that very often have an underlying psychological cause. These automatisms, 'regular and predetermined' (van der Hart & Horst, 1989, p.4), find their expression through conduct and physical actions. However, these automatisms are not always integrated in the personality of a subject. This forms the basis of Janet's theory on dissociation whereby automatisms can reflect the content of traumatic experiences and memories cut off from the rest of the organism that can sometimes develop into independent integrated units, and result in, in extreme cases, what will be later described as dissociative identity disorder. What is important to underline here is how Janet very early on understood how the physiological patterns of the body constitute an access road into the internal emotional life that may not have been integrated into a whole system.

The psychophysiology of human development shows that muscle patterns established in childhood largely determine the posture adopted by the body in adulthood, but also reflect core emotions, experiences, or conflicts that the psyche might defend itself against. The psychoanalyst and founder of body psychotherapy Wilhelm Reich (1897–1957) called this 'character armour' (1980), which Stauffer (2010) describes as 'the pattern of tension we hold unconsciously in our bodies, and that determines, to a certain extent, the shape of our bones and thus our posture, the way we use our limbs, and the expression on our faces at rest' (p.96).

The body therefore, for Reich, is the repository of a very large vocabulary that tells the story of our life's traumas. Traumatic experience gets caught in the body and is encoded in muscles that give it its shape and posture, and affect, as Marcel Jousse would put it, its bilateralism. Memory is stored in muscles that contain feelings which are being implicitly expressed through patterns and automatisms. The whole body is displaying an impressive array of clues that are testimonies of its own history. If the skeletal muscles and body movements are physiologically orchestrated by the somatic nervous system associated with voluntary control, it remains true that muscular action also reflects involuntary patterns that, for Reich (1980), are akin to blocks in body and muscular structure.

More recent somatic therapeutic approaches in the treatment of trauma have suggested similar physiological phenomena. Peter Levine (2010), the founder of Somatic Experiencing (SE), a therapeutic modality that focuses on bodily responses to trauma and on resolving the symptoms of chronic and post-traumatic stress (Payne et al., 2015), describes how an interrupted normal trauma response to a life-threatening situation results in 'frozen energy' held and retained in the physiology of the body (Levine, 2008, p.26). The storage of undischarged energy contributes to the formation of symptoms that directly affect the body in its neurophysiology and in its capacity to move and be mobile. Amongst these, we can especially highlight the constriction of the body, which includes breathing, posture, and muscle tone; dissociation, which can be experienced through disconnection from parts of the body, sensory distortions, or pain; and re-enactment, which can be comprised of repeated actions or patterns of conduct and behaviour that somehow replicate the original trauma (Levine, 2008). It can be noticed that all these symptoms engage the somatic and musculoskeletal nervous system in the body, and provide a justification for 'a treatment approach that directly addresses the effects of trauma on both the body and the mind' (Ogden et al., 2006, p.5).

Ogden et al. (2006) underline the bi-directionality between symptoms held in the physiology of the body as a result of a traumatic experience and the other two levels of information processing, i.e. cognitive and emotional. This is reflected in the formation of 'automatic action tendencies' (Ogden et al., 2006, p.22) that translate the maladaptive ways in which experience is organised in traumatised individuals, and that encapsulates specific patterns of exchange and interaction between the different levels of information processing. Ogden et al. argue for treatments to include somatic techniques integrated with cognitive and emotional interventions so that 'adaptive information processing is increased on all three levels' (Ogden et al., 2006, p.8). This integration is also contained in Levine's SIBAM model (Sensation, Image, Behaviour, Affect and Meaning) that represents different dimensions or channels of experience that can either overlap or be dissociated in traumatised bodies (Levine, 2010). This provides a map or matrix of internal functioning that reveals types of coupling dynamics between elements of the model. The task of the trauma therapist, writes Levine, is 'to provide the somatic tools to free the client from being tangled up in these habituated physiological associations from the past' (2010, p.154).

If SE can be viewed as a form of trauma therapy that specifically engages with dysregulated neurophysiological states, it is nevertheless an integrated model that attends to not only fluctuations in the autonomic nervous system but also in three other subcortical structures and networks, including the emotional motor system, to form a complex dynamical system[2] that 'can enter various discrete functional and dysfunctional states' (Payne et al., 2015, p.3). If Levine famously claimed that 'trauma is in the nervous system and body not in the event' (Payne et al., 2015, p.5), this means that effective treatment involves strategies that directly engage with dysregulated subcortical networks in the brain. In SE, this is achieved by paying attention to inner-body sensations or interoceptive experiences, kinesthetic and proprioceptive experiences, and gestures. As such, Levine, like Merleau-Ponty, relocates perceptions in the experiences of the body.

Awareness of interoceptive and kinesthetic experiences appears to have in SE a double function. First, it enables clients to connect with the felt sense of body sensations of safety and comfort that constitute embodied resources that will be useful and can be returned to when approaching traumatic memories. Second, it serves the body to release and discharge excess activation stuck in the autonomic nervous system, and to eventually complete the normal biological survival response to the traumatic event. Gestures and movements are integral parts in this process of engaging intentionally with subcortical networks. This is because gestures and movements (but also postures and vocal patterns) carry memories, feelings, and emotions that have not necessarily been assimilated by the rest of the organism but have been procedurally encoded and stored in the brain. SE provides the physiological tools to engage with the physical manifestations of procedural memory and inhibited responses, so that an explicit narrative can be constructed (Levine, 2015).

Integrated Psychophysical Strategies for Healing

The language of theatre is far from absent in the literature on trauma-informed therapies. Bessel van der Kolk devotes a whole chapter in *The Body Keeps the Score* (2014) to the therapeutic possibilities of theatre. He mainly discusses theatre practices in terms of collective and ritual action through which individuals can connect with their shared humanity. Peter Levine also mentions 'the theatre of the body' (2010, p.183) as a metaphor to describe how the body stages trauma through sets of postural and gestural imprints. In order to keep considering how theatre can inform trauma healing, I intend now to examine ways in which specific theatre techniques and processes, such as those developed by Chekhov, can be integrated within existing psychophysical trauma-informed modalities to strengthen the body as a resource.

Levine (2008) distinguishes and describes different phases in the healing of trauma that he groups into four main stages. These stages constitute different and successive ways of engaging with the neurophysiology of the body to work towards integration and healing slowly and safely. Levine names them the preparatory phase, tracking skills, discharging activation and completion, returning to equilibrium. I will adopt a similar sequence to also identify four stages that reflect different applications of the psychophysicality of the human body as understood in theatre and that form the basis of a *therapy of gesture* for the traumatised body. The stages will focus on the discovery of (1) the capacity of the body; (2) the language of the body; (3) the possibilities of the body; and (4) the inner wisdom of the body. The aims of the *therapy of gesture* are to nurture and develop the healing and creative capacity of the body, to increase its resources, to regain agency, and to restore a sense of vitality, play, and joy.

The first stage acquaints us with the body and its capacities to receive and radiate. It is a stage whereby we gently welcome, acknowledge, and recognise the body for its capacity to have survived experiences that as human beings we should not have to endure. Trauma severely impacts on the body and can result in feeling disconnected from it, threatened by it, or avoidant because it can be a source of pain and memory. As Levine writes (2008, p.39), 'in order to heal trauma, we must learn how to safely come back into our bodies by experiencing them as a container to our feelings'. The task can be difficult and requires sensitive, compassionate, and radical acceptance of the body. This can involve a slow process of titration whereby we gradually familiarise ourselves with it and (re)discover its internal capacities. As we have seen, Chekhov helps us to reconnect with a sense of presence and the source within ourselves, or the ideal centre. Connecting with the ideal centre enables us to place ourselves in a state of attuned receptivity and deep embodied listening to the internal creative, grounding, and nurturing energy within the body. As the body learns to receive, it also learns to radiate and to send out energy. As such, the body learns different ways of regulating itself and of negotiating the pendulation between receiving and giving depending on its internal demands and needs.

The second stage acquaints us with the language of the body, the forms of sensations, feelings, and gestures. It enables us to familiarise ourselves with the somatic narrative of the traumatised body with curiosity and acceptance. The ideal centre allows us to notice sensations as they arise in the body (Rushe, 2019). As the body gradually learns safety and resources, it also becomes accustomed to its own language. As we slowly focus on sensations within the body, we also become aware of its shape in contact with these sensations, of variations in its bilateralism (Jousse, 2018), of its rhythms and tempo, and of its patterns of contraction and expansion in response to certain stimuli or images. As we have seen, Chekhov helps us to pay particular attention to the feeling of form within the body (Chekhov, 1991). This is most important to develop or regain agency over the body as a moving and moveable form, but also to realise that any shapes adopted by the body through gestures have a clear beginning and ending, and that, as such, they are not loose but rather contained. In accordance with the law of bi-directionality, feelings and emotions also find their expression through body states, physiological patterns, and automatisms. The awareness of this embodied language may help increase the capacity to tolerate emotions (Selvam, 2022), regulate the internal emotional experience, and reduce the sense of helplessness characteristic of trauma (Levine, 2010). Equally, the kinaesthetic awareness of the feeling of form can constitute an additional resource to release some of the frozen energy (Levine, 2008) locked in the neurophysiology of the body as a result of trauma.

In the third stage, we become acquainted with the possibilities of the body. If the previous stage was about discovering the language of the body, this one is about learning a new language or a somatic counternarrative. Here, the traumatised body is not only a receptacle of experiences that we learn to regulate, but also a vehicle for change and a conductor through which energy can freely flow. As the body has gradually regained a sense of agency through the two previous stages by developing an awareness of its own vocabulary, it is now more readily able and available to engage with the content of its traumatic past. This stage is therefore not solely about what the body is doing, but how it is doing it. As we have seen, for Chekhov (1991) the interplay between action and the quality of that action constitutes the essence of the psychological gesture that will help awaken the inner life of the character but also reveal new possibilities for adaptation as the character evolves through the unfolding of the story and vice versa. Bringing attention to the qualities of gestures, impulses, change in polarities and their possible variations in shape, intensity, directionality, sequence, or tempo will not only help cultivate new action patterns (Ogden et al., 2006) but also provide additional resources to enable the completion of the survival response, memory reconsolidation, and the renegotiation of meaning. As in the novel of Simenon (1968), this stage largely enables the inception of audacious gestures.

The fourth stage reunites us with the inner wisdom of the body, its capacity to reorganise itself and to achieve balance. In this stage, the body is rediscovering its own bilateralism and experiences itself as a coherent whole. Chekhov describes this as a feeling of entirety that translates the wholeness of the body where each part works harmoniously in relation to the other parts but also beyond to other bodies and to the natural world (Rushe, 2019). In this stage, we also learn to cultivate mindful gestures and an 'embodied inner sense of self' (Nixon, 2019, p.97) as treading the 'path to freedom' (Rushe, 2019, p.70) requires constant and renewed mindful attention and attunement. This stage is a celebration of the ways in which the body has been able to take effective action to overcome learned helplessness. It is an acknowledgement of embodied acts of triumph, as Pierre Janet suggested, through which the body has been able to demonstrate its resilience and its capacity for survival.

Conclusion

I have presented in this chapter different facets of psychophysicality as outlined in neuro- and cognitive science, theatre and trauma-focused somatic therapies.

These have been integrated into an original embodied practice that provides additional resources to think about trauma and strategies for the healing of the traumatised body. There is no doubt that the psychophysical approach presented in this chapter requires further elaboration and refinement. It does not claim to set the foundations for a new embodied approach to trauma healing. If anything, it reframes some of the existing treatment modalities by integrating learnings from different fields of study, most notably theatre and acting. It also offers new opportunities to think somatically about dramatherapy practice, especially when addressing the needs of traumatised clients. It will be useful to describe in more detail how the *therapy of gesture* has been applied in clinical practice. But for now, I hope to have shown that the applications of artistic and embodied practice in theatre have valuable contributions to make to the somatics of trauma. I also hope that this integration of the artistic with the therapeutic will continue to offer fresh perspectives on healing.

Notes

1 For more on gestures and psychological gestures, also refer to Chapter 10 by Roanna Mitchell.

2 This system is named the Core Response Network (CRN). It includes the autonomic nervous system, the emotional motor system, the reticular arousal system, and the limbic system. Details of how this integrated network organises responses to environmental stimuli can be find in Payne et al. (2015).

References

Bülher, K.-E. & Heim, G. (2001). General introduction to the psychotherapy of Pierre Janet. *American Journal of Psychotherapy*, 55(1), 74–91.

Chekhov, M. (1991). *On the technique of acting*. HarperCollins.

Chekhov, M. (2014). *To the actor: On the technique of acting*. Martino Publishing.

Ciaunica, A., Safron, A., & Delafield-Butt, J. (2021). Back to square one: The bodily roots of conscious experiences in early life. *Neuroscience of Consciousness*, 7(2), 1–10.

Damasio, A. (2000). *The Feeling of what happened: Body, emotion and the making of consciousness*. Vintage.

Damasio, A. & Carvalho, G. B. (2013). The nature of feelings: Evolutionary and neurobiological origins. *Nature Reviews Neuroscience*, 14, 143–152.

Draguhn, A. & Sauer, J. F. (2023). Body and mind: How somatic feedback signals shape brain activity and cognition. *Pflügers Archiv – European Journal of Physiology*, 475, 1–4. https://doi.org/10.1007/s00424-022-02778-5

Feldman Barrett, L. (2017). *How emotions are made: The secret life of the brain*. Macmillan.

Fincher-Kiefer, R. (2019). *How the body shapes knowledge: Empirical support for embodied cognition*. American Psychological Association.

Foglia, L. & Wilson, R. A. (2013). Embodied cognition. *WIREs Cognitive Science*, 4, 319–325.

Gallese, V. & Lakoff, G. (2005). The brain's concepts: The role of the sensory-motor system in conceptual knowledge. *Cognitive Neuropsychology*, 22 (3/4), 455–479.

Glenberg, A. M. (2015). Few believe the world is flat: How embodiment is changing the scientific understanding of cognition. *Canadian Journal of Experimental Psychology*, 69(2), 165–171. https://doi.org/10.1037/cep0000056

Janet, P. (1998). *L'Automatisme psychologique*. Editions Odile Jacob.

Jousse, M. (2018). *L'Anthropologie du geste*. Gallimard.

Kemp, R. (2019). Acting technique, Jacques Lecoq and embodied meaning. In R. Kemp & B. McConachie (Eds.), *The Routledge companion to theatre, performance and cognitive science* (pp. 177–189). Routledge.

Kemp, R. & McConachie, B. (2019). *The Routledge companion to theatre, performance and cognitive science*. Routledge.

Lecoq, J. (1997). *Le corps poétique*. Actes Sud.

Lecoq, J. (2006). *Theatre of movement and gesture*. Routledge.

Levine, P. A. (2008). *Healing trauma*. Sounds True.

Levine, P. A. (2010). *In an unspoken voice: How the body releases trauma and restores goodness*. North Atlantic Books.

Levine, P. A. (2015). *Trauma and memory: Brain and body in a search for the living past*. North Atlantic Books.

Merleau-Ponty, M. (1964). *The primacy of perception*. Northwest University Press.

Merleau-Ponty, M. (2009). *Phenomenology of perception*. Routledge Classics.

Niedenthal, P. M. & Maringer, M. (2009). Embodied emotion considered. *Emotion Review*, 1(2), 122–128.

Nixon, E. (2019). Embodied correspondences with the material world: Marcel Jousse's 'Laboratory of the Self' as a force for creative practice in performer training. *Theatre, Dance and Performance Training*, 10(1), 97–112. https://doi.org/10.1080/19443927.2019.1578821

Ogden, P., Minton, K., & Pain, C. (2006). *Trauma and the body: A sensorimotor approach to psychotherapy*. W. W. Norton & Company.

Okon-Singer, H., Hendler, T., Pessoa, L., & Shackman, A. J. (2015). The neurobiology of emotion-cognition interactions: Fundamental questions and strategies for future research. *Frontiers in Human Neuroscience*, 9(58). Retrieved from www.frontiersin.org/articles/10.3389/fnhum.2015.00058/full

Payne, P., Levine, P. A., & Crane-Godreau (2015). Somatic experiencing: Using interoception and proprioception as core elements of trauma therapy. *Frontiers in Psychology*, 6(93). https://doi.org/10.3389/fpsyg.2015.00093

Reich, W. (1980). *Character analysis*. Farrar, Strauss & Giroux.

Rushe, S. (2019). *Michael Chekhov's acting technique: A practitioner's guide*. Methuen Drama.

Scheper-Hughes, N. & Lock, M. M. (1987). The mindful body: A prolegomenon to future work in medical anthropology. *Medical Anthropology Quarterly*, 1(1), 6–41.

Selvam, R. (2022). *The Practice of embodying emotions*. North Atlantic Books.

Simenon, G. (1968). *La main*. Presses de la Cité.

Stauffer, K. A. (2010). *Anatomy & physiology for psychotherapists: Connecting body & soul*. W. W. Norton.

Tardan-Masquelier, Y. (1993). Marcel Jousse, theorist of gesture. *The UNESCO Courier*, September, p.19.

van der Hart, O. & Horst, R. (1989). The dissociation theory of Pierre Janet. *Journal of Traumatic Stress*, 2(4), 1–11.

van der Kolk, B. (2014). *The body keeps the score: Mind, brain and body in the transformation of trauma*. Penguin Books.

Varela, F. J., Thompson, E., & Rosch, E. (2016). *The embodied mind: Cognitive science and human experience* (2nd ed.). The MIT Press.

Winkielman, P., Niedenthal, P. M., & Oberman, L. (2008). The embodied emotional mind. In G. R. Semin & E. R. Smith (Eds.), *Embodied grounding: Social, cognitive, affective and neuroscientific approaches* (pp. 263–288). Cambridge University Press.

Chapter 6

Playing in Multifaceted Trauma

Reflections on Embodied Drama Therapy in South Africa

Margie Pankhurst and Jessica Mayson

Introduction

In this chapter, we conduct a theoretical and reflective exploration of working with children and multifaceted trauma in a postcolonial context. Multifaceted trauma considers the legacies of chronic and complex oppression, the impact of pervasive social, economic, political, and structural traumas that occur as a result of oppression, and how these influence psychosocial development and attachment patterns. This chapter illustrates this context in South Africa (SA) and considers an embodied approach to drama therapy with children that has emerged in response.

SA is saturated with multifaceted intergenerational trauma. This is the result of decades of institutionalised oppression that was intentional, racial, and patriarchal (Bower, 2014; Gqola, 2015). The current impact of this oppression cannot be underestimated. High levels of chronic poverty (Sulla, 2020) are barely survived by the majority of South Africans, and violent, sexual, physical, relational, and attachment trauma are intensely prevalent.

There is a large proportion of children in their early development, as well as their caregivers, who survived this violence and trauma. After the dismantling of apartheid in 1994, SA embraced an ethic of *ubuntu* ('I am because we are') and stressed an ideal of an African cultural network of care where children are not raised by their parents alone but are the responsibility of all adults in their surroundings. However, this has often been negated by the legacy of historic dismantling of communities and of broken government structures that did not provide quality of care to those in need (Lund, 2016). Statistics paint a bleak picture of the inaccessibility of mental healthcare. Research suggests that up to 60% of South Africans are living with PTSD (Nguse & Wassenaar, 2021), and that treatment is inaccessible to the vast majority of the population with severe mental health needs (Lund et al., 2009; Nwachukwu & Segalo, 2018; Craig et al., 2022). Mental health disorders are third in the national burden of diseases (Lund et al., 2009), and the prevalence of child and adolescent psychiatric need is higher in SA than in any other middle-income countries (Flisher et al., 2012). A recent survey shows that rates of mental health needs are

DOI: 10.4324/9781003322375-8

directly linked to adverse childhood experiences strongly associated with poverty (Craig et al., 2022). The public health system that serves 84% of the population (Docrat et al., 2019) is under-resourced and under severe strain. Only 50% of public hospitals have a psychiatrist whereas only 30% have a psychologist (Nguse & Wassenaar, 2021). Within the public and private mental health sectors, the legacy of racial oppression and its accompanying conscious and unconscious power structures is still alive. This is particularly present within transracial and transcultural therapy relationships which are common in the South African context where many mental health professionals are white (Edwards, 2015).

This chapter seeks to understand how the interplay of chronic poverty, broken systems of care, transracial therapy relationships, and historic and current trauma impacts on the body of clients and therapists. It explores the form of a meaningful embodied clinical approach to drama therapy that is congruent with this specific context and the early childhood trauma that is pervasive within it. We suggest an outline of an approach based on experiences with prepubescent boys who survived early trauma.

The focus is specifically on boys because this population's vulnerability and experience of abuse is often side-lined. This frequently denies them adequate support (Clulow & Van Niekerk, 2021). The impact of trauma can also present differently across genders (Gauthier-Duchesne et al., 2018; Levine & Kline, 2006). For these reasons, this writing is an attempt to give a voice to this population.

South African Context

To be able to get to grips with the depth of trauma and how it manifests in the wellbeing of children, it is necessary to contextualise the history of oppression and violence in SA. Kaminer and Eagle (2010) highlight the need for a profound understanding of inequities in relation to trauma (the impact of which reverberates across generations) before offering support.

Centuries of colonialism and the institutionalised oppression of apartheid systematically brutalised the indigenous majority of the population through impoverishment, displacement, dispossession, deculturation, dehumanisation, and violence by the military force (Gqola, 2015). The early 1990s brought a period of negotiating a true democracy in the country, which brought the hope of a 'rainbow nation' where historic injustices could be healed and diversity celebrated. As Gqola (2015, p.57) states, this was a period which allowed us to project an image of ourselves 'as it would be if we were our best selves'. During the political transition, there was an acknowledgement of the importance of facing the burden of the past. The Truth and Reconciliation Commission (TRC) was established as a space where victims could openly speak in a quest to find resolution and restitution, and where perpetrators could ask for forgiveness. It was a time of deep listening and painful testimony – a process to support the birth of a rainbow nation. That was the hope. The reality is that the legacy of apartheid is still felt today by the majority of black people who continue to experience persistent poverty and racial discrimination (Gqola, 2015).

If the current cycles of trauma are to be interrupted, the African ethic of *ubuntu* necessitates consideration of the impact of trauma on children who are socialised in a world that is constituted by violent interactions. Gqola (2015) suggests that the healing of our collective self will take conscious hard work from all levels of society. As she writes, 'loosening the stranglehold of violence is going to require fewer excuses and more imagination' (p.54).

The Trauma of History

This overall context can feel overwhelming when entering the therapy room with boys who are carrying this burden of history. It is necessary to consider how the complexity of trauma and disruption of nurturing care came to be if we are aiming to offer a different way of being. As drama therapists, we carry the responsibility to understand how our bodies in terms of race (white), gender (women) and age (young adult and middle-aged) impact the therapeutic alliance when working with black and coloured[1] children. We need to hold the history of oppression in mind when working with boys who have impulses for destruction directed at others and often towards themselves.

Race is embodied, produced, performed, and created (Mayor, 2012). This is a universal truth. In SA, race is politically and emotionally loaded because the roles of perpetrator and victim were historically cast along racial lines. Race significantly influences multiracial therapy relationships as it can be the juncture of personal and collective trauma. The client will experience the therapist through the lens of history. As Mayor (2012, p.216) suggests, 'the body becomes regulated and formed by repetitive activity, oppression and trauma'. The bodies of the white therapists carry unconscious meaning for the child based on his ancestors' repeated experiences with similar bodies. Building a trusting therapy relationship is impacted and becomes difficult, as our capacity to act outside of the assigned roles of perpetrators is constantly tested. This can feel like a wrestling match – having to grapple to be allowed to step into a different role.

Atkinson et al. (2010) state that there is a link between colonisation and increased rates of violence in families and communities. Historic trauma is the subjective remembering of experienced events passed from adults to their children in a cyclical process, leading to collective emotional and psychological injury across generations (Atkinson et al., 2010). This is cumulative over time (Duran et al., 1998). If the *ubuntu* ethic is considered, it is impossible not to share the ancestral pain. If a person is a person through others, this includes not only the rainbow nation but also the trauma. Violence becomes internalised oppression that models the release of psychic tension by directing it either inwards to self or outwards to others (Duran et al., 1998). In the context of complex racialised trauma in SA, this violence may have a psychological function when the depth of intergenerational trauma is considered. Therapeutic safety and alliance take on new meaning knowing that what is being worked towards are reparative relationships which include the possibility of forgiveness. Gobodo-Madikizela (2008) writes that the notion of repair does not present a finality but rather a possibility. This could be salient when considering therapeutic repair. Embodied action is the essence of human life, bringing the potential for both destructiveness and its counterpart – creativity. The symbolic destruction within therapy relationships carries with it the possibility of the co-creation of something different: a new way of being.

The Trauma of Poverty

Shonkoff and Garner (2012) posit that the significant stress of chronic poverty is a risk factor for health-threatening behaviours such as poor nutrition, unavailable parents, and substance abuse – all of which impact on attachment formation and healthy development for children. Palacios-Barrios and Hanson (2019) connect psychosocial processes, neurobiology, and the risk for psychopathology, stating that children from lower income families are two to three times more likely to develop mental health problems. According to Statistics SA (Maluleke, 2022), the national unemployment rate during the first quarter of 2022 stood at 34.5%, with 13.6% of the total population living in informal settlements without basic services. It seems reasonable to believe that caregivers who are chronically stressed by food insecurity, recurring health problems, and inadequate access to services are less resourced to support secure attachment formation.

The SA government has attempted to put structures in place to support the psychosocial health of the most vulnerable. However, the government services of care are damaged in fundamental ways. The need is greater than the system can manage. There are barriers of language and marked inaccessibility of services, not to mention vicarious trauma and burnout of clinicians, and backlogs in the provision of services including child protection (Lund et al., 2009). These cycles of trauma and lack of support feed into one another, intensifying the struggles of the majority of the population.

Our Approach

In the following section, we outline an approach of embodied drama therapy that attempts to work meaningfully within this context. This approach emerged from our work with young boys who survived combinations of trauma: social (including poverty), intergenerational, attachment and developmental, physical, and sexual. From this exploration, the potency of embodied and symbolic play became clear. Our approach consists in providing a supportive space for the child to follow their embodied and symbolic needs using play to process trauma.

Why an Embodied Approach?

We work from a standpoint that the body is the home for all that we are: emotions, thoughts, feelings, and spirit. It follows that embodiment expresses the physical manifestation of our conscious and unconscious selves, the tangible indicator of the way we respond to the world, our relationship to ourselves, our identity and others (Jones, 2007). Neuroscience has made vast inroads into how trauma significantly affects the physical development of children's brain and nervous system (Porges, 2011; van der Kolk, 2014). This has shown how specific psychological trauma responses are often communicated physically and how trauma recovery should view the body as integral to how we play, rest, communicate, and heal.

When trauma occurs in the non-verbal period of development, there is a possibility that words will never fully resolve the feelings and experiences, as these are locked into the preverbal limbic brain, unable to be integrated verbally and only finding expression through 'acting-out' (Ramsden, 2011, p.60). Using an embodied approach can be the non-verbal aid to trauma recovery.

However, embodiment needs to be handled sensitively, especially when working with complex trauma. Beginning therapy work can easily overwhelm an already stunned nervous system (van der Kolk, 2014). We witness this physical dysregulation when clients first engage with their body. This activation, often closely associated with infants, such as shaking, vomiting, defecating, or urinating, shows how the body can remember and return to the stage when many of the traumas first happened. Although potentially overwhelmed, the boys regularly rejected working away from direct embodied play, refusing and quickly bored by projected object play. It seems that the trauma held in the body urgently needs to be released through the body.

Despite this urgency, it is crucial to understand how play can feel threatening to individuals who have experienced trauma (Frydman & McLellelan, 2014). Navigating this threat and urgency becomes our first main task where consistency is key. Safety in the therapy room is not to be taken for granted when a child has learnt not to trust that his needs will be met by adults who may be potential perpetrators. As Frydman and McLellelan (2014, p.268) indicate, 'relationships become repeated stagnant encounters devoid of flexibility'. In our approach, we are guided by PACE (Playful, Accepting, Curious and Empathic) to assist in building the client's ability to tolerate these moments of difficulty and to develop trust (Hughes, 2018). In this way, the therapists explore difficult moments with curiosity and playfulness, potentially mitigating the client's beliefs regarding their perceived 'badness'. There is no judgment or direct injunction to change behaviour within this playspace, but rather an empathic curiosity to discover the internal world of the young clients.

Our experiences led us to see how boys' bodies are often stuck in repeating their lived trauma reality. When given the opportunity to engage with their own and other bodies, there can be a tendency to thematically play out scenes from trauma histories. In real life, bodies become weapons for survival, physically needing to fight and defend. As Seebohm writes (2011, p.131), 'as an action organised out of primitive defences expressing the intolerable internal states, destructiveness is an important communication'. Power potentially permeates literal enactments with a need to control. Themes of destruction, violence, and aggression may pervade. This can feel like a therapeutic stranglehold in the creative space, rendering the therapist either hostage or perpetrator, and the client either captor or captive (Seebohm, 2011).

The world of imaginative play can feel inaccessible when complex trauma is present with little confidence or trust to explore it (Frydman & McLellelan, 2014; Malchiodi, 2020). In essence, children become fixed in literal fight responses and their capacity to play beyond this is dulled. They need to learn that they can 'tolerate their sensations, befriend their inner experiences and cultivate new action patterns' (van der Kolk, 2014, Kindle location 4934).

Observations of this complex dysregulation and regression illustrate how deeply and fundamentally the trauma shapes relationships to the body, self, and others. We can feel this rigidity ourselves as therapists, stuck and not knowing how to invite any flexibility, processing, or transformation for clients. We know that our responsibility is to create enough safety to enable reparative experiences of connection, co-regulation, processing, integration, and release. Trust needs to be built to loosen defences for underlying feelings and experiences to be engaged with. We are held by the psychodynamic understanding that by engaging and processing the impact of trauma in ways that allow defences to be safely lowered, moments of reparation, health, and support can be found (Rudado, 2016).

From these initial reflections, it is clear that it is essential to find ways to be guided by pendulation, to support the clients in moving towards and away from the original wounds of trauma, and to gradually widen their window of tolerance for both their nervous system and psyche to engage in healing. Pendulation refers to what Levine and Kline (2006) describe as a natural rhythm inherent to humans: moving between pleasant and unpleasant sensations, allowing for new experiences and meanings to develop. This natural process is compromised by trauma due to an ever-present past needing to be unconsciously defended against. Moving between feelings of helplessness or rage and healthy control and calm can help support the clients. This pendulation between states can support the 'ability of the body to shift out of a state of shutdown, anxiety, aggression, helplessness or feelings of estrangement into a sense of vitality, joy, hope, initiative, and connection [which] is the best resource of all' (Levine & Kline, 2006, p.138). We regularly open sessions with children deciding on a physical warm-up like body stretches or jumping jacks. As rudimentary as this sounds, it is an important part of sessions where children can play with a constructive sense of agency and control. From this initial experience of control, they are more able to let go and experiment with improvised creative expression later.

From this incorporation of pendulation, we now look at ways in which we can help children widen their window of tolerance and move away from destructive and defensive impulses in order to experience creative bodies that hold the potential for health and healing.

Embodied Play and Symbolic Embodied Play

Our work often follows a similar pattern. Clients first engage in embodied play which is often reality-based and repetitive, and only thereafter in symbolic embodied play which is more expansive. This pattern is echoed in other drama therapy literature (James et al., 2005; Haen, 2015b) and is discussed in detail in this section. This movement through phases of embodied play becomes a way for clients to process their trauma through their own personalised creative expression and aesthetic. Influenced by humanistic and developmental psychology, we trust that given the right environment, the clients move towards the healing mechanism unique to themselves which unconsciously strengthens their internal sense of competency (Sigelman & Rider, 2012). This is a potent creative invitation that drama therapists are uniquely positioned to offer. The following sections provide a practical overview of our discoveries.

Embodied Play

We define embodied play as a form of play that engages the whole being and bodies of the therapist and client into the play-encounter. In our approach, embodied play starts in a similar way to how James et al. (2005) approach Developmental Transformations (DvT)[2] with traumatised children: an almost empty therapy space just containing colourful cloths, simple soft toys, paper, and a few crayons. The clients are introduced to the permissiveness of playing out improvised narratives using their own and the therapist's body. They then follow their needs and impulses from within the embodied play, with us following their lead (Zeal, 2011). While the form that play takes depends on each client, what is central is the use of the body. Body is where the play emerges from and where it takes shape. Clients begin to hone the skill of not being caught up in their heads, but rather of responding to prompts suggesting whether the body needs to move and play or needs to shake or shout, be still, or be with another. Given permission to play safely in this way, clients are able to communicate through their bodies in a way that 'the trauma [is] projected out' (Haen, 2015b, p.236). As previously mentioned, when clients are first offered this opportunity, they seem to use it to enact repetitive scenes of destruction, perpetration, and violence with little space for metaphor or symbol. The emerging play is fairly literal. The drama therapy space often becomes a 'designated chaos and destruction zone' (Zeal, 2011, p.77) that illustrates their internal world and capacity of being with another. Stepping into open-ended play can be difficult and it is important to emphasise the permissiveness of the play-space, while also reinforcing its boundaries. We often do this verbally by reminding that, even though we are playing, we cannot harm ourselves, others, or the space.

Symbolic Embodied Play

By being given permission to listen to their bodies and bring them into play in this way, clients are guided to the symbolic story emerging from their embodied impulses. Symbolic embodied play encourages the child to work with their whole embodied being in the world of metaphor and symbol, and to create necessary distance from the hugely emotional content that emerges. Focusing on characters, narratives, and actions that come out of embodied states allows clients to bring their own personal material when they feel safe enough to do so. From the emerging narratives and symbols, clients will identify characters, decide what happens, as well as when and how it happens in the embodied play-space. This kind of play is completely improvised and spontaneous, with the therapist encouraging stories or metaphors for expression. If a child comes into the session wanting to roar with rage, he has permission to follow this impulse. Fear may be present but by staying with it, this embodied need is extended into symbolic embodied play where it may become a roaring animal. As this play develops, the child can find expression for their feelings through their body as they step more fully into the symbolic embodied world of the roaring animal. A new possibility emerges as the fear dissipates and connections are made. Third-person narration can also be a useful reflection tool, a way to validate the clients' play and to name possible underlying feelings. This technique, often used in play therapy, can aid aesthetic distance and psychological safety.

Through intertwining symbol and body, the potency of noticing the story that the body holds, and then moving into and through necessary therapeutic thresholds in a way that supports discovery and connection to self, is increased (Pearson, 1996). This progression takes time, and only seems to happen once clients' repetitive embodiment of destruction have been witnessed and tolerated. We are guided by the drama therapy understanding that underlies many approaches in the field. This is the understanding that 'imagination is central to meaning-making' (Haen, 2015b, p.236), and that because symbolic embodied work engages the whole being, an active focus on this kind of play can restore access not only to therapeutic meaning but also to oneself. The internal stories that trauma survivors create can become rigid, with particular narratives solidifying intergenerational trauma patterns. However, when using symbolic embodied play, the ability to access symbol, imagination, and metaphor is intentionally broadened. Through this re-storying, new perspectives and integration are made possible (Malchiodi, 2020). Being witnessed and responded to by a therapist in this way can be likened to an attuned caregiver responding to their young child, noticing and creating a safe transitional space where new ways of being can be explored (Winnicott, 1971).

The Movement From Embodied Play to Symbolic Embodied Play

As the symbolic embodied play muscle becomes stronger, so does clients' aesthetic distance from the material, which allows for a widening of their window of tolerance for the more vulnerable content. Aesthetic distance (Landy, 1983) provides psychological safety. Metaphor and symbol provide just enough distance from the personal material so that clients can engage fully without feeling overwhelmed. When aesthetic distance is achieved, the client experiences a state of 'me and not me', where their engagement is balanced in terms of affect, cognition, expression, and control (Jones, 2007). This allows them to be with and move through the felt sense of the trauma (Malchiodi, 2020), rather than chronological trauma processing. This symbolic engagement is particularly useful in our work as it affords clients the ability to invest themselves in embodied play with increasing capacity to stay regulated. This approach also creates space for the clients to pendulate between control and surrender in the play. Control and surrender are loaded with meaning for children who have survived trauma. Rehearsing safe ways of control, as opposed to destructive ones, and safe ways of surrender seem to support the embodied sense of safe-enough. It also allows the child to find some repair in the attachment structures that have been initially ruptured. It is this aesthetic distance provided by the symbolic embodied play that, we believe, allows for the widening of the window of tolerance required for trauma healing (van der Kolk, 2014; Levine & Kline, 2006).

Being in a same co-embodied space, we are able to remind clients that playfulness is possible by subtly trying to show them how to bring flexibility to rigidity. It is key to model that alternative stories and alternative ways of exploring them are possible. This is perhaps the most challenging aspect of the work – to be able to hold the consistency through very rigid, aggressive, and often unplayful moments. It is also the most crucial, when clients are testing the resilience and trustworthiness of the therapist and seemingly asking whether they are sturdy enough to contain all that is in them (Gil & Dias, 2014). Through this, the legacies of race and oppression, ever-present in the transracial therapy relationships, can be exposed and played with in fundamental ways (Mayor, 2012). If often children communicate in rigid and unplayful moments that they do not believe that any personal or historical alternative is possible, it becomes the responsibility of the therapist to hold that hope and possibility.

With time, increased trust, ritualised consistency, and capacity to bring playfulness to rigidity, clients' play gradually becomes more symbolic. It is here that the unconscious and vulnerable material underneath their intergenerational trauma responses emerges, such as grief, loss of control, fear, loneliness, abandonment, rage, wishes for belonging, or numbness. A new trust in alternative means of expression develops through finding joy in the beauty of being creative without the need for destruction, whether this is through a dance with colourful cloths, tales of growth and adventure, celebration gatherings, the expression of the grief of death, or a new song that holds multitudes of stories.

Embodied Relationships Within Embodied and Symbolic Play

The centrality of the body in this process also supports the growth of therapeutic attunement and trust. The therapist is within the play with the child, either enrolled in character, mirroring the child's action, or reflecting on the play from within. This physical proximity supports co-regulation, kinaesthetic empathy, and the supportive action of mirror neurons (van der Kolk, 2014; Devereaux & Harrison, 2022). In this way, reparative therapeutic relationships mimic secure attachment with possibilities of 'delight, rupture, and repair' (van der Kolk, 2014, Kindle location 1940). In addition, this intimate presence – consistent, accepting, attentive, and curious – brings a potent 'humaning' to the therapeutic alliance. 'Humaning', a concept used by Erasmus (2017), differs from 'humanising'. It does not impose a particular way of being human, but rather a 'lifelong process of life-in-the-making with others' (Erasmus, 2017, p.xxvii), that encourages deep personal, cultural, social, and emotional engagement on a human-to-human level. This is a crucial therapy practice in contexts of intergenerational trauma and historical colonial oppression.

Being white therapists working with black and coloured children demands an awareness of how power is distributed in the therapy room. It places the emphasis on the essence of what it means to be in a therapeutic relationship with a child and how to navigate it without colluding or perpetuating power dynamics. We believe that the experience of 'humaning' embodied connection provides possibilities for understanding self and others in new ways. The previously powerless victim of oppression gains, through being the co-creator of symbolic embodied play, agency and viscerally experiences mastery and control over the direction that the play takes (Ramsden, 2011). Resilience can be the product of this agency, knowing that what you do makes a difference (van der Kolk, 2014). By engaging in an intimate and embodied therapeutic process with an accepting therapist, the child's body is given an alternative experience of being in relationship with another. In this way, they can step out of the prescribed roles assigned by trauma history and allow for new roles to emerge. The meeting of body memory, therapeutic relationship, and play can be profoundly reparative.

Expression and Integration

Because the therapy is embodied, the embodied memory of trauma can be metabolised (Haen, 2015a). Once the therapy alliance is more established, the children sometimes seem to need the therapist to speak the words they cannot find, to hold the feelings that overwhelm them and, in this sense, to metabolise or digest what they cannot yet. Through this supportive process, the children become slowly more able to begin to independently integrate these felt experiences (Casement, 2014).

Through this, the whole self is present and welcome as new narratives are explored, new parts of self discovered, and alternative ways of being rehearsed (Pearson, 1996; Nwoye, 2006; Theogene, 2018). As Malchiodi suggests (2022), 'it is the starting place to replace distressful memories and body sensations with the imagination of new and hopefully healing narratives'. The type of embodied practices described in this chapter provide opportunities for a 're-membering (bringing together, repairing)' of traumatic experiences and for a 're-embodiment' of new narratives of the self (Theogene, 2018, p.117) without the need for verbalisation. This non-linear integration is often held within the symbolic metaphors of the children themselves. Within the embodied play, all parts of the self can find a place to be expressed and integrated.

Therapy, particularly when engaging with unconscious trauma content, is exhausting. The children may frequently need time to rest. This rest is playfully connected and supported by the preceding symbolic encounters, rather than dissociated from the therapeutic process. The clients often need the therapist to be close and willing to engage with these vulnerable moments. The co-created symbols are flexible enough to encompass integration and therapeutic safety through rest.

Additional Reflections and Evaluation

Through practising this approach, we have reflected on some key areas that serve to fortify the work.

Ritual

A ritual container for the sessions is crucial, with sessions beginning and ending in the same way. The ritual can consist in a sequence of physical exercises co-created by the children, providing predictability within a therapy medium that encourages spontaneity. Symbolically, they offer safety for clients, and stability for the therapist knowing that rituals support the therapy contract. A co-created and firmly held ritualised session structure allows for an experience of constructive control.

South African indigenous ritual approaches to healing often include aspects similar to those used in drama therapy practice. While we are not guided by a psychospiritual frame, these elements enter the therapy space within the SA context. There is complexity within this when the therapists are from different racial, cultural, and religious backgrounds to their clients. Cultural appropriation needs to be seriously considered for all parties to feel safe.

Unconscious Communication

Working in such an embodied way can intensify the unconscious communication in the therapy relationship. This can manifest throughout the work and through the body in experiences such as exhaustion, nausea, tears, hunger, rage, and fear. It is crucial to notice this unconscious communication and use it as insight into the clients' internal world as often clients communicate their trauma responses in non-verbal ways. To avoid the re-enactment of trauma patterns, it is crucial to do this reflective work. Judith Herman's (1992) writing is useful to understand this unconscious communication. Herman explains that it is not only the client and therapist who are present in the process but also the perpetrator(s) who are still invisibly holding some power. This needs to be acknowledged by both the client and the therapist. Within the complexity of SA history, multiple ancestral perpetrators and victims are implicitly present. This demands resilience from the therapist, a deep understanding of the wounds of collective trauma, a sense of accountability, and a willingness to face personal wounds.

Equally, it is essential for therapists to seek collegial support and supervision. As so much of this work is experienced through the body, processing takes time and patience. If ignored, burn-out quickly follows. It is therefore equally important for therapists to find creative rituals for embodied release, regulation, and resource. Self-care becomes an ethical obligation.

Evaluation

We feel obliged to reflect and evaluate the strengths and limitations of this approach. The main strength is that it makes available an additional language for processing trauma. Using the language of embodied and symbolic play in this way makes trauma recovery much more accessible for those in desperate need of support. Because we now know the extent to which trauma is unconsciously held by the brain's physical structure and that words might not be available for intergenerational or early developmental trauma, working with embodiment is crucial. This approach allows for an empowering therapy journey, where the child's agency is honoured and valued. The need to trust the child's innate capacity to recover requires conscious reminders.

However, it is an approach that needs significant time, and this is not always possible. It also requires robust social support from all parties involved, to contain the regression and difficulties that inevitably arise. This includes the institution or treatment team, the caregivers, and the environment to support the child's therapy gains and challenges.

Conclusion

In this chapter we have illustrated the multifaceted nature of trauma in South Africa and how embodied and symbolic play is a potent drama therapy intervention for boys in that context. This chapter has shown how a therapy centred on expression through body and symbol can give children who have survived trauma – and who are often labelled as 'defiant' or 'oppositional' – the possibility to create new narratives and ways of being. It has also shown the critical inclusion of the therapist to 'play in' the multifaceted trauma story with the child, to broaden symbolic engagement (and therefore perspective and distance), and to offer an alternative connection amid historically rigid relations.

This chapter constitutes a significant voice in the limited literature exploring drama therapy approaches in postcolonial contexts such as South Africa. The drama therapy approach outlined in this chapter can be implemented in contexts with similar complexity. However, this should only be considered if the therapist is able to consistently hold in mind the multifaceted nature of trauma and its implications for therapy. We suggest that the multifaceted holding that is required can be represented through a number of concentric circles.

In the inner and core circle is located the child whose fullness, intensity, destructive impulses, bravery, and creative capacity need to be met and held by the therapist with tenacity and compassion. The next circle refers to the therapeutic relationship that acknowledges the historically assigned roles related to race, as well as the issue of trust and unconscious communication. The following circle constitutes the drama therapy approach discussed in this chapter that has outlined how, as trauma is kept in the body, the use of embodied and symbolic play can contribute to an intentional reworking of the trauma responses held in the nervous system, and provide a safe space for recovery. Finally, the outer circle refers to the overall context and how the psychosocial, economic, and historical legacies of trauma and oppression impact on intergenerational trauma, poverty, broken systems of care, and attachment formation. What resides within this circle is the ethical concern that such systemic issues may fail children to heal from their trauma, but also the hope that the reconnection to self and creativity on an embodied level can contribute to the building of resilience to help navigate those broken structures.

Just as trauma is multifaceted, so is the responsibility of the therapist who plays alongside the child. The concentric circles represent this multifaceted responsibility that needs to constantly be held in mind when inviting embodied and symbolic play in contexts similar to South Africa. We believe that if these can be welcomed and played with, there is possibility for meaningful expression, release, integration, and healing.

Notes

1 The term 'coloured' is used ubiquitously in South Africa to describe a population group with ancestry from multiple races and ethnicities.

2 Developmental Transformations is a drama therapy method that intentionally uses improvisatory, dramatic play to allow for unconscious material to be processed. Both therapist and client are in the play together, with the therapist using interventions from within the play to support a deepening of expression and release.

References

Atkinson, J., Nelson, J., & Atkinson, C. (2010). Trauma, transgenerational transfer and effects on community wellbeing. In N. Purdie, P. Dudgeon, & R. Walker (Eds.), *Working together: Aboriginal and Torres Strait Islander mental health and wellbeing principles and practice* (pp. 135–144). Australian Government Department of the Prime Minister and Cabinet.

Bower, C. (2014). The plight of women and children in South Africa. *The Annals of the American Academy of Political and Social Science*, 652, 106–126.

Casement, P. (2014). *On learning from the patient*. Routledge.

Clulow, S. & Van Niekerk, J. (2021). *Caring for boys affected by sexual violence in South Africa*. CINDI.

Craig, A., Rochat, T., Naicker, S., Mapanga, W., Mtintsilana, A., Dlamini, S. N., Ware, L. J., Du Toit, J., Draper, D. E., Richter, L., & Shane, A. (2022). The prevalence of probable depression and probable anxiety, and associations with adverse childhood experiences and socio-demographics: A national survey in South Africa. *Frontiers in Public Health*, Vol. 10.

Devereaux, C. & Harrison, L. (2022). Body, brain, and relationship: Dance/movement therapy and children with complex trauma. In R. Dieterich-Hartwell & A. Melsom (Eds.), *Dance/movement therapy for trauma survivors: Theoretical, clinical and cultural perspectives* (pp. 74–86). Routledge.

Docrat, S., Bedada, D., Cleary, S. D., & Lund, C. (2019). Mental health system costs, resources and constraints in South Africa: A national survey. *Health Policy and Planning*, 34, 706–719.

Duran, E., Duran, B., Heart, M. Y., & Horse-Davis, S. Y. (1998). Soul wound. In Y. Danieli (Ed.), *International handbook of multigenerational legacies of trauma* (pp. 341–355). Plenum Press.

Edwards, S. (2015). Integral approach to South African psychology with special reference to indigenous knowledge. *Journal of Psychology in South Africa*, 24(6), 526–532.

Erasmus, Z. (2017). *Race otherwise: Forging a new humanism for South Africa*. Wits University Press.

Flisher, A., Dawes, A., Kafaar, Z., Lund, C., Sorsdahl, K., Myers, B., Thom, R., & Seedat, S. (2012). Child and adolescent mental health in South Africa. *Journal of Child & Adolescent Mental Health*, 24(2), 149–161.

Frydman, J. & McLellelan, L. (2014). Complex trauma and executive functioning: Evisioning a cognitive based trauma-informed approach to drama therapy. In D. Johnson & N. Sajnani (Eds.), *Trauma informed drama therapy: Transforming clinics, classrooms and communities* (pp. 175–201). Charles C Thomas.

Gauthier-Duchesne, A., Hebert, M., & Daspe, M.-E. (2018). Gender as a predictor of posttraumatic stress symptoms and externalising behavior problems in sexually abused children. *Canadian Institutes of Health Research*, 79–88.

Gil, E. & Dias, T. (2014). The integration of drama therapy and play therapy in attachment work with traumatised children. In C. Malchiodi & D. Crenshaw (Eds.), *Creative arts and play therapy for attachment problems* (pp. 100–120). The Guildford Press.

Gobodo-Madikizela, P. (2008). Empathetic repair after mass trauma: When vengeance is arrested. *European Journal of Social Theory*, 11(3), 331–350.

Gqola, P. (2015). *RAPE: A South African nightmare*. Jacana Media.

Haen, C. (2015a). Fostering change when safety is fleeting: Expressive therapy groups for adolescents with complex trauma. In N. Webb & L. Terr (Eds.), *Play therapy with children and adolescents in crisis* (pp. 239–257). Guilford Publications.

Haen, C. (2015b). Vanquishing monsters: Group drama therapy for treating trauma. In C. E. Malchiodi (Ed.), *Creative interventions with traumatised children* (pp. 235–258). The Guildford Press.

Herman, J. (1992). *Trauma and recovery*. Health Communications Inc.

Hughes, D. (2018). *Building the bonds of attachment*. Rowman & Littlefield.

James, M., Forrester, A., & Kim, K. (2005). Developmental transformations in the treatment of sexually abused children. In A. Weber & C. Haen (Eds.), *Clinical applications of drama therapy in child and adolescent treatment* (pp. 67–87). Brunner-Routledge.

Jones, P. (2007). *Drama as therapy* (2nd ed.). Routledge.

Kaminer, D. & Eagle, G. (2010). *Traumatic stress in South Africa*. Wits University Press.

Landy, R. (1983). The use of distancing in drama therapy. *The Arts in Psychotherapy*, 10(3), 175–185.

Levine, P. & Kline, M. (2006). *Trauma through a child's eyes*. North Atlantic Books.

Lund, C. (2016). Mental health and human rights in South Africa: The hidden humanitarian crisis. *South African Journal on Human Rights*, 32(3), 403–405.

Lund, C., Kakuma, R., & Flisher, A. J. (2009). Public sector mental health systems in South Africa: Inter-provincial comparisons and policy implications. *Social Psychiatry and Psychiatric Epidemiology*, 45(3), 393–404.

Malchiodi, C. (2020). *Trauma and expressive arts therapy: Brain, body and imagination in the healing process*. The Guilford Press.

Malchiodi, C. (2022, September 15). *Can imagination help heal trauma?* Retrieved from www.psychologytoday.com/za/blog/arts-and-health/202209/can-imagination-help-heal-trauma

Maluleke, R. (2022). *Quarterly labour force survey (QLFS)(Q1:2022)*. Retrieved from www.statssa.gov.za/publications/P0211/Presentation%20QLFS%20Q1%202022.pdf

Mayor, C. (2012). Playing with race: A theoretical framework and approach for creative arts therapists. *The Arts in Psychotherapy*, 39, 214–219.

Nguse, S. & Wassenaar, D. (2021). Mental health and COVID-19 in South Africa. *South African Journal of Psychology*, 51(2), 304–313.

Nwachukwu, P. & Segalo, P. (2018). Life Esidimeni tragedy: Articulating ecological justice code branding for social care and mental health practice. *Gender & Behaviour*, 16(2), 11235–11249.

Nwoye, A. (2006). A narrative approach to child and family therapy in Africa. *Contemporary Family Therapy*, 28(1), 1–23.

Palacios-Barrios, E. & Hanson, J. (2019). Poverty and self-regulation: Connecting psychosocial processes, neurobiology and the risk for psychopathology. *Comprehensive Psychiatry*, 90, 52–64.

Pearson, J. (1996). *Discovering the self through drama and movement*. Jessica Kingsley Publishers.

Porges, S. (2011). *The polyvagal theory: Neuropsycholgical foundations of emotions, attachment, communication and self-regulation*. Norton.

Ramsden, E. (2011). Joshua and the expression of make-believe violence: Dramatherapy in a primary school setting. In D. Dokter, P. Holloway, & H. Seebohm (Eds.), *Dramatherapy and destructiveness: Creating the evidence base, playing with Thanatos* (pp. 53–65). Routledge.

Rudado, J. (2016). What do we talk about when we talk about psychoanalysis? *International Forum of Psychoanalysis*, 25(3), 179–185.

Seebohm, H. (2011). On bondage and liberty: The art of the possible in medium-secure settings. In D. Dokter, P. Holloway, & H. Seebohm (Eds.), *Dramatherapy and destructiveness: Creating the evidence base, playing with Thanatos* (pp. 118–132). Routledge.

Shonkoff, J. P. & Garner, A. S. (2012). The lifelong effects of early childhood adversity and toxic stress. *Pediatrics*, 129, 232–246.

Sigelman, C. & Rider, E. (2012). *Human development across the life span*. Cengage Learning.

Sulla, V. (2020). *Poverty and equity brief: Sub-Saharan Africa: South Africa*. Retrieved from https://databank.worldbank.org/data/download/poverty/33EF03BB-9722-4AE2-ABC7-AA2972D68AFE/Global_POVEQ_ZAF.pdf

Theogene, N. (2018). A critique of embodiment. *Strategic review for Southern Africa*, 117–133.

van der Kolk, B. (2014). *The body keeps the score: Mind, brain and body in the transformation of trauma*. Penguin.

Winnicott, D. (1971). *Playing and reality*. Routledge Classics.

Zeal, E. (2011). Chaos, destruction and abuse: Dramatherapy in a school for excluded adolescents. In D. Doktor, P. Holloway, & H. Seebohm (Eds.), *Dramatherapy and destructiveness: Creating the evidence base, playing with Thanatos*, (pp. 66–77). Routledge.

Chapter 7

Integrating Dramatherapy With the NeuroAffective Relational Model™ (NARM) for Healing Developmental Trauma

Danai Karvouni

This chapter introduces the integration – or *league* – of dramatherapy with the NeuroAffective Relational Model™ (NARM) for healing developmental trauma. I use the word *league* inspired by a line in one of Shakespeare's sonnets (2004/1609, p.99), 'Betwixt mine eye and heart a league is took', as this model has been drawn from both my passion for dramatherapy and the vital clarity that NARM has offered me to address and work with developmental trauma. This chapter presents this integrated model of work by unfolding how dramatherapy and NARM developmental theories and practice influenced by embodied and relational healing can be incorporated to support therapists in their work with the traumatised population.

As a dramatherapist working with trauma, I discovered that although dramatherapy provides unlimited creative and embodied means, it does not offer a clear framework to share and build on with clients in trauma-focused work. I have found that this lack of structure may present its challenges in practice, including an impact on the therapists' health and confidence as practitioners support clients with often very complex presentations. On the contrary, NARM is a therapy specifically designed to address trauma symptoms such as nervous system dysregulation, attachment, and identity distortions (Gruber et al., 2021). It thus provides a well-defined theoretical, practical, and relational framework to support clinicians in their work with developmental trauma. NARM is a somatic-oriented method of therapy based on mindfulness interventions including sensing, naming, and learning from one's present somatic sensations. Although mindfulness driven, NARM is mainly a talking therapy restricted to verbal communication. Compared to dramatherapy's creative and expressive means, it offers more limited ways of exploration and expression towards healing. In my practice as a dramatherapist and NARM practitioner, I found that an alliance between these approaches started to develop and that a combination of these filled the gap I encountered if solely relying on one or the other. I discovered that the integration of the two models helped my sense of confidence as a therapist and led to positive therapeutic outcomes for my clients.

DOI: 10.4324/9781003322375-9

Bessel van der Kolk (2014) refers to developmental trauma as 'the hidden epidemic', highlighting how childhood trauma, its effects, and healing have been left unaddressed and unexplored for years. In this chapter, I define developmental trauma as the repeated traumatic experiences, such as neglect or abuse, which occur mainly during early development and childhood, as well as the aftermath of those. As awareness of developmental trauma increases, research findings keep evidencing its effects on the somatic level and biopsychosocial experience. Trauma-specific models which consider embodied experience in healing are therefore becoming more widely recognised and researched (Maercker, 2021). We now know that traumatised children develop into adults with symptoms such as chronic shame, negative view of self, difficulty in managing emotions, relational disturbances, and patterns that are deeply stored in the autonomic nervous system.

As evidence on body and healing from trauma is expanding, it seems essential to review how embodied methods in dramatherapy can inform newer therapy models, and explore how new knowledge on multifaceted topics can enlighten and improve dramatherapy practice further. In the following paragraphs, I present a model of work which I have used as an initial framework that still has room for expansion and growth. I introduce this integrated therapy model by firstly presenting the NARM's developmental framework (Heller & LaPierre, 2012), and by discussing it in relation to dramatherapy's developmental paradigms of Embodiment-Projection-Role (Jennings, 1999) and Neuro-Dramatic-Play (Jennings & Gerhardt, 2011). I then explore the NARM process based on mindfulness and the four pillars in therapy (Heller & Kammer, 2022) in relation to embodiment and non-verbal core processes in dramatherapy (Jones, 2007). I finally discuss the relational aspect of healing in developmental trauma to further explore the therapists' somatic responses and their role in practice.

The aim of this chapter is to contribute to the field of trauma research and practice by sharing how an integration of dramatherapy, especially its embodied-based methods, with a specialised model for healing developmental trauma can offer safer and more effective ways of healing. My hope is to propose how a league between approaches with mutual aims can support a therapist's quest towards healing and to point out key learnings and suggestions for future practice.

Dramatherapy and NARM in Theory

Introduction to the NeuroAffective Relational Model™

NARM is a developmentally oriented and neuroscientifically informed model of psychotherapy developed by psychologist and academic Dr Laurence Heller to support mental health professionals in their work with trauma (Heller, 2018). It was developed in parallel with the ground-breaking theories of van der Kolk (2014) and Levine (2010) on the impact of developmental trauma on the body and the nervous system. Emerging from earlier psychotherapeutic orientations including Psychodynamic Psychotherapy, Attachment Theory, Cognitive Therapy, and Somatic Experiencing, NARM bridges traditional psychotherapy with somatic approaches within a context of relational practice and mindfulness. It is 'a somatically based psychotherapy that focuses on supporting an individual's capacity for increasing connection and aliveness' (Heller & LaPierre, 2012, p.2). By working in the present moment and through somatic mindfulness, NARM aims to support individuals to become more aware of their body and mind experiences, and to disidentify with survival patterns that maintain chronic nervous system dysregulation. Through careful observation and noting physiological shifts during the therapy process, NARM ultimately supports clients to re-connect to their personal strengths and self-healing capacities as a means towards greater nervous system regulation and emotional resilience.

The NARM theoretical framework is based on five core biological needs and developmental stages essential to emotional and physical health and wellbeing (Heller & LaPierre, 2012). These are the need for Connection (0–6 months), Attunement (6–18 months), Trust (18 months–4 years), Autonomy (2–4 years), and Love and Sexuality (4–6 and 11–15 years). Depending on how these essential needs are met in the first years of life, the capacity for healthy attunement and response to these needs as adults is developed. Specifically, a good enough meeting of the above needs supports the development of a greater capacity as adults (1) to be in touch and attune to the body and emotions with the ability to reach out for and take in nourishment; (2) to trust oneself as well as others to find a healthy balance between dependence and interdependence; (3) to feel autonomous enough to set boundaries and say no without guilt or fear; and (4) to live a life with an open heart and to be able to integrate loving relationships with a vital sexuality. In NARM, these capacities are seen as essential in promoting self-regulation, positive self-image and authentic connection to self and others and thus wellbeing.

When the environment or caregivers fail to meet those core developmental needs efficiently, children are faced with a main dilemma between their survival and the authentic connection and expression of themselves. This dilemma leads to recurring painful emotions of anger, shame, and chronic fight-flight nervous system activation extending to physiological collapse. In order to survive such emotional states, children adapt by disconnecting from themselves and from what NARM refers to as their 'life force' (Heller & LaPierre, 2012, p.32). The impact of this ongoing disconnection is observed in the body in areas of tension, weakness, or disconnection. Muscular tightening, bracing, and collapse are some of the physical manifestations of adaptation which further compromise essential capacities for wellbeing. As a result, authentic connection, expression, and response to oneself and needs are being compromised, leading to a limited capacity to attend, sooth, and regulate, and therefore to the development of symptoms.

According to NARM, childhood adaptations will lead to the development of five main patterns of surviving the impact of unfulfilled core needs. Each survival style is named after the associated unmet need and reflects difficulties in the corresponding capacities (Gruber et al., 2021). Therefore, individuals with the Connection Survival Style adapt by disconnecting from themselves, their body, and others as connection has been too threatening or unbearable. In the Attunement Survival Style, sensing and expressing one's own needs is compromised often in favour of others. Individuals with the Trust Survival Style learn to shut down their need for dependence and interdependence in fear of being betrayed. Whereas in the Autonomy Survival Style, they give up on authentic expression or boundary setting in fear of being abandoned. Lastly, people with the Love-Sexuality Survival Style learn to associate love with looks and performance leading often to difficulties in healthy integration of love and sexuality. These adaptive survival strategies are seen as necessary for one's own health and safety as responses to a hostile environment. As life continues and the threat has passed, these adaptations are held in the body and imprinted in the nervous system. A limited awareness of those becomes an obstacle to one's authentic needs and wishes.

Dramatic Development and Developmental Trauma

Following NARM's developmental framework, I continue my discussion exploring its relation to two of the most widely recognised developmental paradigms within dramatherapy, the Embodiment-Projection-Role (EPR) (Jennings, 1999) and Neuro-Dramatic-Play (NDP) (Jennings & Gerhardt, 2011). As EPR and NDP reflect the developmental stages of dramatic embodiment, expression, and play, I intend to explore how the two developmental models may converge, and whether an alliance between those may be beneficial in the healing of developmental trauma.

The EPR and NDP models were developed by Sue Jennings after observations of early years, and the attachment relationship through the lens of children's dramatic development through play. EPR follows the progression of dramatic play from birth to 7 years and is formed by the three stages of Embodiment, Projection, and Role. The stage of Embodiment refers to the time in development when we experience self and others *by and through the body*. The NDP model is an extension of the Embodiment stage which starts six months before birth and lasts until six months after birth. Here, sensory, rhythmic, and dramatic play have crucial importance in children's healthy attachment and wellbeing. Jennings (2015) speaks about the way in which trauma distorts infants' healthy development and suggests that returning to those early play stages can support healing. The stage of Projection, starting from 13 months to 3 years, refers to the play *outside our body*, and includes play with objects, art, and others. Lastly, the Role stage, which develops between 3 and 7 years, refers to *as if* play through enacting roles and creating stories and characters.

As these models have widely informed dramatherapists' work, I want to explore how their integration with NARM as a trauma-focused model of therapy can improve clinical practice.

In my work, I have integrated Jennings's dramatic development paradigms with the NARM theory on developmental needs and capacities. As both are informed by attachment theory, they highlight the impact that the lack of caregivers' attunement has on children's development. EPR elaborates specifically on the importance of all aspects of play for healthy attachment, development, and expression, whereas NARM introduces the five core needs as essential to one's overall capacity for healthy connection to self and others, and for wellbeing. EPR suggests that children or adults will have less capacity in one or all of these dramatic domains depending on which one was interrupted in childhood. NARM, on the other hand, suggests that individuals will develop certain survival strategies that later become obstacles to the fulfilment of needs essential to wellbeing.

A combined theoretical framework can be used to support therapists' working hypotheses and interventions by bringing together body and mind. EPR and NDP offer a structure informed by dramatic development and play, whereas NARM introduces a comprehensive theoretical and practical framework to address developmental trauma. This may be particularly useful when working with trauma due to the complexity of client presentations and how this can affect therapists' responses. For example, when clients present themselves with a limited capacity to name what they feel and to connect to themselves, we can suspect that difficulties stem from the first months of life during the Connection and Embodiment developmental stages. This can form a working hypothesis that the need for connection to self has been too threatening or unsafe. The therapists' attention may shift towards supporting safe reconnection to self and increasing the capacity for the body to become a safe place again. NARM suggests that healing happens when individuals reconnect with parts of themselves that they have been disconnected from because of trauma. This allows reconnection to their self-healing resources and capacities (Heller & LaPierre, 2012). The focus is therefore not necessarily on exploring what happened to them but on how interventions can support the connection to feeling safe again.

In Table 7.1, I introduce the developmental stages and associated needs and capacities as suggested by NARM in relation to the stages of Embodiment-Projection-Role, and their correlated embodied activities to promote associated therapeutic aims. This integrative framework offers an understanding of clients' difficulties under a developmental perspective and a path towards embodied interventions based on dramatic development to encourage re-connection and thus healing. Engagement with embodied activities such as sensory, rhythmic, or dramatic play may offer an opportunity toward restoring a sense of self in the body and inviting clients to remain present in the here and now within a safe and supportive relationship. This may allow moving away from past

Table 7.1 EPR and NARM Integrative Developmental Framework

Developmental stages	*NARM core needs and capacities*	*EPR developmental stages*	*Embodied methods to promote healing*	*Associated therapeutic aims*
0–6 months	Connection	Embodiment (NDP)	Sensory, rhythmic, and dramatic embodied play	To safely start reconnecting with the body's felt sense and others
6–18 months	Attunement	Embodiment (NDP) Projection	Sensory, rhythmic, and dramatic embodied play Play beyond the body, with toys, art, and with others	To develop capacity to recognise needs, obstacles and to overcome those
18 months–4 years	Trust	Projection Role	Play beyond the body, with toys, art, and with others Play through roles and stories	To develop capacity to trust and rehearse healthy dependence and interdependence
2–4 years	Autonomy	Role	Play through roles and stories	To explore capacity for setting healthy boundaries, saying 'no' and developing confidence in self
4–6 years 11–15 years	Love and sexuality	Role	Play through roles and stories	To discover, witness, and embrace all aspects of self, strengths, and flaws; to increase capacity for love of self and others

adaptations and negative associations between the embodied sense of self and safety. For example, clients whose needs were not adequately met during the Connection or Embodiment developmental stages may present with difficulties related to their bodies such as persisting disconnection from their embodied experience, their felt sense as well as others. Interventions that allow them to reconnect with their bodies in safe ways may support these individuals to regain a sense of body and thus self. Due to this being the basis of healthy development, it can be predicted that these clients will experience challenges associated with the following stages. The question of how much progress one may make without resolving or at least acknowledging difficulties in this first stage will be considered when speaking about long-term therapy effectiveness.

Other clients may present in therapy with more capacity to sense their bodies and connect to themselves but with challenges related to one of the other developmental stages. For instance, a client may present in therapy with difficulties in trusting others and maintaining relationships. As these difficulties seem to relate to the stages of Trust, Projection, and Role, therapy explorations can focus on the client's relationship with dependence and interdependence, and conflicts arising between the need for those. Projective play with objects may support clients in that stage to represent their fears and dilemmas, looking at them from a third perspective and from a distance. Storytelling and role further offer other means to experience patterns and rehearse changes and desired new ways of being. A final example to illustrate how this framework can be used is that of a client whose problems are related to setting boundaries or expressing themselves authentically. Here, difficulties may emerge from the developmental stage of Autonomy and Role. This time, the therapist interventions may be more focused on discovering barriers and fears to set boundaries. Clients in that stage may be supported through storytelling or role-based activities to help them discover more about themselves through the embodiment of new possibilities and perspectives. Consequently, in this model of work, it is both the embodied awareness and experience that support clients in disidentifying with old behavioural patterns to promote effective results in therapy.

Having discussed this integrative theoretical framework, it is useful to highlight an element of shared language between the two approaches. NARM speaks about needs, capacities, and survival strategies, shifting from pathologising symptoms and behaviour. It validates and humanises individuals' experiences and supports them to deconstruct outdated responses that have obsolete usefulness. EPR in dramatherapy, on the other hand, discusses basic human needs of play, embodiment, and creative expression. It does not pathologise one's limited capacity for one or the other, but rather suggests revisiting those basic needs as means towards healing. These common concepts may be particularly useful when working with clients who have been chronically stigmatised or shamed about their experiences as they appear to promote acceptance and compassion towards human nature and ways of surviving. Such language may be valuable to therapists who wish to address complicated themes with clients and to invite them to explore those creatively through the safe distance of dramatic play. In that respect, the integration of these theories offers a structure through which chaos can be explored and contained to ensure the safety of both therapist and clients.

Dramatherapy and NARM in Practice

Heller (2018) suggests that all therapeutic approaches are based on an inherent metaprocess, or an underlying method that invites clients to pay attention to certain aspects of their experience more than others. In this section, I discuss NARM and dramatherapy underlying metaprocesses as well as their core approaches towards healing. I then further explore how these may meet and support one another in an integrative method for the healing of developmental trauma.

NARM and Mindfulness

The main process that underlies the NARM model is that of mindful awareness of self in the present moment (Heller, 2018). In recent years, there has been increasing evidence of the benefits of mindfulness in mental health outcomes, and it is now widely used as an intervention (Coronado-Montoya et al., 2016). The NARM method is built on two specific aspects of it: somatic mindfulness and mindful awareness of one's survival styles.

As Levine (2010) suggests, it is through the physical body's awareness that the mind can comprehend. NARM's metaprocess of somatic mindfulness reflects the fact that the body's internal sensations are crucial in the healing process. As we know, exposure to repeated trauma affects the person's nervous system function and relationship with their embodied felt sense (Levine, 2010; van der Kolk, 2014). Traumatised individuals learn to numb or disconnect from their body self to survive unbearable feelings. The implicit cost of this is that their capacity to connect to pure joy, expansion, and aliveness also gets dulled. NARM as a model informed by the tradition of mindfulness and the knowledge of the nervous system invites individuals to stay present, name, and tolerate organised internal states. Somatic mindfulness is used as a method to increase capacity to recognise one's own somatic responses, thoughts, and feelings with the aim of supporting nervous system regulation. It is through this process that the clients' capacity for emotional regulation and experiences of joy and aliveness can grow. Sensing, naming, and identifying internal sensations is considered indeed one of the main steps to recovery (van der Kolk, 2014).

Additionally, NARM supports clients to recognise their adaptive survival styles and organising principles through mindful awareness. As the capacity for re-connecting to internal experience and self-regulation develops, clients start to become more self-aware of adaptations they had to make and to explore identity distortions. They are invited to explore the patterns preventing them from being present in their life and are encouraged to delve into this inquiry on the cognitive, emotional, and physiological levels of experience (Heller, 2018). Through this awareness, they acknowledge the conflicts in their experience and reconnect with their sense of agency to further resolve these.

Dramatherapy and Dramatic Embodiment

Although NARM uses aspects of mindfulness to allow reconnection and expansion, and invites observations on a somatic level, it is limited to verbal means of reflection and exploration. Jones (2007) summarised the core dramatherapy processes that support change within dramatherapy. These active and often non-verbal processes all involve embodied participation to a degree. Amongst the existing dramatherapy approaches (Johnson & Emunah, 2021), embodiment through theatre and drama techniques, or dramatic embodiment, is considered indeed one of the main vehicles to promote change. Langley (2006) suggests that it is the engagement in the dramatic process that promotes self-awareness and leads to transformation. Thus, dramatic embodiment, by inviting clients to shift their attention into the experience of the dramatic process, can be considered as dramatherapy's underlying metaprocess.

As earlier described, due to the impact of trauma on a physiological level, the benefits of dramatic embodiment within therapy will be considered. Through dramatic embodiment, clients are invited to express and encounter material in the here and now, in a way that 'the self is realised by and through the body' (Jones, 2007, p.113). As Levine (2010) suggests, having a relationship with the physical self is critical to connect to oneself and take appropriate action. In dramatherapy, the body is seen as the primary means by which communication occurs between self and other. Traumatised bodies are overexerted in recognising pain and suffering, and often have limited space and capacity to achieve optimal levels of arousal and self-regulation. By allowing healthy reconnection to self through dramatic embodiment, creativity, and play, clients are offered a greater chance to enhance their relationship with their physical self. This subsequently increases their capacity for self and nervous system regulation especially when interventions based only on words have proved not to be enough.

This invitation for engagement with one's own body can be observed in other core dramatherapy processes as well. Those of dramatic projection, play, and role are especially reflected within the EPR and NDP models. Within dramatic projection, aspects of self or experiences are projected into dramatic materials or into enactment. Clients externalise inner conflicts and open a dramatic dialogue between the internal situation and the external expression of that situation (Jones, 2007). Dramatic projection offers clients a safe distance through which they can view aspects of themselves or experiences that have been too overwhelming to process otherwise. In addition, playing is seen as a process which promotes a flexible attitude towards situations and held ideas. Playing allows clients to experiment with new behaviours and take on new roles. It promotes a liberating sense of flexibility that can support clients to move away from survival strategies and maladaptive identifications (Cattanach, 1994). Finally, through role, clients are invited to explore themes in an *as if* dramatic reality, either directly by embodying characters or indirectly through projective objects such as puppets. Similar to play, role offers opportunities to discover new ways of being and expressing oneself. It is a chance to rehearse the desired change, making it less threatening and more visible.

To summarise, dramatic embodiment allows clients to engage and work through traumatic material without relying solely on verbal expression. Dramatic means may then take the lead in allowing clients to reconnect with their physical selves in less direct and thus safer ways.

NARM and Dramatherapy Approaches to Healing

Having discussed the underlying processes for each modality, I will now discuss their specific applications to healing. I will then reflect on how similarities between those support an alliance between the two models leading to an integrative method towards healing.

To begin with, the NARM approach consists of four pillars that provide a structure to the sessions (Heller & Kammer, 2022). The first pillar clarifies the therapeutic contract and invites clients to set their intention for the session. The second pillar continues with exploratory questions, gathering information and inviting clients to explore what gets in the way of their intention in all levels of experience (somatic, cognitive, and emotional) by remaining focused on the present moment. Then, the therapist's attention moves to the third pillar which supports the client's sense of agency and ownership over their life story, by recognising the unconscious identifications and strategies that distort their sense of reality. The fourth and final pillar is a process of anchoring shifts in embodied experience of authentic connection. A conscious awareness of such moments is encouraged by reflecting on psychobiological shifts in all levels of experience. For NARM, it is through this process of connection that the capacity for self-regulation gets developed.

On the other hand, core aspects of dramatherapy practice that promote healing and change have been researched and summarised by Cassidy et al. (2014). Authors found four main processes that seem to underpin dramatherapists' interventions. These are working in the present moment, *the here and now*, establishing safety within the therapy space, working alongside the client by offering them control and choice over their therapy, and enabling clients' active involvement through the creative expressive means.

When comparing both therapies' main approaches to healing, it is evident that they share a common ground. They both remain focused on working in the present moment. They also invite an exploration of themes through curiosity and openness in a collaborative rather than directive manner, although within dramatherapy therapists may be actively involved in creative activities to support clients' explorations. Furthermore, both therapies focus on offering clients control and choice in therapy, thus sharing a commitment to promoting a sense of agency. The main difference between NARM and dramatherapy is the way through which they build on those main processes. NARM does this through verbal ways and by promoting somatic mindfulness, whereas dramatherapy works through non-verbal means that offer more options towards communication and explorations, whereby the body is directly (e.g. play, role) or less directly (e.g. dramatic projection) involved. Lastly, dramatherapy has been developed over the years to help a variety of clients rather than specific client groups. Consequently, dramatherapists who work with traumatised populations have integrated similar principles in their work, yet following a variety of different approaches (Sajnani & Johnson, 2014). NARM on the other hand, by putting forward processes based on mindfulness and the four pillars, offers a comprehensive framework to address developmental trauma.

I suggest that an alliance between the main aspects of the two modalities could effectively promote change and support therapists' practice. This alliance constitutes an original model that can be utilised to guide practice, although I also encourage that interventions remain experimental and informed by mindful presence and curiosity led by the client's needs.

In Table 7.2, I propose an integration of the four pillars structure as outlined by NARM with embodied means proven to promote change in dramatherapy. Following the structure of NARM's four pillars in therapy, I suggest dramatic means to support these pillars and overcome obstacles, specifically through embodied and non-verbal forms. For example, if clients find it hard to clarify and thus connect to their therapeutic intention verbally, therapists can invite them to explore or represent it through dramatic means. As discussed earlier, difficulties in finding one's own wish might relate to one of the very first

Table 7.2 NARM pillars integrated with dramatic processes in therapy

NARM pillars in therapy	*Dramatic processes in therapy*
Setting the therapeutic intention	Representing or exploring intention through dramatic projection
Asking exploratory questions and exploring obstacles	Exploring creatively through dramatic embodiment, projection, play, and role
Reinforcing agency	Offering choice and control within and outside the dramatic activity
Reflecting and anchoring positive shifts	Tracking and reflecting back positive shifts within and outside the dramatic activity Anchoring shifts by inviting dramatic embodiment

survival adaptations. Non-verbal methods may therefore constitute more accessible means to represent and work through obstacles. By encouraging clients to represent aspects of themselves or their wishes in non-verbal ways, such as through movement, imagery, or art, an opportunity is created to re-establish a relationship to themselves and their future. Imagining another possibility, enacting or embodying it, may lead to its emergence and then verbalisation. When the intention is established, therapists can facilitate an exploration of themes or obstacles linked to clients' therapeutic intention through either verbal or embodied methods. Offering this choice is important as it also supports the third pillar in allowing clients to take control over when and which embodied means in therapy feel safe or suitable. It is important that embodied activities are presented in the form of invitations to those who have been violated because of trauma. By choosing or suggesting preferred ways of working, clients learn to regain agency. Finally, noticing positive shifts, such as authentic connection and expansion within or outside a dramatic activity, can support growth and change. An offer to represent such shifts through a dramatic form (e.g. movement) may further anchor and enhance somatic memory and embodied change.

To conclude, the NARM framework of mindfulness, core needs, capacities, and the four pillars can equip therapists with a structure to build on their sessions, while the dramatherapy core processes based on embodiment provide them with flexible tools to address, explore, and anchor moments of positive embodied connection further. With dramatherapy methods, the healing experience does not remain on a mindful somatic level but on an active embodied one to create new somatic memory. These processes promote flexibility and lead to greater emotional resilience. Clients may reach states of greater connection to themselves through dramatic embodiment, which may further enhance the rewiring of neural pathways (Heller & Kammer, 2022). Ultimately, greater tolerance of experience may promote and instil change.

Embodiment in the Relational Aspect of Healing

I now turn my discussion to the relational aspect of therapy as being another significant element towards healing developmental trauma (Herman, 2015). I further discuss its implications as an embodied dynamic process for both client and therapist. It is important to show how this embodied process may manifest within an integrative model and how therapists can manage or learn from their somatic involvement and responses.

The therapeutic relationship has been widely explored and proved to be one of the main factors of effectiveness in psychotherapy (Clarkson, 2003). In the field of developmental trauma, the relational aspect of healing seems of even greater importance. Because trauma has occurred within relationships, healing can only take place within a relational context (Herman, 2015). The therapeutic relationship can therefore be viewed as a co-embodied process and alliance between client and therapist whereby this space in between can also be explored through the integrative approach previously described.

Because dramatherapy is a creative form of therapy that often involves the therapist's active somatic involvement, the impact of this on therapists' wellbeing should be considered. In NARM, the therapist's bodily sensations are carefully examined by inviting therapists to mindfully track these and how they may impact on their practice. Both NARM and dramatherapy address the importance of the relationship between client and therapist in healing. The significance of the relational element of the NARM model is emphasised throughout its theoretical framework (Heller & Kammer, 2022; Vasquez, 2022). Apart from clients' embodied responses, NARM highlights therapists' capacity to use what they feel somatically as another method towards healing. It particularly addresses interventions led by the therapists' survival responses and how awareness of those prevents their interferences with the therapy process. This also refers to therapists' risk of developing secondary traumatisation and burnout. The therapists' wellbeing is addressed through the lens of mindful acceptance of their needs and limitations. In dramatherapy, the therapeutic relationship has been explored through a third element, that of the art form (Jones, 2007). This triangular relationship is seen as a key process within dramatherapy for the opportunity that it offers clients and therapists to explore relational themes that emerge in the therapy space through the dramatic medium. The art form offers another avenue and opportunity for complex or covert dynamics to be embodied and processed, leading to greater chances for relational healing.

Additionally, the NARM relational model describes a dynamic and embodied structure that supports and encourages therapists to remain interested in theirs and their clients' responses, and to use those effectively. Likewise, in dramatherapy, it is suggested that the therapist's capacities to work alongside the client in the present moment and to offer them control and choice contribute to change (Cassidy et al., 2014). In that respect, the therapeutic relationship allows trauma survivors to re-establish their capacity for healthy connection to themselves and others, whilst also enabling a safe encounter within their own body in relation to another.

Within this integrative model of work, I suggest that the same openness and curiosity that are required in explorations with clients are maintained in relation to therapists' own somatic and survival responses. Reflective practice through dramatic methods may be particularly useful as a means for self-care when working with trauma. As embodied means are essential in trauma healing, they might also be vital for therapists to look after themselves whilst engaging in relational healing. This gives an opportunity to model an authentic therapeutic relationship built on respect and care for both self and the other.

Conclusion

I started this chapter with the first line of a Shakespearean sonnet that has a personal resonance for me and my journey to become a therapist. It has allowed me to reflect on the league that has been formed between NARM and dramatherapy, and how it can support 'being with' traumatised clients. In this chapter, I have explored how dramatherapy as an embodied therapy can be integrated with NARM as a modality specifically developed for healing developmental trauma. My aim was to especially address how dramatic embodiment alongside a comprehensive theoretical and practical framework on trauma may support clients and therapists in their quest towards healing. Additionally, it seemed of vital importance to address the relational aspect of healing and how integrative models of work may support therapists to feel confident, contained, and safe in their work.

As a dramatherapist, I felt prepared to enter the professional world with many creative tools and a great capacity to reflect on my work in both verbal and non-verbal ways. During my first years of practice, I lacked a clearer framework to support me with very complex dynamics whilst working with traumatised individuals. Interestingly, therapists from various backgrounds and experiences have suggested that NARM provides the essential knowledge and skills to be able to work with clients in a way that is 'enjoyable, effective, and may be more sustainable' (Vasquez, 2022, p.98).

Having presented this integrative model of work, it will be interesting to assess the application of this framework and its impact in practice. Due to its emphasis on the main processes in dramatherapy, this model has been developed to support practitioners trained in dramatherapy through its integration with a developmental trauma framework. It may be useful to explore further this integrative model's efficacy in clinical practice in three main areas. Firstly, by considering the way in which its structure may improve clinical outcomes. Secondly, by looking at how its application supports dramatherapists' confidence and wellbeing. Lastly, by examining its application in groups since it has mainly been used in individual work.

To conclude, I hope that, as valuable dramatherapy processes and new concepts in NARM have been brought together in this chapter, the connections between trauma healing and embodiment will keep evolving and expanding further.

References

Cassidy, S., Turnbull, S., & Gumley, A. (2014). Exploring core processes facilitating therapeutic change in dramatherapy: A grounded theory analysis of published case studies. *The Arts in Psychotherapy*, 41(4), 353–365. https://doi.org/10.1016/j.aip.2014.07.003

Cattanach, A. (1994). The developmental model of dramatherapy. In S. Jennings, A. Cattanach, S. Mitchell., A. Chesner, & B. Meldrum (Eds.), *The handbook of dramatherapy* (pp. 28–40). Routledge.

Clarkson, P. (2003). *The therapeutic relationship* (2nd ed.). Whurr.

Coronado-Montoya, S., Levis, A. W., Kwakkenbos, L., Steele, R. J., Turner, E. H., & Thombs, B. D. (2016). Reporting of positive results in randomized controlled trials of mindfulness-based mental health interventions. *PLoS ONE*, 11(4), Article e0153220. https://doi.org/10.1371/journal.pone.0153220

Gruber, S. M., Stein, P. K., Kammer, B. J., & Heller, L. (2021). Perceived effectiveness of NeuroAffective Relational Model Therapy in treating characteristics of complex trauma. *NARM Training Institute*. Retrieved from https://narmtraining.com/articles-research/

Heller, L. (2018, December 26). *Introduction to the NeuroAffective Relational Model™ [NARM]*. Dr Laurence Heller. Retrieved from https://drlaurenceheller.com/narm-introduction/

Heller, L. & Kammer, B. J. (2022). *The practical guide for healing developmental trauma*. North Atlantic Books.

Heller, L. & LaPierre, A. (2012). *Healing developmental trauma: How early trauma affects self-regulation, self-image, and the capacity for relationship*. North Atlantic Books.

Herman, J. L. (2015). *Trauma and recovery: Aftermath of violence from domestic abuse to political terror*. Basicbooks.

Jennings, S. (1999). *Introduction to developmental playtherapy*. Jessica Kingsley.

Jennings, S. (2015, September 15). *Trauma: The body, the play and the drama*. British Association for Counselling and Psychotherapy. Retrieved from www.bacp.co.uk/bacp-journals/bacp-children-young-people-and-families-journal/september-2015/trauma-the-body-the-play-and-the-drama/

Jennings, S. & Gerhardt, C. (2011). *Healthy attachments and neuro-dramatic-play*. Jessica Kingsley.

Johnson, D. R. & Emunah, R. (2021). *Current approaches in drama therapy*. Charles C Thomas.

Jones, P. (2007). *Drama as therapy: Theory, practice and research* (Vol. 1). Routledge.

Langley, D. M. (2006). *An introduction to dramatherapy*. Sage Publications.

Levine, P. A. (2010). *In an unspoken voice: How the body releases trauma and restores goodness*. North Atlantic.

Maercker, A. (2021). Development of the new CPTSD diagnosis for ICD-11. *Borderline Personality Disorder and Emotion Dysregulation*, 8(1). https://doi.org/10.1186/s40479-021-00148-8

Sajnani, N., and Johnson, D. R. (2014). *Trauma-informed drama therapy; Transforming clinics, classrooms, and communities*. Charles C Thomas.

Shakespeare, W. (2004). *Shakespeare's sonnets* (original work published 1609). (Edited by B. A. Mowat and P. Werstine). Simon & Schuster.

van der Kolk, B. (2014). *The Body keeps the score: mind, brain and body in the transformation of trauma*. Penguin Books.

Vasquez, J. A. (2022). *Meaning making: Understanding professional quality of life for Neuroaffective Relational Model trained trauma therapists* (Publication No. 29069087). [Doctoral Dissertation, Our Lady of the Lake University]. ProQuest Dissertations & Theses Global.

Part II

Intersection

Chapter 8

In the Shadow of Oppression

Nora Amin's *Theatre of Crime*

Noha Bayoumy

Amid the international #MeToo movement, Egyptian playwright Nora Amin brought to the stage the sexual assault of a woman at the gate of a theatre. In her 2019 play *Theatre of Crime*, a group of people arrive to see a play but are barred from entering by two security guards. The crowd is given the absurd reason that the theatre is already full and that the VIPs among the audience will get angry if it is overcrowded. The crowd grows in numbers and so does their anger. As a result, some of them lash out at each other. A man takes advantage of this chaotic situation and sexually assaults a random woman. The play shows the ensuing police investigation where the investigator treats the female victim with hostility. His investigation techniques reflect misogynistic views and the failings of the authorities when tackling reports of sexual assault. *Theatre of Crime* demonstrates that violence against women does not happen in a vacuum but is the result of powerful forces of oppression. Amin dramatises the increasing tensions and absurd conditions that allow the assault to happen. When the molester eventually walks free towards the end of the play, the dramatic world collapses. In the final scene, the characters step out of the experience of the play and back into reality. They re-enact the events of the play and invite the audience to assist the Woman in her ordeal. The play dissolves into the real and invites an analysis based on Brazilian theatre practitioner Augusto Boal's Theatre of the Oppressed.

Augusto Boal (1931–2009) formulated the concept of the Theatre of the Oppressed (1979) by combining different dramatic techniques that serve to highlight the mechanisms of exploitation and oppression in everyday situations (Coudray, 2017). According to Boal, the Theatre of the Oppressed aims to dismantle authoritarianism and give power back to the audience. He states that the main objective of the poetics of the oppressed is to change the spectators from watching passively to being actors and transformers of the dramatic action. He hypothesises that in order to transform the spectator into an actor, theatre has to go through four stages: 'knowing the body', 'making the body expressive', 'the theatre as language', and 'the theatre as discourse' (Boal, 1979, p.102). The first stages of the Theatre of the Oppressed consist in involving

DOI: 10.4324/9781003322375-11

both actors and spectators in exercises designed to better understand that the body is socially conditioned. They learn to understand the body's potential of expression as well as its limitations, and to make it expressive in new ways. Forum Theatre follows on from these first stages. It is a fully developed form of performance where the spectators are encouraged to participate and change the events of the play at a point of crisis (Boal, 1979). Amin adopts Boal's method of Forum Theatre to liberate her audience from the shackles of oppression, by transforming the potential of the body from a site of trauma to a tool for socio-political change. The play conveys how that socio-political change is embodied in people's intervention to undo the injustice against the Woman and to provide potential healing for the victims of sexual violence.

In this chapter, I will analyse the oppressive forces which foster violence against women as depicted in *Theatre of Crime*, namely classism[1] and misogyny. I will also analyse the moment of traumatic impact and the potential for healing that the play suggests.

The Oppressions

Amin presents classism and misogyny as the forces of oppression in the play. These overlapping and interconnected forces are shown both in the events leading up to the assault and in the investigation that follows. From the beginning of the play, Amin showcases the segregation between the world of the play and the crowd that arrives to see it. The young theatre makers Ahmad and Walid who first arrive at the theatre wonder how their friends have been able to secure a production at this A-list venue, where VIPs are expected to attend. Amin specifies that the crowd represents different walks of life, such as theatre makers, lecturers, or nurses. The guards closing the gate and their silent dismissal of the crowd reinforce the symbolism of theatre as a classist venue. It is a silence that illustrates the relational dynamics between them, representing a state-run establishment, and the people. The guards enforce a power that is arbitrary, unnecessary, and has devastating consequences. Therefore, the crowd feels dehumanised, like Ali, one of the people waiting at the gate protesting:

> They always enjoy humiliating us. There may not even be an audience in the auditorium, and then they complain that no one goes to the theatre.
>
> (Amin, 2019, p.25)

This remark is implicitly supported by the arrival of the stage manager, the only character whose attire is described, wearing a shiny, smart suit with an overall air of elegance. Before saying a word, his polished appearance contrasts with the agitation of the crowd. Worst of all, the guards and the manager exert their power in the interest of the 'big names' whom the manager fears will get angry. Furthermore, the divide between the unseen, privileged audience inside, and the underprivileged one outside is made clearer with the nonchalant and dismissive attitude of the manager and his reference to the 'big names' who do not want the crowd to be admitted. The security guards and the manager therefore represent the means of oppression that crush everyone indiscriminately. The explicit violence of the closed gate and the implicit violence of the guards' hostility fester and spread into the crowd. As the crowd grows, they redirect their anger and frustration at one another and suspect that there is corruption. As the infighting continues, crossing the gate and seeing the play becomes a privilege that the audience is denied.

Amin interweaves the scenes at the theatre gate with the investigation scenes, drawing the threads of classism and misogyny together. The Investigator, espousing misogynistic views, employs different tactics of questioning that put the Woman in a position of culpability. He insinuates that she acted 'obscene' scenes and suggests that she is mentally ill, and exaggerated what happened. The Investigator's accusation and dismissal of her mental health are reminiscent of early trauma theory. His attitude recalls the early days of psychiatry, when women who exhibited a wide range of symptoms, such as mutism, motor paralysis, hallucinations and nightmares, were collectively branded as hysterical. The work of French neurologist Jean-Martin Charcot (1825–1893) helped validate the experiences of women and dispel the misconception that their mental distress was caused by their gender (hence the term 'hysteria', which derives from the Greek *hystera*, meaning womb). He concluded that their symptoms were a response to psychological trauma, with psychologist Pierre Janet (1859–1947) and neurologist Sigmund Freud (1856–1939) uncovering the root cause of trauma to be childhood sexual abuse (Herman, 1997; Ringel and Brandell, 2012). To this day, hysteria is often used in derogatory and misogynistic attitudes to indicate women's alleged inability to control their emotions. This historical root of misogyny is helpful in our understanding of the play as it contextualises the hostile attitude of the Investigator and of several members of the crowd.

Furthermore, the Investigator suggests that the Woman imagined the assault during one of her panic attacks. In response, the Woman explains the frequency and severity of street harassment and assault that women face:

Woman: What if the woman you are investigating now is your wife?
Investigator: My wife would never be in your situation.
Woman: Why? Doesn't she walk in the street? Doesn't she walk in crowded places? We live in a reality full of violence and harassment. There hasn't been a girl or woman that has not experienced it. Our society, sir, is the worst environment for the lives of women and their safety. We no longer know what 'safety' is. And now you are investigating me as if I am guilty. And if I am not guilty, then I must be mad or imagining things.

(Amin, 2019, p.39)

While the assault is a one-time occurrence within the action of the play, Amin situates it within the wider context of habitual violence against women. The assault is severe, but Amin also draws attention to the unstated and routine aggressions that women face in public spaces. Feminist theorist Laura S. Brown (2008) and postcolonial trauma theorist Stef Craps (2015) draw attention to this constant sense of danger based on one's gender. Brown describes the 'normative, quotidian aspects of trauma in the lives of many oppressed and disempowered persons' (2008, p.18). Craps similarly refers to attempts by different academics and feminists to expand the concept of trauma to 'assist in understanding the impact of everyday racism, sexism, homophobia, classism, ableism, and other forms of structural oppression' (2015, pp.25–26). As the Woman in the play suggests, continuous harassment can destabilise and isolate the victims, and leave them feeling permanently unsafe. It would therefore be unlikely to think of trauma as a matter of the past but as a constant threat to the victim's wellbeing. Trying to spin his web further, the Investigator insinuates that the Woman is presenting a fictitious account since she is an actress. He even goes as far as accusing her of being 'an agent of sorts' who is seeking fame (Amin, 2019, p.40). The investigation scenes convey how the state apparatuses and police investigations can re-traumatise the victims of sexual assault.

It becomes evident that the Investigator's misogynistic views are not isolated when several characters are invited to give their testimony and share similar attitudes. The witnesses are categorised into two groups: the majority, who represent a reserved and regressive view of women, and a progressive, rebellious minority who defend the right of women to be safe in the public sphere. The majority of the characters show contempt for the Woman based solely on her gender. This includes the theatre staff whom Amin portrays as perpetuators and enablers of the abuse of women. The theatre manager, for example, plays an integral role in the assault on the Woman because he gave the order to shut the gate. A female staff member is portrayed as a cog in the machine of oppression. She reveals that she has been a victim of abuse and harassment herself but does not admit it or condemn the men responsible for her ordeal. She embodies a form of traumatised experience whereby the perception of abuse is distorted to the point where she does not realise her own position as a victim. Ironically, when the Molester gives a statement, he does not express sexist views. This further strengthens the argument that the crime is a product of the circumstances that allowed it, and that sexual offenders will be emboldened by bystanders who are complicit due to their own misogyny and passive compliance.

The Trauma

Amin makes the dramaturgical choice of showing the sexual assault clearly on stage. The dynamics between the security guards, the manager, and the female staff member on the one hand and the entire crowd on the other reflect both visible and invisible violence. As a result, the crowd gradually becomes aggressive, culminating in the assault of the Woman. The assault is not shown until Scene Seven. The first six scenes thereby lay the groundwork for the conditions that facilitate and allow it to happen. The play text describes the assault graphically, arguably leaving no room for denial or questioning its effect on the victim. Furthermore, the scene shows the array of emotions that the Woman experiences and that precludes words or action at the time of the trauma:

> The tall man starts to sexually assault the Woman from behind. We see him repeatedly moving his waist as if he is anally raping her, except that their clothes are in the way. He repeats this movement four times continuously and more aggressively in the dense crowd without anyone noticing. She turns around suddenly and with difficulty, so she is adjacent to him. He stops. She is shocked and truly horrified … Her eyes dilated as she looks at the [tall] man's chest, unable to look into his eyes. She seems paralysed. Her left hand is raised towards him and her fingers set apart as if they are screaming. She turns her gaze with difficulty toward the gate, crying. Her eyes meet two women standing behind the security personnel.
>
> (Amin, 2019, p.49)

Amin's focus on how the Woman's body responds (her shakiness and fighting for breath) suggests that she is unable to process the attack verbally. The suddenness and unexpectedness of the traumatic event, as in most cases of assault, can leave victims in a state of shock, feeling as if what is happening is unreal, rendering them speechless. It is this speechlessness that trauma causes that psychiatrist Bessel van der Kolk calls speechless horror (2014). He shows that traumatic experience effectively *shuts down* the area of the brain responsible for speech, contending that 'all trauma is preverbal [and] by nature drives us to the edge of comprehension, cutting us off from language based on common experience or an imaginable past' (van der Kolk, 2014, p.43). Even when traumatised people piece the events together and form a story, 'these stories rarely capture the inner truth of the experience' (2014, p.43). This scene, however, arguably shows that theatre can be an effective medium in communicating this silent blow. If a story of trauma cannot capture the truth of the experience, as van der Kolk suggests, Amin's play proposes that theatre can be the closest possible reflection. Furthermore, the dramatisation of the assault could be key in shaping the audience's reaction in the final scene when they are invited to take part in the action.

The scene of the assault demonstrates the body's response to trauma when the mind cannot process it verbally. If traumatic experience cannot be narrated because of its suddenness, theatre has the potential to represent it in various other forms. This is what Amin emphasises and utilises in this shocking scene. She provides a visual testimony of the event, showing how theatre has the ability to transcend language. Through the series of images and actions, it shows violence and its catastrophic effects on the victims without using a single word. The Woman's paralysed body, dilated eyes, and gaping mouth are a testimony of her trauma or indeed of any woman's trauma. Furthermore, the Woman understands well what has happened to her. Her speechlessness is not a sign of miscomprehension and does not preclude the theatre's ability to communicate suffering. She exhibits an awareness of her situation as she chooses to prosecute immediately, and also to put her experience within the wider context of violence against women.

By dramatising the assault instead of having it narrated, Amin puts into theatrical images what cannot be put into words. Her choice recalls van der Kolk's argument that traumatic experience is significantly preverbal. On that basis, narration is inherently unable to capture the assault in its immediacy. Amin places the audience in position of witness alongside the fictional crowd so that presumably there will be no room for contention on what happened, or whether the Investigator is justified in his string of accusations. It therefore becomes a case of seeing and believing.

It can also be argued that Amin's choice to show the assault naturalistically and graphically is an implicit comment on society's denial that these assaults happen or severely impact the victim. Watching the assault prompts the actual audience to see for themselves and assess the experience and all the circumstances that led to its occurrence. The undeniability of the assault in the play extends beyond the walls of the theatre, as Amin invites the audience to witness what can happen to a random woman on a random day especially as a result of the interplay of classism and sexism. The building up of emotions of anger, hurt, or shock is, however, not without release. The final scene is an opportunity for the audience to act on these emotions.

The Potential for Healing

In my view, healing takes the shape of transforming the body from a site of trauma to a tool for resistance. Theatre becomes a vessel for this change, both within the drama and for the spectators. *Theatre of Crime* opens the stage, literally and metaphorically, to its audience to intervene at the point of crisis. The oppression that the play presents runs parallel to the theatre makers' profound belief in the power of theatre to subvert the status quo. Their tool for subversion is to utilise their own bodies to protect the Woman and remove the gate. The play explores the relation between the theatre makers and the society in which they live, particularly how artists perceive society and vice versa. To illustrate this, the Woman expresses how safe she feels in the theatre and does not anticipate that anything can go wrong. The theatre, as she puts it, heightens her awareness of the world around her. Another witness among the theatre makers in the crowd, Mahmoud, uses his anger as a fuel for change:

> I adore the theatre […] The actor who trains and gains experience in the theatre can do anything.
>
> (Amin, 2019, p.62)

This statement can be understood literally as well as figuratively to describe how the actor can help change society. Similarly, another witness and theatre maker, Heba, who helps rescue the Woman from the assault, gives a touching testimony, acknowledging an affinity with the Woman that gave her the power to break the cycle of abuse:

> When I freed you from the claws of that female staff from hell, I felt like I was doing the first revolutionary act in my life. I faced these monsters alone and caught you. […] and I realised how strong we are!
>
> (Amin, 2019, pp.71–72)

Heba likens herself to a woman who gave birth. In essence, she invokes the physical strength a woman needs to give birth to describe her ability to save the Woman from her distress. The analogy creates new personalities for both women. They are re-born as women who have the ability to throw off the shackles of their oppression. If harassment constrains feminine power, reclaiming it would be an effective method of fighting this aggression. However, this newfound strength requires the physical solidarity and support of other women as well as wider sections of society. The support comes in the following scene when the audience is invited to rewrite the Woman's story.

In a dramatic moment that mixes despondency and hope, the actors step into the reality and breathe life into it. They present themselves specifically as theatre makers. They express a solidarity that cuts across social class and gender:

Mahmoud and Heba: (*Together*) We are the product of theatre; we are theatre makers. We are the ones who can change the ending.

The Woman: We must change reality first. Reality is not a play.

Mahmoud: But sometimes, reality and plays converge. This is our only chance to get out of this play and this memory. This time Heba will join us. We must change the ending. The crowd of 70 people has now become 170, and they will not be silent or deluded this time.

(Amin, 2019, p.74)

Amin arguably gives her audience the key to release themselves from their passive compliance after calling attention to their own silence, at best, and complicity, at worst, in this cycle of violence. These final lines of the play recall Boal's assertion in *Theatre of the Oppressed* that 'spectator' is a bad word (2008). He argues that traditional theatre, which is run by the powerful, 'has imposed finished visions of the world' (2008, p.135) which do not inspire or encourage the spectators to subvert the status quo. The aim of the Theatre of the Oppressed is therefore to regain the spectator's ability to act: 'The spectators in the people's theatre (i.e. the people themselves) cannot go on being the passive victims of those images' (2008, p.135). The key that the spectators need is the theatrical performance, and it is the same key that Heba, Mahmoud, and the Woman announce as their means of emancipation from the experience they witnessed and respectively went through.

Amin puts the potential of trauma healing in the hands and the bodies of the audience. Her proposition differs from the predominant trauma therapy approaches in the Western world that emphasise the need for narrating the traumatic event and for finding emotional release in order to heal (Herman, 1997; van der Kolk, 2014). As Stef Craps (2015) notes, Western trauma theory often focuses narrowly on the individual and does not question the forces of oppression and misogyny which are the root causes of traumatisation. In *Theatre of Crime*, it is clear that individual salvation is not a viable healing mechanism when the trauma is caused by widespread misogynistic violence. There is rather a communal and collective need to dismantle the tools of oppression if healing were to take place. The audiences, fictional and actual, embody social change. They are called upon to resist the physical cue of oppression with their own bodies.

The open ending makes it clear that it is up to the audience to undo the damage and traumatisation that oppression creates. Boal and Amin demonstrate that the best response is to utilise the body to protest and subvert the status quo. The effects of traumatic experience, as the play suggests, cannot be undone. However, people who are empowered to stand up to their oppressors are capable of intervening and limiting the incidence of traumatisation by defying the patriarchal values of society. The ending, therefore, has a significance beyond protecting the Woman from the molester. Amin hypothesises that some audience members will remove the iron gate, thereby undoing the situation that left the Woman vulnerable in the first place.

Conclusion

Theatre of Crime shows the oppression of various sections of society under the double threat of misogyny and classism. The mechanisms of oppression transform the theatre from a space of freedom and opportunities to a nightmarish embodiment of the violence of oppression. The trauma of sexual assault is seen as an extension and result of the mass traumatisation caused by oppression and the disregard for people's welfare, especially women. The investigation scenes suggest that a political solution to the crisis of violence against women alone does not suffice, but that it is the responsibility of everyone to resist violence against women.

Nonetheless, the play also promotes theatre as a tool for resisting oppression and subverting the status quo. After revealing the layers of socio-political oppression that contribute to sexual assault and abuse, the shattering of the dramatic form paves the way for the spectators to take action. Amin dissects society while putting faith and hope in the hands and bodies of theatre makers and the wider public to acknowledge and combat sexual assault. Theatre therefore becomes a space for healing through resistance.

Note

1 Classism defines the 'unfair treatment of people because of their social or economic class' (Encyclopedia Britannica, 2023).

References

Amin, N. (2019). *Theatre of crime*. General Organization of Cultural Palaces.

Boal, A. (1979). *Theatre of the oppressed*. Translated by C. A. McBride & M. Leal McBride. Pluto Press.

Boal, A. (2008). *Theatre of the oppressed*. Translated from Spanish by Charles A. McBride, Maria-Odilia Leal McBride, & Emily Fryer. Pluto Press.

Brown, L. S. (2008). *Cultural competence in trauma therapy: Beyond the flashback*. American Psychological Association.

Coudray, S. (2017). *The theatre of the oppressed*. Retrieved from www.culturematters.org.uk/index.php/arts/theatre/item/2455-the-theatre-of-the-oppressed

Craps, S. (2015). *Postcolonial witnessing: Trauma out of bounds*. Palgrave Macmillan.

Encyclopedia Britannica (2023, April 3). *Classism*. Retrieved from www.britannica.com/dictionary/classism

Herman, J. (1997). *Trauma and recovery: From domestic abuse to political terror*. Pandora.

Ringel, S. & Brandell, J. R. (2012). *Trauma: Contemporary directions in theory, practice and research*. Sage Publications.

van der Kolk, B. (2014). *The body keeps the score: Mind, brain and body in the transformation of trauma*. Penguin Books.

Part III

Practice and Research Perspectives

Chapter 9

The Girl at Christmas Cottage

An Embodied Experience of Making Theatre in Individual Dramatherapy with an Adopted Child

Sarah Mann Shaw

Introduction

In my practice as a dramatherapist and child and adolescent psychotherapist with adopted children, I work creatively to unlock and explore a child/young person's somatic experience of trauma.

Trauma can be defined as a deeply felt pervasive experience, the response to which can majorly impact a child's ability to cope with and manage relationships (Crenshaw, 2014; Perry, 2009; Schore, 2013; Siegel, 2001; van der Kolk, 2005, 2014). It can cause feelings of helplessness and fear, diminishing a sense of self and the ability to trust that others are available to help manage distressing feelings.

This chapter will focus on the development of a piece of theatre in dramatherapy sessions with an adopted young person. It will explore the interplay between the embodied experience, current research on neuroscience (in particular the role of mirroring and engagement of the polyvagal system), metaphor and theatre as a way of processing trauma. Theatre can safely capture, through metaphorical or dramatic distance, our earliest experiences, and enable an exploration of feelings and unhelpful belief systems that are too difficult to express directly in speech. Creating theatre within a dramatherapy context offers a containing and aesthetically distanced method of engagement. The case study presented in this chapter will examine how the bodies of the dramatherapist and the client in communication with one another enhance co-regulation, help negotiate risk, and enable the exploration of affects through the process of creating theatre.

Theatre making in dramatherapy will also be linked to current theories in neuroscience, and how change is created in the embodied material and the client's relationship to it. I will present three vignettes from the case study that will link theory to practice and explore the complexity of our craft in working with somatic trauma in dramatherapy.

DOI: 10.4324/9781003322375-13

Preliminary Thoughts on Neuroscience, Early Trauma, the Body, Metaphors and Theatre Making

Trauma experiences are tied to our bodies, our minds, and thus to our relationship with the world.

The co-construction of theatre in dramatherapy engages the traumatised self in a safe and exploratory way. It engages implicit and explicit memory through metaphor (Wilkinson, 2010), activates mirror neurons in the development of resonance and empathy (van der Kolk 2014), and stimulates the social engagement function of the polyvagal system (Falletti et al., 2017).

Memory signifies an event in the past that we can draw upon. Neurologically, memory is complex. It involves the activation of neurons and the ability to store and recall information with some sense of sequence, cohesiveness, and narrative. This is referred to as explicit memory which begins when the hippocampus develops in the second year of life. The hippocampus encodes and stores factual and autobiographical memory. In the event of preverbal trauma or when dissociation has been caused by a traumatic event, our memory is stored as implicit. Implicit memory includes our perceptual, behavioural, emotional, and body sensory memory. It encodes our earliest experiences. However, when our embodied memories are triggered by current events, they 'can emerge in our experience without our knowing that it is from the past' (Siegel, 2012, p.30).

Research by Bosquet Enlow et al. (2017) indicates that the prenatal brain develops rapidly and is negatively impacted by the level of stress experienced by the mother. They argue that the level of stress and trauma a pregnant woman is exposed to directly corelates to increased infant distress and their subsequent ability to recover from stressful experiences. Davis et al. (2007, p.12) write that,

> prenatal cortisol exposure is hypothesized to program the foetus's hypothalamic–pituitary adrenal axis (HPAA) and other neural systems involved in the stress response (e.g., amygdala). Thus, functioning of the maternal HPAA in pregnancy may have a critical influence on infant negative affectivity.

Maternal HPAA undergoes dramatic changes during pregnancy and postpartum. Elevated cortisol during pregnancy is associated with adverse birth outcomes and may alter foetal development and subsequent mental health (Evans et al., 2008).

Perry (2009) supports this premise, writing that in-utero and infant trauma has a more fundamental impact than later trauma experiences. My understanding of the relationship between a stressed maternal woman and the impact on her developing infant was key to working with my adopted client.

To safely manage early traumatic experiences, the therapist's focus on the regulation of anxiety and impulsivity is key. The significance of mirroring and empathy in the therapeutic relationship is crucial in supporting the client to experience relational safety (Solomon & Siegel, 2017; Watt, 2003; Wilkinson, 2010). If a client feels safe, they can tolerate arousal with greater capacity. Regulation can be achieved through repetitive movements, simple rhythm creation, and sensorimotor experiences such as clay, water, sand, or bubble painting. Awareness and development of attuned and non-verbal communication, and the tempo of that communication, also contribute to relational regulation (Siegel, 2001). Regulation is also achieved through the therapist's capacity to notice a client's arousal. Schore (2007) writes that, like the securely attached mother, the psychobiologically attuned therapist's awareness of the client's arousal state is critical in facilitating a more stable internal state. In dramatherapy this is engaged in the therapeutic relationship but also in our methodology. We would not invite a client into role and theatre making without first working to enhance their capacity to regulate.

Cozolino (2006) suggests that metaphors connect our minds to our bodies. As he writes (p.190), 'our ubiquitous use of physical metaphors to describe our inner experience may betray the sensory-motor core of both our subjective experience and abstract thought'. Metaphors allow for the expression of the intangible and reveal meaning through words and form. Metaphors in dramatherapy combine creativity and imagery, and in doing so engage the right hemisphere of the brain. The right hemisphere develops earlier and includes 'images, sensations and impressions' (Fosha, 2003, p.229) which constitute rich material to create metaphors and give form to experience. The metaphors emerging from the right hemisphere are often those deeply connected to embodied (implicit) trauma (Wilkinson, 2010). Dramatherapists pay particular attention to the expression of these metaphors that requires attuned work (Cozolino, 2002). Curiosity about and empathy towards these emerging metaphors are key. It is through the skill of attunement that the dramatherapist can become aware of any defences present in the telling of the trauma story. Defences are unconscious resources used to decrease internal stress and conflict, and can take the form of denial, displacement, projection, or repression. When defence to a metaphor is activated, it may be because the metaphor hasn't generated enough aesthetic distance to support safe emotional engagement. The nuance of a metaphor, or the image it creates, may readily activate a deeply rooted trauma memory. It is the dramatherapist's responsibility to ensure that the memory does not become overwhelming, and that it is safely managed.

Falletti et al. (2017) suggest that most neuroscience literature relates consciousness to an explicit process associated with declarative memory and knowledge, whereas it defines procedural knowledge and memory as a predominantly unconscious process. Actors develop a consciousness of self in performance and yet this is not always declarative. If it was, they argue, actors would be distracted from the craft and quality of their performance. The trained actor can refine their sensitivity to their part at a more elusive level of consciousness. Stanislavski (2012) spoke of actors understanding their craft based on feelings and accessing an emotional memory to inform their relationship with the part played. Meyerhold talked of the actor being able to hold a mirror to themselves to understand expressiveness, rhythm, and responsiveness through the actions of the body (Braun & Pitches, 2016). Grotowski (2012) latterly became interested in the actor's capacity to have a higher level of consciousness that would then enable them to enter role with an increased awareness – linked not to conscious understanding and language but to presence.

Theatre is a relational process. In individual dramatherapy, the reciprocal relationship between actor and audience is different. Peter Brook (1968) outlines the significance of the spectator in creating theatre. The audience not only bears witness, it also develops individual identity in the actor. Through the activation of a complex sequence of mimetic movements shared between actor and audience, both parts experience a sense of belonging and a sense of difference (Wilshire 1982). Pitruzzella (2009) writes that the gaze of an *other* establishes theatre. He likens it to the early developmental gaze between mother and infant. Stern (1985) suggests that the early relational gaze supports the development of a sense of agency, physical cohesion, continuity, affectivity, organisation, subjective self, and the ability to transmit meaning. In individual dramatherapy, to endow action with a sense of theatre, an imaginary audience, at least, must be evoked. In evoking an audience, dramatherapy makes use of the therapist and/or client to bear witness to the action; in doing so the function of the early relational gaze is replicated.

Creating a fictional character is an important aspect of theatre making. Stepping into character in therapeutic theatre can empower the client to explore and express both familiar and unfamiliar experiences, sometimes noticing the motives of their own actions in relation to the world, other people, or their own embodied self. Enactment promotes creativity and flexibility, and therefore the opportunity to rehearse more regulated responses to ourselves and the world (Emunah, 2020).

During theatre making in dramatherapy the client as actor comes to 'know' the character they are portraying, and perhaps to know themselves as a result. In the creation of theatre, a coherent metaphorical narrative of experience can be shared and responded to. Metaphor and theatre enable a safe exploration of traumatic experiences.

Case Study

In the following sections, I will offer some history of my client and share three practice vignettes. Each vignette will link the dramatherapy intervention to theories of trauma, embodiment, and neuroscience. In the first vignette, I will explore the traumatised imagination and the activation of the social engagement system. In vignette two, I will explore the importance of the process of creativity and relationship through engagement of mirror neurons to enhance a sense of agency, organisation, continuity, and communication. I will argue that it is through the process of developing intersubjectivity with another that my client was able to engage with her sense of internal loneliness and abandonment. This will be further explored in vignette three which looks at how the experience of trauma can be decoded through theatre and therapeutic relationship.

Background

Jess was an 11-year-old adopted girl of white British descent[1]. She was referred for dramatherapy through the UK Adoption Support Fund which provides funding for adopted children and young people to access a range of psychological therapies. She was referred with difficulties in self-regulation, perpetual negative thinking, low confidence and self-esteem, and an anxious attachment style. During the initial assessment interview, her adoptive parents reported that Jess presented as developmentally younger than her 11 years and was not resilient to life experiences.

Jess was impacted by prenatal trauma and early infant relational loss. Her mother experienced domestic violence and used class A drugs whilst pregnant. She was removed from her biological mother's care at birth and placed in a stable foster home for nine months after which she was adopted by a heterosexual white couple who had a birth child four years later. Jess would claim that her sister was everything that she was not and that crucially she 'belonged'. I wondered how this might be connected to Jess's early trauma experiences and to her relational understanding of adoption. She had not 'come from' her family but rather she had 'come to' it. In adopted children, this difference can feel profound. During the first assessment session, her adoptive mum described Jess as 'bruised from the inside'. I was struck by that description of Jess's body and wondered about the marks and feelings of soreness that in-utero experience may have left her with. I suggest that the traumatic prenatal experience had been encoded into her body as implicit memory.

Initial Considerations

Trauma is a 'psychophysical experience' (Rothschild, 2000, p.5). It inhabits the very sinews of our being. The experience of trauma floods our bodies with the stress hormone cortisol. This shuts down the part of the brain that encodes memories, leading to explicit recollection and verbal narrative. In the case of Jess, trauma had been experienced at such an early developmental stage – the brain had no way of 'making sense' of experience – that it was left held in the body. Jess's narrative was one based on fear, on not feeling *good enough*, separate from the world around her, and finding connection and relationship difficult. She experienced the world as a frightening place, felt unsettled and alone.

I deliberated on how Jess's amygdala, the emotional centre of the brain, had been affected by her early prenatal experience and how this impacted on subsequent development and her sense of self. Rothschild (2000) writes that although emotions are interpreted and named by the mind, they are inherently experienced in the body. Each emotion has a unique way of expressing itself through the body, whether this is facial expression, muscular tension, or body posture. Each reflects a distinctive somatic experience. I considered the potential of those neurological pathways that had been created in fear through Jess's early somatic experience. I wondered whether they were still wiring and firing, thus creating meaning that was based on the early experience of 'I am not safe', 'I am not loveable', 'I am not worthy of relationship', 'Others are better than me'.

In my work with traumatised children and adolescents, my observation has been that negative embodied experience often becomes translated into negative self-beliefs that are then subconsciously 'proved' through relational patterns and behaviours. Jess had trouble making friends and maintaining them. She had experienced bullying all through primary school. She told me that this was 'proof' of the above negative and inhibiting self-beliefs.

Finding a Dramatherapy Structure

Children who have experienced trauma do not necessarily follow a sequential model of human development. Trauma and attachment styles interrupt development. Each stage can only proceed normally if the preceding ones have been successfully navigated. In choosing a dramatherapy structure, I needed to think about how it matched Jess's developmental needs. In the assessment sessions, Jess demonstrated a love for stories. In starting with simple word exchanges, using story dice (Rory's Story Cubes), story jigsaw pieces, archetypal cards (Myss, 2003), then moving on to more complex storyboard structures, I provided a developmental framework of dramatherapeutic engagement. In doing so, I hoped that Jess could externalise some of her internally held narrative in a safe, relational space. Jess was able to play with the initial story-making processes and in a subsequent session created a story board. At the time, I wondered whether the story would contain relevant 'here and now' questions from Jess's subconscious, and what it would reveal in terms of the developmental stage it emerged from.

It felt important that Jess's stories engaged her body. She wanted her selected story to become theatre created in the dramatherapy space. She wanted me to be her co-player. Steve Mitchell (1996), writing about the theatre of self-expression in dramatherapy, argues that theatre is intrinsically connected to health and healing. He uses a particular methodology to explore character development, teaching clients ways of entering and stepping out of character. I invited Jess to explore her characters in the same way, finding a neutral stance and then stepping into a sculpt which embodied the character physically, vocally, and relationally. In stepping out, I invited Jess to interview her characters, to flesh out their personality, motivations, their function, and contribution to the story. In individual dramatherapy, the therapist offers a relational approach to the client's development of character and to the process of dialogue between two characters. Mitchell uses the phrase 'substitution' to refer to this process. The therapist witnesses the client play the character and then steps in to copy this, so that the client can witness, develop, and respond to the character being substituted. Jess became artistic director, script writer, stage manager, and actor as we worked to develop and refine the interaction between her characters.

As we rehearsed stepping in and out of embodying the characters, their physicality became extended and melodramatic in essence. In melodrama, all motions and gestures are dramatically exaggerated, and facial expressions heightened. As Clausen writes, 'actors concentrate on "showing" emotions more than feeling them' (Clausen, 2016, p.119). I wondered if initially showing rather than feeling could offer Jess an emotional distance to her somatised experience and enable a freedom for greater theatrical expression. Jess's characters developed into stereotypical stock characters, another feature of melodrama. Characters were given stereotypical roles, deriving from the six stock characters: the villain, the sensitive hero, the persecuted heroine, the clown, the faithful friend, and the villain's accomplice. Jess's story used three of these six characters: the persecuted heroine that was described as innocent, beautiful, and vulnerable; the faithful friend as loyal and sometimes providing comic relief; and the villain as immoral, evil, greedy, dishonest, and corrupt.

The use of these melodramatic features became crucial in the telling of Jess's story. Melodrama's use of an exaggerated characterisation style, archetypal themes of good versus evil, betrayal, sacrifice, and redemption contained and allowed an expression of Jess's early trauma and somatic experience.

The Girl at Christmas Cottage

Jess's story evolved through the process of creating theatre. As Jess became aware of her felt experiences rehearsing her piece of theatre, scenes were replayed, changed, additional scenes added, and characters' development changed. Through engagement in theatre, Jess began to experience and rehearse a different way of being safely held in the therapeutic relationship and metaphorical narrative.

The story moved into a collection of acts and scenes to structure, rehearse, and create coherence. We used a screen to differentiate between being on and off stage. Jess wrote the scenes down and told me that we needed to be prepared for each one. It was important to her that each character knew their entrances and exits. It is worth noting that as an adopted child, she had experienced the exits and entrances of significant people in her early narrative that had been out of her control.

I discuss here three vignettes to integrate the theory and practice of making theatre in dramatherapy and its relation to the embodied trauma story. Jess's story was structured as follows:

Act 1: Christmas Cottage

Scene 1
Bryony lives alone in Christmas Cottage in the middle of the woods, but no one visits. At Christmas, Santa does not remember her, so there are never any presents under the tree. She is forgotten, even though she is good. She feels anger, despair, and distress, and drowns in tears. Santa flies above the cottage. Once again, he cannot locate Christmas Cottage as it is hidden deep in the woods.

Scene 2
Bryony has one friend, a snowman called Jeff. Jeff is optimistic and sometimes Bryony cannot bear this. Jeff thinks that Santa needs a light to find his way to the cottage. Eventually, Bryony agrees and they create a magical fluorescent carrot nose for Jeff.

Scene 3
Bryony waits for her mum to return and claim her as her own. At Christmas, everyone else is being thought about but not Bryony. Her mum never sends a present.

Act 2: Christmas

Scene 1
It is Christmas eve. Jeff turns on his magical illuminating nose. Bryony has lost hope. She argues with Jeff and goes to sleep.

Scene 2
Christmas Day. There are presents under the tree – presents for all the years Bryony believed she had been forgotten. She insists that it is a cruel joke and that they are for Jeff. Jeff gets cross and shows her a gift with her name. Slowly she believes that she has been remembered. The gifts include magical seeds that can always grow, illuminated noses to guide Santa, and a refrigerator so that Jeff can stay all year. There is also a notebook to help Bryony document her difficult feelings, and a scarf from Mum which had been in the cottage, but not seen, for the last seven years.

Act 3: The Awakening

Scene 1
This Christmas, Mum returns but Bryony notices that, even when she is there, her mum does not really notice her. She becomes angry and tells her mother that she is selfish and asks her to leave Christmas Cottage forever.

Act 4: The Future

Scene 1
It is seven years later. Jeff and Bryony see Bryony's mum on the TV. They watch as Mum is accused of fraud and impersonation.

Scene 2
Mum is tried for her crimes. The judge orders a prison sentence for pretending to be someone that she was not.

Scene 3
Later Bryony is a Broadway star. She makes a speech thanking her mum and reiterating that she will be a different kind of mum, one who will love her children.

Scene 4
Bryony and Jeff perform the song 'This Is Me' (Pasek & Paul, 2017). The audience loves her.

Discussion

Vignette 1

Jess spent time rehearsing the embodiment of her characters. She was keen to make props for her performance and for a couple of sessions we focus on making the presents Bryony would open on Christmas morning. Jess dedicated herself to making Jeff's fridge. Jeff was only present in the winter but making a fridge would enable him to be there for her whenever she needed him.

Making sense of the helping character is psychologically significant in dramatherapy. It communicates that the client is simultaneously able to resort to self and other when needed. Jess delegated the task of sewing an orange felt carrot nose for Jeff to me. She was determined that we should work to make Jeff robust. Potentially, Jess's internal world was more full-bodied, perhaps she was more aligned to her feelings, her actions, and ability to express herself than she was aware of. She had an inner strength previously unexpressed.

As we created props, Jess talked about her life's story. Our comfortable co-creation enhanced safety and stabilisation in our therapeutic relationship and enabled us to prepare for the difficult first scene of her play – a scene in which Bryony delivers a monologue exploring the experience of being alone in the world. In preparing her props, she had an embodied and conscious awareness of safety and of being held in mind by others – me as her therapist and Jeff in his robustness. Without experiencing safety, expressing loss and grief may have been too risky.

Reflections

Dramatherapy invites clients to work with their body to enable an exploration of their relationship to the somatised material. It also challenges and engages our imagination. A traumatised imagination can present through numbness, shutting down, or anxiety as excessive adrenalin is caught in the body (Porges, 2017). The sympathetic nervous system responsible for arousal, including the fight or flight response, is activated to prepare the body to defend or avoid. Polyvagal theory identifies a third type of nervous system, the social engagement system, constituting a balanced mixture of activation and calming (Dana, 2018). The social engagement system helps us navigate relationships and tolerate hyper- and hypo-arousal.

For Jess's social engagement to be activated, she needed to feel that her dramatherapy space and relationship with me was safe enough. In co-creating props, I worked to reassure Jess's autonomic nervous system. I offered attuned therapeutic presence and my own cues of social engagement to bring her into a sense of safety. Jess's vagal nerve could read my open physical gestures, lightness of tone, open eye contact, and socially motivated facial expressions. Our bodies were in communication with one another.

The experience of presence is important. The Oxford English Dictionary (Hawker & Soames, 2012) defines presence as 'being at hand'. The most obvious element of this for Jess was that I was in proximity in space and time. If she needed help with her prop making, I was immediately available. I was in the 'here and now'. Whilst being 'at hand' is important, presence also has a relational component. I was a presence in her life both in and outside of the therapeutic space. She held her dramatherapy and our relationship in mind in between sessions and so had, to a certain extent, internalised the quality of our relationship. Jeff also offered a presence, an ability to stay available. Presence is much more than occupying the same space and time together. It implies a mutuality, an awareness, a rhythm between one another. Bryony and Jeff played their role according to their melodramatic function. Jeff was a constant support, held hope by lighting his nose and as a result impacting Bryony's internal narrative.

Vignette 2

In working on character development and expression, we began with the persecuted heroine who was intrinsically good, innocent, and yet alone, abandoned, and forgotten. We explored how we might present this state of being to our imaginary audience. The imagined audience enabled Jess, as actor, to think about relationships with others. It also held a self-reflective role. Our intention was for our imaginary audience to 'feel', and in feeling to make sense of Jess's theatre making. This was significant given that feeling had previously been unsafe for Jess.

As a dramatherapist, I also bore witness to Jess's process. In using Mitchell's theatre of self-expression model (1996), Jess was able to develop a contemplative relationship with both the characters and the unfolding of her piece of theatre. I shared a sheet of melodramatic poses related to the heroine as charted by Victorian researchers to aid the 'true' expressions of feelings and emotions. As she rehearsed these, I asked her whether she would like them represented back to her, to see what they might look and feel like to our 'audience'.

I held the poses Jess rehearsed. She reflected that they needed to be more exaggerated. We played with this. Jess held the poses first and I then represented them back to her. I mirrored her and in part she then mirrored me back, expanding the mirror to fit theatrical purpose. We acted as both audience and witness, and in doing so were neurologically and relationally interactive.

In her reflection, Jess noticed that the dramatic expression of Bryony had become larger – even an audience member at the back of the auditorium could not fail to understand how lost and alone Bryony felt. Jess reflected that, as an actor, she could experience the despair of the character in her body. I wondered how it was to notice this. Jess was able to reflect on Bryony's experience by giving it a more cognitive and emotional content. The implicit experience of feeling lost and alone had become explicit and tolerable. Once we had de-roled, Jess talked about Bryony, her internal state and external representation. She noted how powerful it was. I reflected on her skill as an actor to portray this, offering a frame for the importance of emotional expression. Emotions did not need to be repressed but could be safely expressed through the medium of theatre. The imaginary audience had also understood this phenomenon.

Reflections

Current research into mirror neurons points to an intrinsic link between expression and reception of emotions. Fuchs and Koch (2014) argue that mirror neurons create an 'interbodily resonance or intercorporeality' (p.6). They suggest that, in every social encounter, the embodied affectivities of two persons become intertwined, and that this experience continually modifies each other's affective experience as well as the future range of potential emotions.

Rizzolatti and Sinigaglia (2008) put forward that mirror neurons register movement, emotional state, and intention. They argue that mirror neurons can note and make internal adjustments in relation to what we notice. Rizzolatti and Sinigaglia (2008, p.9) wrote that 'mirror neurons regulate at a pre-reflective, pre-cognitive level, interpersonal relations via a process of simulation, which generates in the "actor" and "spectator" a shared space of action, the same state of motor, corporeal and emotive change'. This means that we understand because we mirror what we see before us or see what is mirrored in front of us.

In mirroring the characters' states as described in the above vignette, I was hoping to show that it was safe to explore difficult feelings. Mirror neurons are the basis of the core mechanism for learning and growth. Once learning and growth is established, other functions branch off and can be explored (Wilkinson, 2010). One of these is imitation. In imitating the expression of a difficult emotion, the mirror neurons still process and interpret actions so that they can be stored and reused later (Falletti et al., 2017). Mirroring Bryony increased her capacity to explore and understand difficult feelings without activating a fear-based trauma response. It is a relational process which requires the therapist to have an interpersonal and attuned intention at an embodied level. This acts to create resonance. Jess was able to reflect on how she felt it was like to be Bryony. She was beginning to explore and experience those parts of her internal world that had been split off or denied for fear that they would emotionally overwhelm her.

In stepping into role in theatre, there is an awakening of the sympathetic nervous system as we may feel a sense of anticipation or nervousness reflected in somatic experiences, such as a dry mouth, sweating palms, or a beating heart. Whilst trauma impacts on our capacity for spontaneous involvement in our lives and our imagination, theatre enables us to step into that space and to manage the experience knowing that we have managed the arousal. Stepping into role in a safe therapeutic space acts as a regulatory process for the client. We acknowledge the felt sense of arousal, but we have rehearsed the process, know that we are safe and aware of the beginning, middle, and end of the action. In knowing that the arousal can be tolerated, a different relationship with it can develop.

For Jess, the risk, and potential engagement of the sympathetic nervous system, was activated through the stepping into role. This was carefully rehearsed and prepared for in the therapeutic relationship. Relational attunement enables a more resilient experience of self. In having a greater sense of resilience, the polyvagal system becomes more regulated, the sympathetic nervous system less heightened and the parasympathetic more prominent. Stimulating the social engagement system enables clients to experience a greater degree of regulation and so an increased capacity to manage risk taking. Jess, in being Bryony, stepped out of herself into 'another' only to return and know herself differently.

As our sessions continued, we used mirroring as a core process to develop the characters on embodied and emotional levels. Jess became confident with this process and expanded both her emotional vocabulary and spontaneity. She developed a consciousness of self in and through performance, and a subjective experience of knowing what it was like to be her. Jess's metaphorical narrative was intrinsically connected to her life story and to her neurological and embodied experience.

Vignette 3

Bryony's mother's return had initially been constructed as a scene of confrontation, an opportunity for Jess to express her anger at the mother's abandonment. However, as we approached the scene, Jess paused. We stepped out of the performance space and Jess wondered whether she wanted the scene as originally designed, or as a scene expressing reunion and integration in which Bryony could experience a sense of belonging.

Jess played with both ideas. We rehearsed embodied sculpts of reunion and connection, and confrontation. I invited Jess to notice how her body felt in both and whether this attention to her embodied experience would help her decision.

Jess noticed a sense of unease with the first scenario, expressing a sense of discomfort and irritability in her body. With the second one, she noticed a rise in heat and energy. There was no naming of this as an emotion but Jess was able to work with it. She explored the role of the mother and played her as a melodramatic villain. In embodying the villain, Jess said that Bryony was now able to fully challenge her. I substituted for the villainous mother and Jess, playing Bryony, became the heroine who found her voice. We rehearsed and played the scene several times over. Jess decided that an additional scene needed to be added in which the mother found herself in court for the crime of impersonation. I thought about the potential relationship to Jess's birth mother having a limited capacity for presence, due to her own ongoing trauma, and Jess's capacity to experience Bryony as less of a victim.

The more Jess rehearsed, the more aware she became of different emotions present in her body. She was angry and used theatre to express this internally held conflict. I was reminded, from conversations with her adoptive parents, that Jess simultaneously experienced and avoided expressing conflict. Fenichel (1945), adopting the psychodynamic point of view on conflicts, argues that 'the neurotic conflict, by definition, is one between tendency striving for discharge and another tendency that tries to prevent this discharge' (p.129). Jess's work enabled her to safely discharge her internal tension around conflict. In a later scene, Bryony was able to thank her mother, acknowledged that she did what she could but also expressed that it had not been enough. She told her mum that when she was older, she would be a different mum who would love and care for her children. Bryony accepted her bruises and self-identified with a previously unexpressed strength and resilience as she became able to sing in the final scene the words, 'I am brave, I am bruised, I am who I'm meant to be' from the song 'This Is Me' (Pasek & Paul, 2017).

Reflections

James et al. (2005) write that a client's trauma needs to be 'translated into an explicit form (including words) for desensitisation to occur' (p.83). There are many ways to decode trauma and create an externalised form for the meaning of the embodied experience to emerge. This can be done through a process of gaining explicit consciousness through a declarative, sequential, and coherent narrative, or through a story in which words and meanings are held within metaphors. It can also be about noticing shifts in the embodied sense of self, about feeling 'better' or 'different'. Explicit does not always need to be verbal. The felt sensation has often been neglected despite its clinical importance.

In the final scene, Jess as Bryony was able to express what she had never spoken about – her rage, disappointment, acceptance – and reflect on her internally held relationship with her abandoning mother. She made no explicit connection between the metaphor and her life. In using metaphor Jess was allowing one thing to stand for another. Metaphor is a powerful vehicle through which the self may achieve greater integration and change (Wilkinson, 2010).

Conclusion

This chapter has explored my work with Jess through integrating theories of neuroscience, metaphor, and theatre in dramatherapy to process and heal from the experience of embodied trauma.

Trauma for adopted children often occurs in the context of interpersonal relationships which, in some ways, have had boundaries violated. As a result, they can present with a restricted range of emotional connection to self and others. Jess experienced an internal loneliness and avoided emotions of distress, rage, and vulnerability. My work with her consisted in supporting her growth towards emotional and psychological well-being, autonomy, and self-regulation.

To explore this, I used a process of creating theatre in dramatherapy. This engaged Jess in creating a metaphorical story that gave her an emotional distance and a way of creating order, sequencing, and coherence. Her story had a beginning, middle, and end. She knew what she wanted to say and through the course of her dramatherapy changed, developed, and amended her story to fit her purpose. I have shown how working with the body initially helped engage mirror neurons to increase a felt sense of safety, and subsequently supported the social engagement aspect of the polyvagal system to increase Jess's capacity to explore risk and step onto a stage in front of an imagined audience. The intricacy and subtlety of therapeutic attunement was a core component of this process that helped develop resonance and supported Jess's greater capacity for intersubjectivity. As a result, Jess was less alone with her story.

The weaving together of theatre, metaphor, core theories in neuroscience, embodiment, and dramatherapy provided Jess with a safe form to explore her somatised experience of early childhood trauma. In making theatre, Jess was able to project her internal embodied experience into a metaphorical form that she then explored. She found a way to live with her bruises.

Engaging in this work with Jess has been a thought-provoking journey that has raised further research enquiries around embodiment, trauma, the function of gaze in therapy and theatre making, and the role of the imagined audience.

We know that trauma, embodiment, attachment, emotion, action, and neuroscience are inextricably linked, and that to ignore one or the other may reduce the efficacy of our work. This chapter hopes to contribute to an ongoing clinical conversation on the efficacy of embodiment and its relationship to individual theatre making in dramatherapy, even though it has limitations as it only offers one client's experience and one therapist's reflections. Nevertheless, it was a wonderful journey to be a part of.

Note

1 For the purposes of confidentiality, all names and distinguishing details have been changed.

References

Bosquet Enlow, M., Devick, K. L., Brunst, K. J., Lipton, L. R., Coull, B. A., & Wright. R. J. (2017). Maternal lifetime trauma exposure, prenatal cortisol, and infant negative affectivity. *Infancy*, 22(4), 492–513.

Braun, E. & Pitches, J. (2016). *Meyerhold on theatre*. Bloomsbury Methuen Drama.

Brook, P. (1968). *The empty space*. Penguin.

Clausen, M. (2016). *Centre stage*. Cengage Learning Australia.

Cozolino, L. (2002). *The neuroscience of psychotherapy: Building and rebuilding the human Brain*. Norton.

Cozolino, L. (2006). *The neuroscience of human relationships: Attachment and the developing brain*. W.W. Norton & Company.

Crenshaw, D. (2014). Play therapy approaches to attachment issues. In C. Malchiodi & D. Crenshaw (Eds.), *Creative arts and play therapy for attachment problems* (pp. 19–31). Guildford Press.

Dana, D. (2018). *The polyvagal theory in therapy: Engaging the rhythm of regulation*. W.W. Norton & Company

Davis, E. P., Glynn, L. M., Schetter, C. D., Hobel, C., Chicz-Demet, A., & Sandman, C. A. (2007). Prenatal exposure to maternal depression and cortisol influences infant temperament. *Journal of the American Academy of Child and Adolescent Psychiatry*, 46, 737–746.

Emunah, R. (2020). *Drama therapy process, technique and performance*. Routledge.

Evans, L. M., Myers, M. M., & Monk, C. (2008). Pregnant women's cortisol is elevated with anxiety and depression – but only when comorbid. *Arch Women's Mental Health*, 11(3), 239–248. https://doi.org/10.1007/s00737-008-0019-4

Falletti, C., Sofia, G., & Jacono, V. (2017). *Theatre and cognitive neuroscience*. Bloomsbury Methuen Drama.

Fenichel, O. (1945). *The psychoanalytic theory of neurosis*. Retrieved from http://books.google.at/books?id=r1zmhbjEAn0C

Fosha, D. (2003). Dyadic regulation and experiential work with emotion and relatedness in trauma and disorganised attachment. In M. F. Solomon & D. J. Siegal (Eds.), *Healing trauma, attachment, mind, body and brain*, (pp. 221–281). Norton.

Fuchs, T. & Koch, S. C. (2014). Embodied affectivity: On moving and being moved. *Frontiers in Psychology*, 5(508), 1–12.

Grotowski, J. (2012). *Towards a poor theatre*. Routledge.

Hawker, S. & Soames, C. (Eds.) (2012). *The Oxford English Dictionary*. Oxford University Press 7th Edition.

James, M., Forrester, A., & Kim, K., (2005). Developmental transformations in the treatment of sexually abused children 4. In A. M. Weber & C. Haen (Eds.), *Clinical applications of drama therapy. Child and adolescent treatment* (pp. 67–86). Brunner-Routledge.

Mitchell, S. (1996). *Dramatherapy. Clinical studies*. Jessica Kingsley Publishers.

Myss, C. (2003). *Archetypal cards*. Hay House.

Pasek, B. & Paul, J. (2017). This is me. *The greatest showman* [Film]. Atlantic Records.

Perry, B. (2009). Examining child maltreatment through a neurodevelopmental lens: Clinical application of the neurosequential model of therapeutics. *Journal of Loss and Trauma*, 14, 240–255.

Pitruzzella, S. (2009). The audience role in theatre and dramatherapy. *British Association of Dramatherapy Journal*, 31(1) 2–27.

Porges, S. W. (2017). Vagal pathways: Portals to compassion. In E. M. Seppala, E. Simmon-Thomas, S. L. Brown, M. C. Worline, C. D. Cameron, & J. R. Doty (Eds.), *The Oxford handbook of compassion science* (pp. 189–202). Oxford University Press.

Rizzolatti, G. & Sinigaglia, C. (2008). *Mirrors in the brain. How our minds share action and emotions*. Oxford University Press.

Rory's Story Cubes (2022, January 4). *The creative hub*. Retrieved from www.storycubes.com/en/

Rothschild, B. (2000). *The body remembers: The psychophysiology of trauma and trauma treatment*. W.W. Norton and Company.

Schore, A. (2007). Psychoanalytic research, progress, and process: Developmental affective neuroscience and clinical practice. *Psychologist-Psychoanalyst*, 27(3), 6–15.

Schore, A. (2013). Relational trauma, brain development and dissociation. In J. Ford & C. Courtois (Eds.), *Treating complex traumatic stress disorder in children and adolescents*. Guildford Press.

Siegel, D. J. (2001). Towards an interpersonal neurobiology of the developing mind: Attachment relationships, 'mindsight', and neural integration. *Infant Mental Health Journal*, 22(1–2), 67–94.

Siegel, D. J. (2012). *The developing mind: How relationships and the brain interact to shape who we are* (2nd ed.). Guilford Press.

Solomon, M. & Siegel, D. J. (2017). *How people change. Relationships and neuroplasticity in psychotherapy*. W.W. Norton and Company.

Stanislavski, C. (2012). *An actor prepares*. Routledge.

Stern, D. N. (1985). *The interpersonal world of the infant. A view from psychoanalysis and developmental psychology*. Routledge.

van der Kolk, B. (2005). Developmental trauma disorder: A new rational diagnosis for children with complex trauma disorders. *Psychiatric Annals*, 35(5), 401–408.

van der Kolk, B. (2014). *The body keeps the score: Brain, mind and body in the healing of trauma*. Viking.

Watt, D. F. (2003). Psychotherapy in an age of neuroscience: Bridges to affective neuroscience. In J. Corrigal & H. Wilkinson (Eds.), *Revolutionary connections: Psychotherapy and neuroscience* (pp. 79–115). Karnac.

Wilkinson, M. (2010). *Changing minds in therapy. Emotion, attachment, trauma and neurobiology*. W.W. Norton and Company.

Wilshire, B. (1982). *Role-playing and identity. The limits of theatre as metaphor*. Indiana University Press.

Chapter 10

Gesture in Actor Training and With Survivors of BPD Diagnosis

Finding Communication Towards Relational Thirdness

Roanna Mitchell

This chapter considers how certain tools that were originally developed for actor training can inform a practical, psychophysical approach to 'being with' and relational repair with both ourselves and others in the presence of trauma. Specifically, it examines embodied principles from Michael Chekhov's psychophysical technique and play-based training practices – drawing on the author's teaching experience in UK universities and conservatoires over more than a decade – and the ways in which these principles have translated across into the project *'Inappropriate' Anger* (IA). The latter is a UK-based and artist-led project, investigating the use of creative tools and participatory performance practices in the provision of support for survivors of a diagnosis of Borderline Personality Disorder (BPD) or Emotionally Unstable Personality Disorder (EUPD).

BPD/EUPD is a highly stigmatising and contested diagnostic category that disproportionately affects survivors with complex attachment and trauma histories (Aves, 2022; Porter et al., 2020; Rye et al., 2021), for whom, following Judith Herman's seminal work on recovery from trauma, the possibility for recovery is based on empowerment of the survivor and restoration of relationships (Herman, 2002). In light of this, the IA project focuses, in essence, on creating conditions from which relating to ourselves and each other can begin to happen: a safe-enough place from which to express, listen, and be heard. The BPD/EUPD diagnosis is also closely associated with iatrogenic harm, limited access to appropriate support services, and frequent instances of being disbelieved or framed as 'manipulative', 'attention-seeking', or 'demanding' (Aves, 2022). Therefore, one of the key elements to create the conditions for relating in the IA project has been to provide the experience of being believed, and also, importantly, to recover the experience of believing oneself. Both of these resonate with Jessica Benjamin's recognition theory which highlights the radical potential of acknowledgment in healing individual and social trauma (Benjamin, 2018). This chapter outlines how we can understand 'believing' as a psychophysical, gestural process, involving attention to and movement through the relationship between the 'outer' body and the 'inner' life of sensations, feelings, thought, and imagination. It does so by first discussing Michael

DOI: 10.4324/9781003322375-14

Chekhov's notion of gesture as psychophysical from the starting point of actor training, followed by examples of how Chekhov's understanding of gesture is put into practice in therapeutic, applied, and participatory practice. Building on this, the chapter examines how gestures of radical believing are activated in the IA project through the improvisatory tool of 'yes, and'. Using this example, it reflects on how engaging traumatised bodies in practising and playing with gestures of believing can support a re-connection with self and others, acting as a driving force for our ability to both relate to what is and creatively generate new possibilities of relating.

Michael Chekhov's 'Gesture' in Actor Training

The notion of gesture is a key aspect of the technique developed by Russian actor, director, and teacher Michael Chekhov, for use by actors, acting teachers, and other artists (Fleming & Cornford, 2020). In 1953, long before cognitive science entered the field of performance studies, Chekhov wrote, 'it is a known fact that the human body and psychology influence each other and are in constant interplay' (Chekhov, 2002, p.58). Exploring this interplay is the foundation of his whole technique, and within this, gesture – our action or attempted action towards the world around us – is understood as inherently psychophysical. Chekhov's gesture involves the movement of the 'outer' body along with the 'inner life' of thoughts, feelings, sensations, imagination, and can manifest in the expression of body and voice, as well as through extension into another form such as drawing, painting, sculpture, writing, or music.

In life, we are constantly making psychophysical gestures towards one another, and can find them reflected in 'our common language of movement … Our hearts go out to others, or they *break*, our chins *drop*, we rise to the occasion, and *swell* with pride, we *shrink* in fear, or firmly *stand our ground*' (Petit, 2010, p.7). As cognitive linguists and philosophers Lakoff and Johnson (1999) observe, such examples demonstrate how we draw on embodied experience to help us conceptualise more abstract ideas – our thinking is structured through our experience of movement. The task of the actor is to harness such gestures as a conscious activity, to develop a highly attuned awareness of the relationship between the movement of the body and the 'inner life', and to explore how the gestures we make activate and are activated by our will, our desire; while the quality with which we make the gesture awakens or expresses our feelings (Chekhov, 2002).

One process used to develop this highly attuned awareness in Chekhov's technique is to begin first by moving the body, noticing what this changes in us and our relationship to the world. What, for example, are the inner sensations that arise from the movement, the gesture, of opening a fist, a ribcage, perhaps the whole body? What are the sensations, imaginations, or meanings that come into awareness from this act of expanding into space? What are the sensations that arise if this gesture of opening is done staccato or legato, or with a quality of softness or strength? How does the sensation of opening change if it is done with a more specific intention: to dazzle, to intimidate, to impress, to welcome? While exploring in this way, the actor 'must be aware every time they discover a new sensation or reaction during the movement exercises', thereby developing a rich vocabulary of embodied experiences through which the body becomes 'a wise body' (Chekhov, 2018, p.27).

The process of developing such an awareness of sensation may, however, not automatically be a benign experience and requires care in its facilitation. As Chekhov writes in the very first sentence of the first chapter of *To the Actor*, 'Our bodies can be either our best friends or worst enemies' (Chekhov, 2002, p.58). While he is here referring to the problems that an untrained body can present to the actor, the statement resonates in another way when we realise that in any context we may be working with individuals whose body holds fear and trauma, and does not in itself feel like a safe place to be. I have discussed elsewhere (Mitchell, 2022) that while the intention of actor training is not therapeutic, we need to nonetheless consider that a conscious awareness of inner sensation can be a very new experience for many. This means that for some students the initial psychophysical work with certain gestures can be overwhelming, if the unaccustomed contact with their bodily sensations unlocks a flood of feelings and emotions, perhaps 'bringing some of what is kept in the shadows into consciousness' (Brantbjerg, 2020, p.57). With this in mind, it can be useful to carefully consider what in body-based psychotherapy would be termed the 'dosage' of the gesture work (Brantbjerg, 2020, p.57). Collaborating with the students to test the size and pace of movement, the engagement of breath, and the location of the gesture in the body can allow them to find the 'sweet spot' of where the inner life becomes activated so that a movement is no longer just made but felt – but also not felt to a degree that is overwhelming.

Another part of facilitating such training with care, accompanying the developing awareness of dosage, is the return *out of* the gesture and back to a relatively regulated place and rhythm of being in the body. Chekhov offers the imagination of a 'threshold' across which we can step into, and back out of, an exercise, a rehearsal, or a character (Langman, 2014, p.264). This can be usefully supported with exercises that re-set the nervous system, such as the 'physiological sigh' (Huberman, 2021) or Susana Bloch's breath patterns designed to avoid 'emotional hangover' for actors (Angelin, 2010). These step-out techniques can help the students realise that they have choice and agency about making a gesture, engaging with its sensations and for how long. Once they realise this, students can experience the sensations of the gesture as 'real', while knowing that they were caused by a movement they made of their own choosing, and that it is in their power to develop – with time – the tools to regulate and return to what we might call a 'home' state of the nervous system. In this way, the psychophysical training of gesture work not only develops students' skills and expression for the purpose of acting, but also more generally helps them to relate to themselves, to trust and believe their own responses, and – if facilitated to do so – to modulate or 'dose' their work in order to keep themselves safe. As Brantbjerg notes, 'it is sensations in the body that tell me when my boundaries are crossed, or when they are respected. It is sensations in the body that tell me when to say STOP' (Brantbjerg, 2007, p.2).

In this process of exploring the relationship between movement, sensation, thought, and imagination, we are of course also beginning to explore how we relate to the world, as the two are always in dialogue. In fact, Chekhov's technique as a whole can be understood as 'a pedagogy of rhythm and gesture' (Mitchell, 2020b, p.110), thereby activating what psychoanalyst Jessica Benjamin (2018) identifies as the key ingredients for relational exchange. For Benjamin, relational exchange happens through a shift from the 'twoness of opposing doer and done to' to a 'doing with' that 'suggests that shared state of [...] purposeful negotiation of difference that will be called thirdness' (2018, p.5). Benjamin describes how, in the first relationship between baby and primary caregiver, relational 'thirdness' is co-created in the rhythmic dance of gestures between them, a reciprocal exchange that appears as 'a dynamic coordination, in which matching, mismatching, and return to matching of shared direction can be charted as a non-linear relation far from an exact mirroring or synchronicity' (2018, p.5). This improvised dance is very familiar to performers as I have discussed elsewhere (Mitchell, 2022). Benjamin herself uses the example of musical improvisation to illustrate the 'thirdness of attuned play' that arises from it, where 'to the question of "who created this pattern, you or I?", the paradoxical answer is "both and neither"' (2018, p.31). By not just using rhythm and gesture as exercises, but also consciously centring them as key pedagogical principles for structure and facilitation, Chekhov's technique constitutes a fundamentally relational practice (Fleming, 2021) which, in its psychophysicality, brings ideas about relational exchange concretely into the body.

Chekhov's technique can thus become not just a technique to teach, but also a technique *for teaching*. In the same way that students do, a Chekhov teacher may also develop a sensitivity to gesture and rhythm, providing them with a tool for the kind of 'engaged' pedagogy that bell hooks describes as a process of '*being with people*' (hooks, 1994, p.165, emphasis in original). The inner gesture we are making towards our students, our listening for, and acknowledgment that we will be changed by their gestures in turn, are a vital part of the relational dynamic in the classroom, enabling the 'attuned play of thirdness' (Benjamin, 2018, p.31). As Chekhov emphasises in his *Lessons for Teachers*: 'If you are really teaching with your whole being, you will understand at once whether your students have understood you or not. [...] You must always feel what is going on in your pupils. This is most important' (Chekhov, 2018, p.9).

Michael Chekhov's 'Gesture' Beyond Actor Training

Beyond the pedagogical space, the potential of Chekhov's technique to be harnessed in participatory and therapeutic contexts has become a topic of exploration and discussion over recent decades, though there are few, currently mainly anecdotal, publications to chart this work. Caoimhe McAvinchey begins to do so by surveying applications of the technique in these fields as part of the research project 'Michael Chekhov Technique in the Twenty-First Century: New Pathways' (McAvinchey, 2020). Her examples include drama-therapist Zoe Brook's use of the technique for 'embodied empowerment' with Glasgow-based participatory arts organisation Bazooka Arts. Brook describes the powerful impact of Chekhov's psychophysical exercises on traumatised bodies, increasing participants' ability to be present and to exercise self-awareness: 'Chekhov's techniques seem to work for people that have been removed from themselves for a long time [...]. It allows them to access body and emotion' (Brook quoted in McAvinchey, 2020, p.164). Brook notes that it does so not by diving into traumatic events, but by using 'sensory imagination' as an agent for movement and change (2020, p.164).

McAvinchey also introduces director and psychotherapist Martin Sharp's integration of Chekhov's tools in his therapeutic practice where, for example, exchange of gestures and visualisation of felt sensations are used to support his clients 'to find ways to embody, reflect and move through physical manifestations of trauma' (McAvinchey, 2020, p.168). In relation to gesture in particular, McAvinchey examines applied theatre practitioner Hartley Jafine's work in healthcare education where Jafine draws on Chekhov's techniques as part of training 'medical residents who have been identified as requiring communication support' (2020, p.168). Jafine emphasises, in a scoping review of the use of drama in Canadian and US undergraduate medical education, that the strong non-verbal skills needed by physicians can be developed by permitting students to 'connect or move with their bodies to understand the role their body, movements and expressions play in communication' (Johnston & Jafine, 2022, p.6). McAvinchey highlights that Jafine's training addresses 'the reading of the patient's embodied gesture as well as their symptoms', and also encourages healthcare staff to reflect on the way in which their own body 'speaks volumes' to patients and affects how they in turn feel able to engage (2020, p.169). The close link that Chekhov highlights between gesture and rhythm becomes important here, especially when considering autistic patients and clinicians, for whom attending to embodied gesture may feel close to the idea of interpreting body language. The latter is a complex and often painful subject in the context of autism, connected to the social pressures to mask certain behaviours and the risks of misinterpreting social situations, even while movement itself can have a role in 'enhancing divergent and convergent thinking' (Shaughnessy, 2022). Gesture in Chekhov's understanding, however, is not just about body language in the sense of a social code, but also more broadly about dynamics and rhythm. Attending to rhythm can thus offer another, equally powerful entry point into the 'thirdness of attuned play' (Benjamin, 2018, p.31) in embodied communication (Morris et al., 2021). Returning to Benjamin's definition of relational thirdness, developing a heightened awareness and embodied listening through gesture and rhythm may thus shift the relationship between patient and health worker from 'doing to' to 'doing with' (Benjamin, 2018, p.5).

To further reflect on such encounters through gesture towards relational thirdness, I interviewed Patrick Bailey, Chekhov-trained actor, teacher, and collaborator at The Chekhov Collective UK, about his work with Crisis Intervention Team training for the US police and other public safety workers. In programmes designed to give police officers tools to de-escalate situations where someone is in a mental health crisis, Bailey takes the role of the person in crisis, and is able to observe from this vantage point what gestures of 'listening' the trainees are making in the enacted moment. He notes for example that in some instances, 'They're interrupting, they didn't introduce themselves, I just said I feel really terrible and I want to die and they didn't even acknowledge that, they're not saying "yes I understand"' (Bailey, 2022). The inner gestures that Bailey perceives the trainees to make in those moments include the striking image of a door closing: 'They're turned away. Something in them is not… It's like the door was shut before they got there, and now it's even more shut' (Bailey, 2022). Conversely, he describes the moments when the trainees slow down and give space to the encounter as a kind of arrival: 'Suddenly you're not alone. It can be really challenging [for the trainees] in some situations, but it's possible. You've let somebody know that you're there and you hear them. And that's where the de-escalation can start' (Bailey, 2022).

Bailey notes how crucial this work feels in the US, not least because officers are armed. Referring to body-psychotherapist Resmaa Menakem's (2021) work in this area, Bailey observes that 'there is starting to be more recognition among [US] Public Safety agencies that many working peace officers experience ongoing, unresolved embodied trauma' (Bailey, 2022). These questions also become increasingly active in a UK context where serious concerns have been raised – for instance by the survivor-led StopSIM campaign – about the involvement of police as part of community mental health teams, and about punitive responses to calls for help especially from individuals holding a BPD diagnosis (StopSIM, 2021).

The examples above indicate that the use of Chekhov's technique in community and health contexts so far often relates to facilitating thirdness in embodied encounters with self and others. They also illustrate that by expressing a reaction that does not emerge out of the recognition of seeing the other, the 'dance' of rhythm and gesture to co-create relational thirdness is disrupted. In the following section I will discuss the role that 'gestures of believing' might play in facilitating or repairing this dance, through examples drawn from the *'Inappropriate' Anger* project.

Towards Being With Ourselves and Each Other: 'Yes, And…' as a Gesture of Radical Believing

As outlined in the introduction, the creative collaboration with survivors of a BPD/EUPD diagnosis through the IA project has starkly highlighted the importance of being believed as a precondition for relational exchange. IA was instigated in 2020 by myself – a performance-maker and pedagogue specialising in psychophysical practice – and writer and psychodynamic counsellor Louisa Harvey, in response to our witnessing of the high levels of injustice and iatrogenic harm, and dearth of available support affecting individuals given a BPD diagnosis. Our aim in launching the project was to co-create safe-enough spaces for survivors to express, listen, and be heard, through creative activities and exchange with others. The project was opened to individuals who held a diagnosis of BPD/EUPD and who had an interest in creative activities. Between 2020 and 2022, the IA project involved three groups and a total of 20 participants aged 19–65, who discovered the project via Kent-based peer support groups, the charity Porchlight, Kent and Medway Recovery and Wellbeing College, social media survivor groups, and word of mouth. The project's activities include year-round online creative workshops and discussion groups, and annual in-person performance projects. After an initial five-week programme with each new group, designed by the facilitators to establish a shared collaborative language, creative tasks and themes for exploration and discussion are then chosen and developed by participants with facilitator support.

The title of the project, *'Inappropriate' Anger*, refers to one of the 'symptoms' used to diagnose BPD, as well as being a critical commentary on the particular way in which an individual's justified response to adversity and trauma can be framed as symptomatic of a 'disordered' personality. As has been extensively documented, individuals labelled with a BPD diagnosis are often heavily stigmatised within the mental health system, deemed 'attention seeking', 'manipulative', and 'demanding', and refused care with the reasoning that this might cause 'over-dependency' on services (Aves, 2022). Emotional reactions and opinions about the (lack of) care available once the diagnosis has been given are frequently re-framed as symptomatic of something being inherently wrong with the person, leading to a silencing through what clinical psychologist and psychotherapist Jay Watts identifies as 'testimonial injustice' (Watts, 2018). The experience of not being heard and believed is thus a recurring theme for many who live with the impact of this diagnosis, and can also erode trust and belief in one's own perceptions (Aves, 2022). This presents particular challenges for a project that invites participants to creatively explore and articulate their experience. Thus, a central focus of the project has become to establish tools and processes that nurture participants' capacity to believe themselves – an action that is slightly different from the more motivational notion of believing 'in' themselves. This capacity is then expanded into relational thirdness, through creative exchanges that give participants the important experience of being believed by others. To help us do so, we looked for ways to understand believing as a psychophysical, gestural, and playful activity, which is practised and strengthened through a variety of ways of playing a 'believing game' with oneself and others.

The believing game is mentioned in the context of feminist approaches to 'trauma treatment strategies for empowerment' (Brown, 2004, p.469), and is outlined in the field of pedagogy and writing by Peter Elbow (2009). Elbow proposes that there is much to be gained by practising systematic believing rather than seeing that the only way to advance knowledge is through systematic scepticism, doubt, and critical thinking. While neither doubt nor believing can demonstrate that anything is actually true, systematically choosing believing allows us to 'enter into *different* ways of thinking or points of view' (2009, p.7). In doing so, the believing game can help us relate to others by 'finding virtues in a position that the doubting game seems to disqualify' (2009, p.9). It also invites the individual 'to listen and take seriously her own experience and point of view—even if it looks crazy—and not feel that one must subordinate one's perceptions or experience or thinking to that of the group' (2009, p.12).

Elbow emphasises that the believing game is not only about thought, but also about action – i.e. about gesture – noting that 'images and sounds and body movements are particularly helpful for entering into alien ideas' (2009, p.11). As most of us are far better versed in the scepticism of the doubting game, the believing game takes practice and there are tools that help us play it. Performer training offers one such tool in the form of the improvisational principle of 'yes, and'. To move an improvisatory exchange forward, one person makes an offer, the other accepts it (yes) and then offers a response (and), which is in turn accepted (yes), and so on. As discussed above, such improvisation with its dance of rhythm and gesture can lead to co-created relational thirdness. 'Yes, and' is thus a principle of collaborating and relating. I suggest that it is also a gesture: it is an action, a psychophysical enactment, of believing.

The gestural nature of 'yes, and' becomes especially clear when we position it next to its more frequently used counterpart 'yes, but'. Where 'and' extends the direction of travel, 'but' presents a U-turn, reversing the direction and often negating what was said before. Using 'and' instead of 'but' creates another offer, an expansion rather than a shutting down. Within this, it is important to note that working with 'yes, and' does not mean blindly consenting, which would be a dangerous training for exploitation. Rather, it means really seeing and believing another's offer – which may not always be benign – in the knowledge that our 'yes, and' response can also lead to a 'no'.

Playing the Believing Game With Oneself

In the IA project, the creative 'yes, and' was used to first of all practise playing a believing game with oneself. Participants took part in, and invented, a variety of solo creative tasks where the principle of 'yes, and' provided the impulse and impetus for each new creative response. A simplified summary of such a task series might look like this. We choose a theme and create a drawing. We then look at the drawing as though we have never seen it before, and we notice as much as we can about it and pay attention to what makes us curious or interested in it (YES). At this point we do not try to understand or analyse our creation because, as Chekhov notes, this closes down important parts of our listening: 'dry reasoning kills your imagination. The more you probe with your analytical mind, the more silent become your feelings, the weaker your will and the poorer your chances for inspiration' (2002, p.25).

The image and text in Figure 10.1 show one IA participant's process of meeting their own artwork in this way. The notes that this participant, Bunny, made during the process of 'Yes' suggest first an attempt to 'make sense', and then a process of noticing. Finally, a poetic realisation emerges that may provide the impulse for the next creative response, as Bunny writes: 'Everything rains down on us it should come from the bottom and go out the top'[1]. Having looked, received, and believed in this way, we then begin from what made us curious and interested, and let this be the starting point for our response, which might be another drawing or a piece of writing (AND).

This version of playing the believing game with oneself is inspired and influenced by both Michael Chekhov's and art therapist Shaun McNiff's (2004) writings on dialoguing with one's images and creations. For Chekhov, our 'creative images are independent' and 'will require your active collaboration… You must ask questions of these images, as you would ask questions of a friend' (2002, p.23). Similarly, McNiff proposes that what emerges from our creative

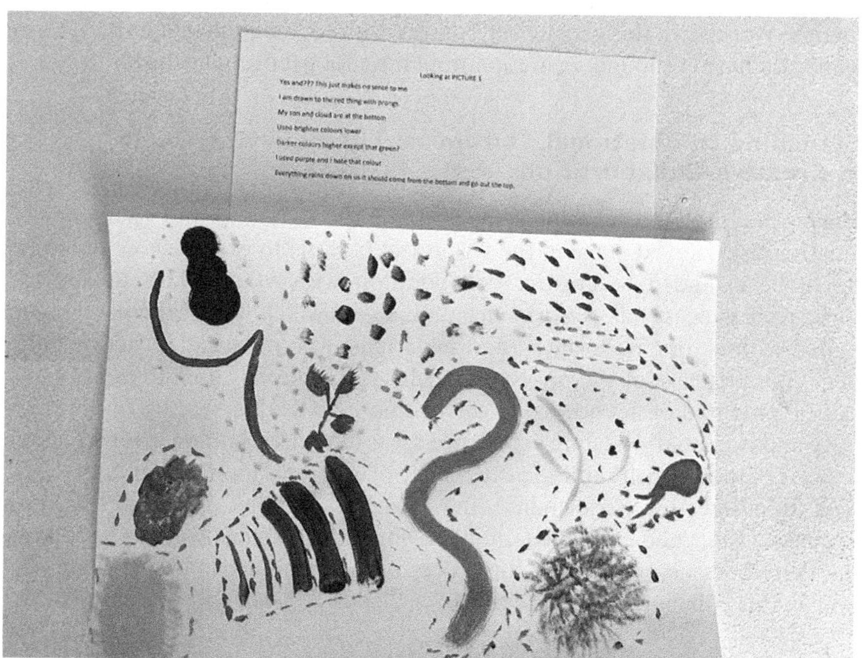

Figure 10.1 An IA participant's dialogue with their own creative work

© Bunny (2021)

activities should be respected as an entity in its own right which we are able to have an exchange with. On the one hand, we might find in this process a way to dialogue with other parts of ourselves, such as our critical inner voices, our imagination, or our unconscious. On the other hand, McNiff suggests that we can go further, tempering 'the tendency to see images as part of the artist who made them' (2004, p.83), so that the process can become more than purely self-referential:

> It is imperative to liberate images from ourselves, give them more creative autonomy, and restore the reality of imagination as a procreative and life-enhancing function [...] Personifying images, gestures, and other artistic expressions enables them to act as 'agencies' of transformation rather than simply as 'illustrations' of the psyche of their makers.
>
> (McNiff, 2004, p.84)

The tool of 'yes, and' can help to navigate this process. It enables us to relate to our creativity, showing us that what we have created is an entity in itself that can surprise us, and at the same time exists in its particularity only through our participation: it is both 'not me' and 'not not me' (Schechner, 1985). This echoes the thirdness that can arise out of improvisation with others and suggests that such thirdness can also be found through improvisation with one's own creative imagination. Working in this way, we can connect with what our imagination offers us while also having enough separation from it to not get overwhelmed by it.

Extending to Relational Thirdness: The Believing Game in Creative Collaboration

Having practised the believing game over a series of months and via a range of creative tasks, a next stage in the IA project became to explore how the game might be extended to creative collaboration with others. This took place through a process of performance-making in which IA participants were paired with actors, performers, and musicians, whom we called 'acting partners'. In this phase of the project, the believing game was used to explore 'the radical potential of acknowledgment' by another (Benjamin, 2018) as a generative and potentially healing experience for traumatised bodies, involving both creative empowerment and the experience of improvisational relational thirdness. In co-creating performance, the process of finding relational thirdness becomes visible and embodied, in other words three-dimensional. The following describes one example of the process of gestural exchange through 'yes, and' in this collaboration phase of IA.

The Offer

Taking the theme of 'This is what I want you to believe about me', an IA participant creates a piece of writing, and then two images in response to re-visiting their writing. They then present these creations to their 'acting partner', along with some verbal context. By choosing how to display their creative work and what additional information to give, they are already giving a small, informal performance that has a very particular gesture and atmosphere. This is their offer.

The 'Yes'

The acting partners, in this example a dancer and a musician, receive the gesture and atmosphere of the offer. They are asked to believe it, without opinion or analysis, to be curious about what is in front of them, and awake to the sensations it stirs within them. The impulse to try to 'understand' in this 'yes' phase is great. An acting partner might, for example, struggle for a while with some paradoxes and contradictions in the offer, and then realise that of course the contradiction itself was the thing that was captivating them. Crucially, they realise that they do not need to solve it.

This believing is a temporal act. We believe the moment for what it is, which in turn allows us to be in it – where doubting or analysis always already displaces us from the present moment. Considering believing as a moment-by-moment activity releases us from the pressure to build 'a belief' or to know, fix, or provide an answer. As Elbow notes, playing the believing game 'invites an individual [...] to say, "Stop arguing with me; just listen for a while. If you can, help me make my position clearer and better"' (2009, p.12). Doing the activity of believing through this 'yes' moment is, in this sense, a gesture of space-making. It creates a space in between the other and myself, gently separating their offer from my own 'stuff'. This in-between space is where the co-creation of thirdness can begin to happen.

The 'And'

Having received and believed the offer made to them, the acting partners' task is to translate the offer into performance. This requires them to have identified a 'poetic essence' of the offer – key elements and dynamics that can be retained when translating the creative expression from one form (for example writing, painting) into another (for example music, dance). Here, while the acting partners are looking to capture faithfully what they have received and believed, the performance they create will also inevitably express something about their own individuality. In creating a performance that says 'This is what I heard when I heard your offer', they are revealing information about their own curiosities, creative impulses, and way of perceiving the world.

To initiate the 'and' phase of the creative process, the acting partners are first of all asked to embody the strongest echoes of the offer they received in one physical movement – what in Chekhov's terms we might call the 'psychological gesture' of the offer (Chekhov, 2002). Psychological gesture in the theatrical world, building on the concept of inner gesture discussed earlier, is a way for the actor to find an embodied understanding of a character's fundamental inner movement over the course of a scene, play, or the character's whole imagined life. In that sense, it is a distillation of the key dynamics of the character's being-in-the-world expressed in movement (Mitchell, 2020a, p.262). The movement of a psychological gesture has a beginning, a middle, and an end. It has particular movement qualities, rhythmic qualities, and directionality. Regarding the latter, where the simple gestures used for initial training have a clear direction of travel – for instance a push travels from back to forward, an opening expands from inward to outward, a lift travels from down to up – a psychological gesture could do the same but often also involves the tension of moving in multiple directions at once. Embodying this complexity is a way to feel our way through the messiness of human experience which so often involves the ability to hold and bear contradictions. Beginning from this felt experience of the offer made to them, the acting partners create a piece of movement and music. The performance that results picks up on certain 'gestures' in the IA participants' artwork, and mirrors these back in a response that is inevitably filtered through the individuality of the acting partners. The 'and' thus becomes a new offer, taking the form of a draft performance.

The IA participants' responses to these first performance drafts already made it clear that seeing someone engage so deeply with what they were trying to express could provide a deep feeling of being acknowledged, respected, and validated. Participants noted that 'We weren't seen as curious oddities but as adults with something to bring', and 'It was so enjoyable to be with creative people who listened and gave your story respect'. However, it was important that the cycle did not end there, but rather could provide an impulse for further exchange, an opening up. Now the IA participants in turn were invited to offer 'yes, and' feedback to their acting partners' first performance-sketches. From here, a buzzing phase of collaboration ensued, with IA participants gradually becoming director-dramaturgs, co-writers, and set-designers for their acting partner; moving, demonstrating, and making props; suggesting and testing different endings; occasionally stepping back to watch and reflect, then re-joining the space to make adjustments. In this way, each pair worked together in cycles of 'yes, and', activating the dance of relational thirdness to refine and develop the performance together.

The Embodied Experience of Being Believed

This extended 'believing game' through repeated processes of 'yes, and' was experienced by the participants as a genuine collaboration that held within it the ingredients of empowerment and relationship building that Herman highlights for their potential to heal individual and social trauma (2002). One IA participant reflected that: 'It was a really special experience, I absolutely had space to give input and mould [my acting partner's] original ideas. It felt co-created which was empowering'. Another noted that 'We very quickly had a very good working relationship. It was very two way. [My acting partner] listened, was interested and showed respect'. The tools of the believing game, and the experience of being believed, provided a safe-enough space for interaction despite the potentially overwhelming experience of meeting new people in the unfamiliar space of a drama studio. This manifested in participants' embodied experience, where symptoms of trauma in the body gradually softened and dissipated. One participant describes this as:

> although I had a frozen feeling, it didn't lead to flight. So, when I'm threatened in some way, whatever way, I usually freeze and then I scarper. But I didn't do any of those things. I could feel the frozen bit, but it just melted, really.

Another observed that:

> I haven't been able to empathise with people in that way. Like, genuinely. To actually take on board the emotion of what they are sharing and react to that in myself and then be okay. Because normally I run away from this. That was really quite profound. So many things happened that [usually] just do not happen for me. [...] I somehow created a barrier for the hallucinations I experience, I think it was mainly because of the safety I felt, and the way we came in and out of the activities.

Being believed also strengthened participants' courage to trust and articulate their own responses and needs, with the element of performance-creation allowing each individual to experience the important step of watching themselves being believed in three dimensions. One participant noted that: 'What would normally happen is, somebody would say "do you want to change something" and I'd say no it's fine, even though it's not fine, I'm feeling something but I daren't say in case I'll be in trouble'. In the case of this collaboration however, the participant felt that: 'The whole space and the whole two days in the end made me feel able to say: "actually, could we change that". And it allowed me to risk holding it as my own story'. Through this, IA participants also found ownership and recognition in the final performance outcomes where, as one wrote: 'There was so much about me that [my acting partner] captured… the thoughts, feelings and words buried deep within!'. There was a sense of having been able to articulate something that moved beneath the surface, as the process of performance-making had unfolded further meanings: 'The final performance was spot on, it communicated on a deeper lever what I had written and created'.

Finally, not only did the process allow participants to articulate their experience, it also enabled them to experience themselves differently in the world. They articulated a shift from arriving with fear: 'The first day looking at the big empty space and thinking holy shit. Oh my god, I can't do that', to finding curiosity and openness: 'The second day looking at the space and going: wow, this space is full of possibilities. And maybe I'm full of possibilities. That's what it really made me feel'.

Conclusion

The above discussion hopes to illustrate that certain principles and techniques that are used in actor training, such as the example of Gesture and the improvisational 'yes, and', can also offer concrete psychophysical tools to help facilitate relational 'thirdness' in other contexts. As such, they can be invaluable for facilitators in participatory creative practice involving trauma, informing all aspects of the work including the set-up of the physical space – a building can also make a gesture – the rhythm and 'dosage' of exercises and interactions, the feedback language, and the rituals and boundaries that provide entry and exit points into different phases of work.

In the example of the *'Inappropriate' Anger* project, these tools came to constitute a key aspect of 'being with' a person suffering the effects of trauma, as well as a key aspect of that person's ability to explore 'being with' themselves. In the process of experiencing what it is to be believed by others, and of practising believing themselves, the elements that were felt by IA participants to be healing included feeling safe, heard, respected, connected, valid, capable, curious, and creative. This resonates with Herman's observation of the psychological faculties that must be re-built in the wake of trauma, which include 'trust, autonomy, initiative, competence, identity and intimacy' (Herman, 2002, p.98).

It is perhaps important to note that while the presence of trauma was deeply respected in the process, it was not approached directly or centralised for the participants. In an early draft of his 'Chart for Inspired Acting' (1991, p.xxxvi), Chekhov draws a circle, marking on its circumference the different elements of his technique. In the centre of the circle he writes: 'Never try to touch the heart itself'. In a similar way, the IA project touched the heart indirectly. The psychophysical creative processes were carefully set up to establish safe-enough conditions for body, mind, and imagination to come into dialogue with each other and with others. This was a process of space-making that supported agency, made offers and invitations, but did not prescribe the level of participation or demand recovery. In the absence of pressure, and with the back-up of being believed and respected, participants found the courage to move, speak, and interact in ways they had rarely done before and which they experienced as generative and healing.

Acknowledgements

I am deeply indebted to my collaborator Louisa Harvey and all IA participants for their creativity, generosity, and insight in our work together.

Note

1 All IA participants go by 'artist names' – pseudonyms that they have chosen for the project, which allow us to credit their work while preserving anonymity. The full text for Bunny's process of meeting their artwork reads as: 'Looking at PICTURE 1: Yes and??? This just makes no sense to me / I am drawn to the red thing with prongs / My son and cloud are at the bottom / Used brighter colours lower / Darker colours higher except that green? / I used purple and I hate that colour / Everything rains down on us it should come from the bottom and go out the top.'

References

Angelin, P. (2010, September 26). *A revolution in emotion: The Alba Technique*. Retrieved from www.albatechnique.com/blog/2019/5/27/a-revolution-in-emotion-the-alba-technique

Aves, W. (2022, October 31). *Fact or fiction? Dissecting BPD healthcare mythology*. Retrieved from www.psychiatryisdrivingmemad.co.uk/post/fact-or-fiction-dissecting-bpd-healthcare-mythology

Bailey, P. (2022, September 23). Personal interview.

Benjamin, J. (2018). *Beyond doer and done to: Recognition theory, intersubjectivity and the third*. Routledge.

Brantbjerg. M. (2007). *Caring for yourself while caring for others*. Retrieved from http://moaiku.dk/moaikuenglish/englishlitterature/articles_pdf/us_letter/Caring.pdf

Brantbjerg, M. (2020). Widening the map of hypo-states: A methodology to modify muscular hypo-response and support regulation of autonomic nervous system arousal. *Body, Movement and Dance Psychotherapy*, 15(1), 53–67. https://doi.org/10.1080/17432979.2019.1699604

Brown, L. S. (2004). Feminist paradigms of trauma treatment. *Psychotherapy: Theory, Research, Practice, Training*, 41(4), 464–471.

Chekhov, M. (1991). *On the technique of acting*. Harper.

Chekhov, M. (2002). *To the actor*. Routledge.

Chekhov, M. (2018). *Lessons for teachers* (expanded ed.). Michael Chekhov Association.

Elbow, P. (2009). The believing game or methodological believing. *Journal for the Assembly for Expanded Perspectives on Learning*, 14, 1–11.

Fleming, C. (2021). 'A constant process of expansion', Michael Chekhov: Imagination and community, performing arts in times of crisis (II). *FAP Revista Científica de Artes* Journal, Brazil: Faculty of Arts of Paraná (FAP) of UNESPAR.

Fleming, C. & Cornford, T. (Eds.) (2020). *Michael Chekhov technique in the twenty-first century: New pathways*. Bloomsbury, Methuen Drama.

Herman, J. L. (2002). Recovery from psychological trauma. *Psychiatry and Critical Neurosciences*, 52(S1), S98–S103.

hooks, b. (1994). *Teaching to transgress: Education as the practice of freedom*. Routledge.

Huberman, A. (2021, April 7). *How to reduce anxiety and stress with the physiological sigh*. Retrieved from www.youtube.com/watch?v=rBdhqBGqiMc

Johnston, B. & Jafine, H. (2022). Applied theatre and drama in undergraduate medical education: A scoping review. *McGill Journal of Medicine*, 39, 1–13.

Lakoff, G. & Johnson, M. (1999). *Philosophy in the flesh: The embodied mind and its challenge to western thought*. Basic Books.

Langman, D. (2014). *The Art of acting: Body – soul – spirit – word, A practical and spiritual guide*. Temple Lodge.

McAvinchey, C. (2020). 'If the new theatre is to have its meaning, the audience too must play its part': Chekhov technique in applied, therapeutic and community contexts. In C. Fleming & T. Cornford (Eds.), *Michael Chekhov technique in the twenty-first century: New pathways* (pp. 153–173). Bloomsbury, Methuen Drama.

McNiff, S. (2004). *Art heals: How creativity cures the soul*. Shambala.

Menakem, R. (2021). *My grandmother's hands: Racialised trauma and the pathway to mending our hearts and bodies*. Penguin Random House.

Mitchell, R. (2020a). Something in the atmosphere? Michael Chekhov, Deirdre Hurst Du Prey, and a web of practices between acting and dance. *Theatre, Dance and Performance Training*, 11(3), 255–273.

Mitchell, R. (2020b). 'The Moment you are not inwardly moving and inwardly participating, you are dead': Chekhov technique in actor-movement and dance. In C. Fleming & T. Cornford (Eds.) *Michael Chekhov technique in the twenty-first century: New pathways* (pp. 153–173). Bloomsbury, Methuen Drama.

Mitchell, R. (2022). Not *not* doing therapy: Performer training and the 'third' space. *Theatre, Dance and Performance Training*, 13(2), 222–237. https://doi.org/10.1080/19443927.2022.2052173

Morris, P., Hope, E., Foulsham, T., & Mills, J. P. (2021). The effectiveness of mirroring- and rhythm-based interventions for children with autism spectrum disorder: A systematic review. *Review Journal for Autism and Developmental Disorders*, 8, 541–561.

Petit, L. (2010). *The Michael Chekhov handbook for the actor*. Routledge.

Porter, C., Palmier-Claus, J., Branitsky, A., Mansell, W., Warwick, H., & Varese, F. (2020). Childhood adversity and borderline personality disorder: A meta-analysis. *Acta Psychiatrica Scandinavica*, 141, 6–20.

Rye, E., Anderson, J., & Pickard, M. (2021). Developing trauma-informed care: Using psychodynamic concepts to help staff respond to the attachment needs of survivors of trauma. *Advances in Mental Health and Intellectual Disabilities*, 15(5), 201–208.

Schechner, R. (1985). *Between theatre and anthropology*. University of Pennsylvania Press.

Shaughnessy, N. (2022). Learning with labyrinths: Neurodivergent journeying towards new concepts of care and creative pedagogy through participatory community autism research. *Critical Studies in Teaching and Learning*, 10(1), 127–150.

StopSIM (2021). *StopSIM: Mental illness is not a crime*. Retrieved from https://stopsim.co.uk

Watts, J. (2018, February 15). Testimonial injustice and borderline personality disorder. *Huffpost*. Retrieved from www.huffingtonpost.co.uk/dr-jay-watts/testimonial-injustice-and_b_14738494.html

Chapter 11

Hands

Their Rhythms, Gestures, and the Portal They Offer in Therapy

Emma Westcott

The awareness of and attendance to the body and movement in therapy are a vital element to working with the effects of trauma with clients. The body and its movements are a vast landscape, many parts of which could be explored at length. However, in service of narrowing the gaze, I am choosing to focus, in this chapter, on hands to explore how their expressive qualities can suggest a pathway towards a felt understanding and connection with the self of the client. Our hands are a particular and vital contact point with self and others throughout our lives. They carry an instinctive action and expression of connection such as reaching, pushing, pulling, grasping, boundary making, self-soothing, communicating, greeting, lifting, holding, touching, and healing. These elements will be explored in this chapter. I will weave threads of my own experience and link it to the story of *The Handless Maiden* (Pinkola Estés, 1992) which speaks eloquently to the symbolism of our hands. I will introduce and discuss four different case studies from my work with clients where the pathway to addressing trauma has been illuminated by noticing and exploring the metaphoric or symbolic gestures of the hands.

In this chapter, the body is not discussed as an entity separate from our mind and our thinking, as Descartes would have had us believe, nor as something to be controlled and manipulated because it is carrying experiences, memories, and symptoms which should be fixed or changed. The aim is to see the body as a wise and rich resource which supports the understanding and compassion that clients can develop for themselves, lending more regulation of their nervous system. I aim to explore ways in which dramatherapy can be included as a somatic embodied modality for the treatment of clients who have suffered trauma. My intention is to welcome and to take seriously the messages the body speaks. I will be exploring how interpersonal neurobiology (Siegel, 1999) informs and supports experiential therapy, by which I mean a therapy wherein the client is facilitated to be in touch with the felt, embodied experience of their body and aspects of themselves. In the weaving of this thread, I am particularly indebted to the work of a strikingly vibrant and clear trainer

DOI: 10.4324/9781003322375-15

and therapist, Juliane Taylor Shore (2021, 2022), whose teachings I have benefited from enormously.

A Personal Image and Its Symbolic Link to the Story of *The Handless Maiden*

I recently uncovered a self-portrait from when I was in my twenties. I noticed an anomaly about my hands in the image. I had painted them claw-like, undeveloped. The rest of the painting was figurative and anatomically correct. As I noticed the hands, I wondered about the story of *The Handless Maiden* or *The Girl Without Hands* collected by the Brothers Grimm (1984). In this tale, a young girl allowed her father to chop off her hands with an axe because of a deal that he unwittingly made with the devil. Grief stricken, she forsook the wealth that her father tried to appease her with and left home to wander alone in the forest in search of healing. Years later, after she has had a baby, she was at a well and her child accidentally fell from the papoose into the water. In one version of the story (Pinkola Estés, 1992), as the young woman thrust her arms into the well to save her precious child, her hands grew back. In her instinctive action to reach and save her child, her hands miraculously reappeared. At the time I painted my portrait, I had been sleepwalking, out of touch with my instincts and needs for safety and self-care. I see retrospectively that I unconsciously depicted my deficit of self-care in my painting by showing my hands undeveloped. In the tale of *The Handless Maiden*, there is a symbolic link between hands and self-value. The story begins with the ignorant or naïve sacrifice by the maiden of her hands, of her own agency. Neither she nor her father value her wholeness, agency, or autonomy. That agency is eventually recovered by prioritising the vulnerable child when she thrusts her arms into the water, wherein her hands are regenerated.

In my therapeutic practice with clients who experienced abuse and trauma, their sense of agency has often been denied or undermined by other people or by circumstances, leaving them ‘handless’. They are left disabled in their ability to grasp or connect with their vulnerability or needs. And just as the maiden’s hands reappear when she thrusts her arms into the water to save her baby, a client’s psychological and physical system begins to come back into balance when they connect to their vulnerability and value. This retrieval is enabled by acknowledging and having compassion for the vulnerable parts within themselves. Our hands often signpost this. They tell a tale or hint at an avenue to be explored in the therapeutic encounter.

Hands can touch parts of the body as well as being touched. Notions of self-care can seem quite abstract to many clients and physically modelling direct contact between a hand and one’s own chest, belly, or shoulder can be a safe introduction to self-connection. As we will explore in the client case material to follow, hands can also reveal unconscious beliefs or hitherto unnoticed experiences. If the therapist can accompany the client in gently giving attention to the gestures of the hands, they offer a portal of entry to help understand current or historic experiences and facilitate an exploration and discovery of meaning. Hands are also used in the creation of art. As we shall see in a case study, the use of hands in art making can be an unconscious process made conscious by giving attention to the object made, to help understand on a deeper level the personal material to which it pertains. In what follows, I show how dramatherapy can contribute to healing the legacy of trauma in clients' lives, and how they can find integration and make sense of their experience by attending to their bodies' gestures and their hands.

Case Material

The following vignettes illustrate some metaphorical signposts where hands have indicated the direction of the therapeutic journey, as well as the use of movement, touch, and sound within it. I will discuss four clients I have been working with in private practice. There has been, in each case, a long-established working alliance. The case studies reflect different ways in which the hands can serve our work in connecting with the self and in building a coherent and meaningful narrative. The first study describes steps from helplessness to agency. The second explores a new and compassionate perspective on a long-established survival strategy. The third study shows how a client developed a compassionate insight into a vulnerability which had hitherto been scorned by them. Finally, in the fourth study, the hands provide an image of a new ground on which to walk for the client. I would like to thank the clients discussed for their permission to reflect on the work. Their names and identifying details have been anonymised.

Anna: 'I Can't Believe Such a Tiny Thing Could Be Noticed'

Anna spent a couple of years in therapy with me, slowly gaining trust and working on the day-to-day challenges of her current life. We attended to layers of grief regarding the loss of a dearly loved friend, the losses of a home and career when she moved as a new mother to a new area to live, and the loss of what she thought her future would hold. She moved locally and was now a single parent having separated from her partner who had been violent and remained financially controlling. She shared and explored her earlier life's chapters before venturing towards her deeply buried earliest trauma. Following sexual abuse by two family members as a young girl, Anna was dismissed and ignored when she attempted to tell her experience to her mother, a teacher, and her GP. In later years, in trying again to find a place to be met in her experience, a previous therapist had let her venture too far outside her window of tolerance (Siegel, 2010). This resulted in Anna dissociating, becoming frozen and unable to move or leave the room at the end of their session. Over time, this exacerbated her experience of abandonment and neglect. Although she had managed to build a functional and successful life, recent life circumstances had taken her legs from under her. Her feelings of helplessness and despair had entrenched and brought her to seek therapy again.

In the face of chronic abuse, people often employ numbing coping mechanisms. Besides, shame is often the unbidden companion of the victim of abuse. It could be said that the victim, metaphorically speaking, walks around in a cloak of shame[1] which paradoxically serves for a whilst as a cloak of protection against the pain of betrayal, abandonment, and exploitation. With an unmet need to be seen, heard, and believed beyond the cloak of shameful hiding, Anna led me through some of the experiences she endured. Within the sharing of her layered history, there was a particular moment when a portal opened and with it, a capacity to punctuate and begin to structure and make coherent her experience. Anna, folded over in a chair in a bound physical state (Laban, 1988), moved her index finger to make an almost imperceptible pulse or tap. It was as if that finger had poked against the cloak of shame. In response to me gently drawing attention to it, there was some curiosity and a return to stillness. I wondered if I could move and sit next to her. I described what I saw, mirrored the gesture, and then, with permission, placed my hand onto hers and invited her to move her finger against mine to have a felt sense of the tiny muscular action. I made the quiet sound of the double tap that sounded a bit like a drum. We valued the gesture, explored its qualities and, in inviting repetition, eventually found some words to accompany it and to match with the rhythm. We could hear its voice and its message. Anna used the words 'no more, enough!' Together we could hear the pulse, its language, acknowledge the boundary it was setting and listen to its clarity. Unused to being seen, Anna was incredulous but shyly smiling through tears. She commented that she couldn't believe such a tiny thing could be noticed. This felt sense of being seen, of existing, and then of valuing the wisdom of her body and her instinct to self-care, seemed to open a new room in the house of our therapy. This tiny pulse, initially from her hand, grew into an embodied stance. Beginning with noticing the movement from a finger slowly broadened into a capacity to sense and communicate the boundaries she needed to hold for herself and for her own child.

Trauma can be described as a broken connection to self, other, or spirit. Healing trauma is a process of becoming more connected, and more embodied, leading to a greater sense of presence. Our memories of trauma reside in the body and in our pains. The interrupted fight or flight response or the need to create a boundary reside there too, as was the case for Anna. She expressed a tiny gesture that held a much larger message. That gesture was there in her body. She had been unable to express and fulfil that message when she was abused as a small child, as to do so would have likely further exacerbated her vulnerability and loneliness. In the here and now of her therapy, alongside another witness, she realised that she did have that clarity and boundary making capacity within her, and that she could see, feel, value, and expand it into action to support her autonomy.

Carl: 'When My Father Shouted "I'll Kill You If ...", I Believed Him'

Carl came to therapy hoping to explore and heal a painful self-image. He could not accept his body as it was and could only see imperfections. He was also a new parent and wanted to be different from his own parents. Carl grew up with an unpredictable and violent father, and a loving, capable but emotionally closed mother who was not able to protect her children or attune to their experiences. Carl functioned well in the world. He had created a rich work and family life but frequently felt stuck in an unreachable and thwarted ideal image of home and self. Through the years of our therapy, we recognised links between his family dynamics and his sense of self, the latter profoundly influenced by the former. Carl brought examples of how he believed that there was something essentially wrong with him whilst growing up, identifying with characters in various TV shows or films. We examined the inherent inequality of power within a family, and how it is very difficult and risky to see the parents on whom we depend as being deficient, even when their behaviours and attitudes are out of control. It was as if the scrutiny he held his body under was driven by an unconscious need to find the fault that justified his experience of being attacked and treated as flawed or wrong. In addition, the invitation to 'be with' himself in a relaxed state of flow was thwarted by Carl's embodied lived experiences in the home. For example, when as a child he played quietly on the carpet and engaged with his toys in a state of quiet focus and peace, he had been violently lifted and thrown across the sitting room. Letting life and himself be just-as-it-is could feel unpredictable and dangerous. Vigilance seemed to have become a constant companion, and the target of his scrutiny was often himself.

As we explored some emotional discomfort in a session, I asked Carl if it could be found in the body. Carl indicated that his throat was hurting. As I invited Carl to feel the sensation in his throat, I wondered if the feeling had a shape or a colour. Carl described an image of 'a hand like an axe' moving swiftly towards the throat as if to stop him from saying anything. We stayed with this image and movement with curiosity and compassion and recognised that it had value by engaging with it. I suggested for Carl to be the voice of the hand. I asked the 'chopping hand' how old Carl was and whether there was anything it felt he should know. It said that it thought Carl was under 12 years old and that it had been stopping him from speaking up to protect him. It also felt that it was a matter of life and death if any words were addressed to the father. Carl shared that when his father shouted 'I'll kill you if…', Carl had believed him. When he was under 12, Carl was clearly particularly vulnerable and reliant on the care of his family in a period when it was far safer to silence himself than trying to confront his father. He had to sacrifice authenticity to protect the attachment and make certain choices for survival. Such implicit beliefs lasted well into adulthood and unconsciously influenced perception and attitude beyond any rational understanding. Carl's sense of having 'something wrong' with him and the feeling that 'speaking up could be dangerous' had continued beyond the family years.

Carl had felt thwarted in trying to stand up for himself and speak up to his father. He had carried some shame for that feeling of ineptitude for a long time. He observed that he could stand up for others articulately and authentically, but that his capacity to stand his own ground verbally had often eluded him in adult life. The process of listening to the part of himself that habitually silenced him and understanding its protective intentions offered Carl a more compassionate take on his self-editing, and a broader insight into the survival strategies he adopted. His self-criticism and contempt for his lack of capacity to speak up could begin to soften. The image of the hand chopping at the neck to cut off speech was valued as meaningful. The understanding which arose out of that exploration offered Carl a coherent sense of the impact of his earlier years. He saw how the emotional conviction that it was dangerous to speak up continued to unconsciously play out in his life despite his adult experience, professionalism, and enormous capacity for empathy for others. Some weeks later, Carl was able to voice to me an irritation towards something I had said within moments of that response arising. At the end of that session, he reflected on the shift in acknowledging his experience and of using his voice. More recently, Carl was able to clearly articulate a response to his father whose language and attitude had been aggressive and explosive. Carl's instinctive boundary making was active. He was able to trust and act according to his integrity. No axe prevented him from speaking up.

Ella: 'I Will Always Be Vulnerable, but It Need Not Diminish Me'

Ella was prompted to seek support following a depression and debilitating rheumatoid arthritis in her hands. Ella was an artist, and yet in our first meeting it became clear that she had been advised by a mentor that she should not make art if she wanted to get better, as art was seen as a defence. I offered an alternative suggestion of bringing whatever she wanted creatively both within the room and into the room. She could bring her art and her artistic self. The next session she arrived with two sculptures, the following one, with three. Imagery in sculptural form, drawings and paintings, dream and metaphorical images became the satellites of our work and relationship as they developed. We played with these images verbally and through enactment in the room. For example, Ella explored in dialogue the embodied relationship between characters from a sculpture she had been working on. She physically moved between these, making active use of her hands, supporting, and being supported, giving and receiving, and moving back and forth between different physical states.

Ella experienced a profound family loss early in life. It became clear that this was part of a pattern of chasms in the family history over many previous generations, whereby a child lost their mother, or a mother lost their child. The loss of a family member when Ella was very young meant that parental attention was distracted and terribly inhibited by grief and depression. This clearly affected her experience of feeling cared for and her capacity to care for herself when vulnerable. An overarching theme through our work became the necessary development of a nurturing capacity for herself and in interpersonal relationships. Early on in our sessions, Ella explained that she had been 'creating art all these years for Mummy to see; ironically, it hasn't been seen much by anyone'. At first, my reparative therapeutic role was that of a mother, seeing and bearing witness, and valuing her work created with her own hands. James Hillman described how 'the support of the good positive mother is indiscriminately nourishing. It puts a positive sign on every emotion and every feeling in order to redeem it from exile in guilt and shame' (Von Franz & Hillman, 1971, p.142). Ella's quest 'to find subjectivity', as she put it, was supported and facilitated through the recognition of her vulnerability.

In one session, Ella presented feeling uncared for, unimportant, and disrespected by a colleague, whilst also confused when that same colleague complimented her work. In describing the incident her arms repeatedly shaped a pattern in the air. The pattern was of her hands and arms moving in a boxing type stance: arms bent, forearms upwards, and hands in fists. Noticing the fight/flight response, I guided Ella's attention to her arms and invited her to put her mind inside them. As I wondered what colour they felt and what they might have to say, we discovered that the arms were of a grey colour and thought that Ella was 2 years old. When dialoguing with these arms, we found that they had provided safety and protection for Ella and were still doing so all these decades later. I thought of the flailing arms of a small child desperate to be picked up and of the boxing stance arms ready to protect and create some safety. I hypothesised that she was enacting and completing a fight survival response which had not been possible to complete as a vulnerable child. Being supported to piece together the past and the present by paying attention to the body in movement and to the memories of the past, Ella found a coherent narrative that included meaning and understanding.

It was in her early years that Ella generated the belief that others mattered more than her. Whilst speaking to the internal part which played out this boxing stance, another aspect of her suddenly and impatiently said that it was 'time to grow up'. When I asked Ella what her response to this was, she said: 'I have arthritis, I can't change'. I asked Ella to repeat this sentence several times. On the fourth repetition she burst out laughing, threw her head back against the sofa and announced: 'I change all the time!' The invitation to experience her body to speak allowed the discovery of a new truth and the refutation of the old belief or myth that she couldn't change. This surprising and energetic discovery, according to Ecker et al. (2012), is the stuff that allows an actual shift in the neural network, so that old beliefs which influence our style of interaction with the world can be revised and our responses to life's challenges change.

Ella brought to our sessions a series of 'inner life' paintings created a decade earlier but that she had now returned to and was willing to explore and understand more consciously. The storylines in the painting series were themes of her own journey which we explored through dialogue, enactment, and improvisation. There is one image that Ella suggested I could use when I told her about the theme of this chapter (see Figure 11.1).

Her painting series, like her therapy journey, investigates in Ella's words 'woman becoming a subject in her own life', and explores whether there 'could be such a thing as a female image of the divine'. I would suggest that our many years of connecting with her physical experience and her artistic expression enabled the creation of a safe ground from which she could embark on such depth work. The characters depicted in her paintings are archetypes of her own personal myth. We paid receptive and vigilant attention to their gestures and details.

One character in the painting sits on a stiletto legged stool on a cloud with no ground beneath her. She is ungrounded and undernourished. A minimal plate of food sits in front of her. She firmly holds her left arm ahead of her and her hand makes a stop sign to the huge, seated figure opposite, denying the life it represents. Her other hand grips a tiny cup, contrasting dramatically with the

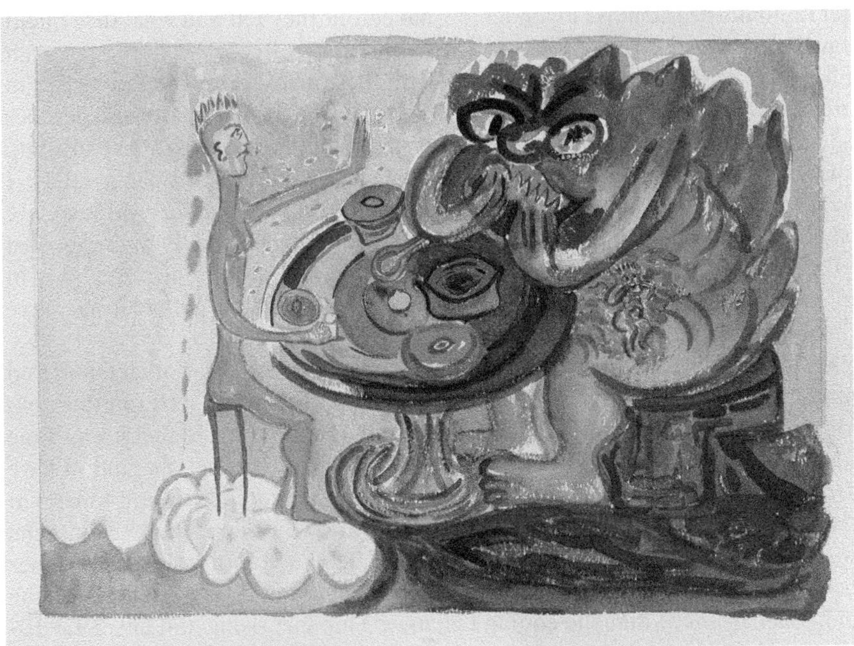

Figure 11.1 Virtuous Cloud Woman meets Grounded Greed. Reproduced with permission of the client

larger food bowls on the other side of the table. The large figure, monstrous with sharp teeth, yellow eyes, and a spiked back, sits on a solid stool on substantial ground and eats vociferously. This character uses their two hands at once to feed themself. The woman on the stiletto stool firmly puts her hand between her and, what can be interpreted as, the denied unconscious and feared part of her. She refuses to look at her companion, blocking the sight-line with her hand, as erect and inflexible as her very thin undernourished body.

As we explored the gestures and the symbolic images, Ella discerned that what she called her 'cloud raft' protected her from experiencing and feeling her real conflicts. She was not feeding herself with sufficient nourishment and was holding her shadow at bay. There is another figure sitting on the lap of the large figure. It is a small green female also using her hands to touch her face and nourish herself. When I look at this small green figure, I recall Ella's descriptions of herself as a 5-year-old freewheeling fearless young girl unfettered by shame or rejection with an appetite for life. This contrasts with the self-denial illustrated in the stiletto stool figure. We interpreted the 'eating' figures as engaging with different aspects of life that Ella had allowed herself to connect with. These figures were living and digesting the aspects of herself that she consistently projected outwards, refusing, with her hand as a block, to see as her own. Ella could see in retrospect that the denied aspects were of experiencing and allowing her breadth and depth of feelings, and of accepting and valuing herself. As she said in one session, she had been expecting the value to come from outside and was furious when it didn't. Reflecting on the time when we looked in depth at the series of paintings, including the one above, Ella noted that:

> this was the point when my projection onto you as my mother came back to me. We were two women with different backgrounds enjoying a story we could share in. I felt separate from you and equal – as if I'd come of age in some way.

She had reclaimed the connection with herself.

Nearing the end of this phase of the therapy, a spontaneous gesture in Ella's hands and arms allowed a return to a deep understanding within her work. In describing an unwelcome interruption to her creative process and comparing herself to a bonded labourer who could never pay off their debt, she held her arms firmly across her torso. In drawing her attention to her physical impulses, Ella commented: 'This is my neurotic self who negotiates life by avoiding it'. She then spontaneously opened her arms into a wide-open stance adding, 'but now I have determination'. As I invited Ella to physically move between the closed and the open arm positions, to trace their felt shape and to allow them to speak to one another, she named courage and fear. Courage said to Fear: 'Come on sweetie you can try, you now have tangible evidence that if you have a shot and fall over, things can come'. And Fear responded, arms opening from the bound position, head a little back and chest lifted: 'I will always be vulnerable, but it need not diminish me'.

In subsequent sessions, this re-vision of her beliefs went deeper. Via an explorative process attending to the body's sensations and felt emotions, Ella connected deeply with the 'unfairness' of her early family trauma. Her hands located this feeling in the chest, which she described metaphorically as 'being under the floorboards'. This emotional description connected her memory to the felt senses in the here and now of her body. In concluding this process, Ella observed: 'I was squashed down and couldn't perform…and yet, I did!'. Both of us laughed in recognition of that truth and acknowledged moments in her childhood of vitality and creativity. She continued, 'I wasn't seen and yet [laughing] I am by … [she named the people who value her]'.

Whilst her process unfolded, Ella continued to connect to her vulnerability with compassion. The rheumatoid arthritis in her hands, with which she arrived in therapy, diminished and medical tests at that time showed a balanced system with no inflammation.

Nathan: 'You're Not Going to Die If You Take that Step'

I am struck that in addition to the hands offering a portal into therapy via their gestures expressed through the body, hands are also a symbolic image that arises from the psyche and the imagination of the client. The hands in the following study are in the service of connecting, holding, and supporting from within.

Nathan, a 60-year-old man, came to therapy to attend to a long and debilitating depression. He experienced a long stint in hospital with pneumonia as a young child, at a time when parents were not allowed to visit. He grew up brown skinned in a non-diverse white community. His parental care was unreliable and moved between being neglectful and invasive. He generally felt unmet, with his name consistently mispronounced by those around him. As an adult, he was able to work in creative teams and fulfil his role in managing creative projects but appeared less able to act on his own behalf. He experienced insurmountable difficulty in doing what he knew would be helpful for him. He described his frustration at how his knowledge and his ability to act were so far apart. We contracted to explore this gap.

Nathan's image for the space between intention and action was a lilac-coloured bottomless blancmange. He knew that if he stepped onto the blancmange, it would be 'like stepping off the edge of a cliff'. Working with the image, Nathan noted that it now had hands underneath the surface. Nathan saw the hands as steppingstones as they told him: 'You're not going to die if you take that step'. As I asked Nathan how he felt towards this blancmange, he found that he was impatient. This impatience was felt in the chest and was shaped like a tight rib cage. As Nathan bore witness to this impatience, the rib cage image turned into hands with long fingers. Curious about these hands, we found that they had been protecting his heart and lungs. This made sense to

Nathan as he had been feeling very vulnerable due to asthma attacks that felt life threatening. Nathan made the connection between this fear and his inability to take a step towards action, as this felt like stepping off a cliff into a bottomless blancmange. I invited Nathan to imagine connecting the inner hands to his physical hands and to move them across his body to track the sensations therein, and to explore afresh the shapes, contours, and size of his limbs. He observed that he was more relaxed than he thought he would be. We noted together how both areas of his dilemma, when attended to, had become hands. We looked again at the space between the self-care intention and action. Nathan observed that the 'steppingstone hands' had now transformed into grass, and that the 'rib hands' held his lungs and heart gently, knowing that Nathan could take a step without dying. We contracted to revisit this landscape and to reinforce the new connectivity. By starting to differentiate and link these two states, Nathan began to find some understanding and trust via a newfound integration.

A memory of a cliff edge recalled whilst exploring the above image was from a trip to Sri Lanka as a child, when the family had returned to his parent's home for a one-off visit. This enquiry revealed Nathan's experience of his younger life with his sibling, observing that his parents 'had no insight into kids being mixed race', and that there was 'no safety net from our parents at all'. This significant deficit had impacted Nathan's capacity to step freely across the thresholds into what he deemed straightforward activities. The embodied exploration and discovery of the hands image loosened this hold of this unconscious belief and allowed grief for the lack of holding in his childhood. In the weeks after the 'steppingstone hands' session, Nathan's procrastination lessened. He took steps to take more care of himself and to attend to his home environment. The images of the cliff, the hands and the green grass became frequent references in our work, as he sustained a connection to his inner world whilst engaging more with his outer one. He has since returned to Sri Lanka and is keen to go back with his children, placing more value in this aspect of his heritage.

To Conclude

Those who have suffered trauma have been 'done to'. They have had their sense of agency, autonomy, and safety often violently and repeatedly thwarted or utterly neglected. Furthermore, in the aftermath of traumatic experience the acknowledgement of the trauma can often be non-existent or aggressively denied. I have shown in this chapter how important it is to support clients to connect with their felt experience in the here and now. As I have discussed, this can be facilitated by noticing and valuing the expressions of the body, such as through the hands. The therapeutic explorations that dramatherapy facilitates, with its alertness to the body, image, and movement, open a powerful safe space to explore and potentially heal the experience of trauma in our clients.

As we have seen in this chapter, the body holds memories and wisdom. The client may not recall everything, but the body remembers and expresses memories in physical and emotional forms (Maté, 2019). It seems important to notice the fleeting messages that the body reveals and to give these messages space to be explored and made sense of. As discussed, clients will often use their hands metaphorically. Their movements will help them become aware of the rhythm, speed, direction, and intensity of their experiences. I am reminded of the hands of the *Handless Maiden* reforming when she rescued her vulnerable child. In this symbolic tale, her compassionate and instinctive movement to retrieve her baby from danger brought a new integration and wholeness to her actual body. Equally, our aim is to help clients experience themselves as valued with a meaningful, coherent, and compassionate understanding of what brought them to therapy.

Being receptive to the body and its expressiveness is vital. I have focussed my gaze on the hands to explore what a vigilant awareness of the body can offer. Hands are a wonderful portal through which the therapist and client can pay attention to vital symbolic, unconscious, unrehearsed, unspoken, or even unspeakable expressions. Further exploration and development of this theme, beyond the limits of this chapter, will be fascinating.

Note

1 James Fitzgerald, Jungian analyst, has kindly given permission for me to use his eloquent image of a 'cloak of shame', from one of our wonderful and consistently insightful conversations.

References

Ecker, B., Ticic, R., & Hulley, L. (2012). *Unlocking the emotional brain: Eliminating symptoms at their roots using memory reconsolidation*. Routledge.

Grimm, J. & Grimm, W. (1984). *The complete illustrated stories of the Brothers Grimm*. Chancellor Press.

Laban, R. (1988). *The mastery of movement*. Northcote House.

Maté, G. (2019). *When the body says no*. Penguin Random House UK.

Pinkola Estés, C. (1992). *Women who run with the wolves: Contacting the power of the wild woman*. Rider.

Siegel, D. (1999). *The developing mind*. The Guilford Press.

Siegel, D. (2010). *Mindsight*. Random House Inc.

Taylor Shore, J. (2021). *Neurobiology with heart*. Retrieved from https://learn.therapywisdom.com

Taylor Shore, J. (2022). *Understanding your client's brain: Incorporating neuroscience into treatment planning and clinical interventions*. Retrieved from https://learn.therapywisdom.com

Von Franz, M. L. & Hillman, J. (1971). *Lectures on Jung's typology*. Spring Publications Inc.

Chapter 12

The Voice and Anger

Experiences of Healing Through Performance

Greta Sharp

I've been angry for a long time. It can't find its way out.
It gets caught in my throat like an unfinished sentence. Like the tiny
bit of vomit that you swallow back down and the taste
of acid stings in your mouth.
I swallow my anger back down.
I push it down, back into my stomach, back into my limbs. I let it sit
in my pelvis, hardening there and turning it numb.
I won't let
it escape.
I try to suffocate it instead inside of me
without oxygen. I don't want to give it life. If I let it out of me
it will breathe in the air and it will expand and get bigger and
grow
and
take on a life of its own and
I won't be able to control it
anymore.
It will become nasty and stale and mouldy when
the air touches it. It will rot and become a
bad thing
that no one wants to touch.
I must contain it inside of me, where it can't breathe, where it can't
grow and
turn stale. Where it sits lifeless, manifesting
and ruminating
and stewing. It chews on old wounds and picks
at them with nothing else to do. It is confined to the shape of my
insides. I am scared of it.
I am scared of what it will do if I unleash it. So I keep
it bound and
contained. I swallow it back

DOI: 10.4324/9781003322375-16

down and keep it stifled inside
of me.
Anger (Sharp, 2021)

Introduction

This chapter explores using the voice as a tool for somatic trauma healing, discussing my performance practice as a starting point. The focus of this practice is on developing a physiological felt sense of safety within the nervous system by using the voice as a tool for healing. I primarily focus on developmental trauma as this is my experience of a nervous system that did not know safety until it started feeling and healing.

Much of my own healing journey has been informed by practices such as Internal Family Systems (Schwartz, 2021) and Somatic Experiencing (Levine, 1997), both of which position the self and the body as having an innate wealth of wisdom which intuitively allows healing to unfold when we make space to listen to what they have to say. By taking what I have learned on my own journey and sharing with others my creative practice, I seek to explore additional opportunities for healing within alternative community spaces, and briefly touch on what purpose these spaces occupy between art, healing, and social practice.

I draw on research into the nervous system, more specifically Polyvagal Theory (Porges, 2017), and the way our bodies and voices are impacted by trauma to explore why using our voice in safe relationship can be such a profound tool to regulate our nervous system and help heal from relational trauma. I refer to Vocal Psychotherapy as developed by Diane Austin (2008) and relevant ongoing research into the voice and trauma by the *Voice and Trauma Group*, a non-profit organisation founded by specialists to create a platform for conversations in this young and growing field of research. In particular, I connect the voice to the expression of anger, as a valid self-protective response to trauma that couldn't be expressed and resulted in a dorsal vagal override of the nervous system (Porges, 2017). I discuss how expressing our anger and using our voice within safe relationships support us in moving out of a freeze response where our emotions and experiences are silenced and numbed. I also draw on Pete Walker's (2013) understanding of complex PTSD, to add further detail into the specific difficulties of healing from early relational trauma and explain why grief work is so important. Where anger teaches us boundaries and self-protection, grief teaches us vulnerability and love. These two emotions co-exist and support one another. By feeling our grief, we connect to our innate wholeness which supports us in knowing that we are worthy of our boundaries and of protection, as boundaries are the protective membranes that allow us to softly connect to our grief.

Screaming at The Sea

A Ritual of Screaming

When I first screamed, it was because a sound needed to come out of me that I hadn't been able, or allowed myself, to express before. I had spent a year or so screaming into pillows, muffling the noises my body could make. I felt as though all these sounds had been trapped in my body for years. When I screamed, they were finally being released. These vocal sounds were my 'No', my rage, my pain, and grief.

This became a ritual of screaming and I chose the beach as my place for this. A large portion of my developmental trauma took place in a small seaside town in Kent. I had since associated the seaside with that trauma, avoiding it wherever possible. I believe my avoidance of the seaside was a contributing factor to my diagnosis of PTSD at the age of 14. My bodymind (Price, 2015) made a connection between visiting any seaside town or beach and the abuse from my perpetrator. As a result, the mere thought of a day trip to the beach made me feel viscerally unwell and anxious.

The sea was synonymous with the trauma I experienced for many years and, in some ways, still is. I had spent 15 years avoiding the British coast as the sound of seagulls, seeing worn out arcades and the smell of the sea salt air would trigger me into a flashback. Perhaps surprisingly as an adult, I decided to move to the seaside to take up a place on a year-long artist programme. Somewhere inside, I was driven by the sense that if I could have a relationship with the sea, then my relationship with it could be healed as well as part of the trauma I associated with it. Having previously experienced the re-traumatisation of being asked to talk about traumatic events before I was ready with counsellors I did not trust, this appealed to me as I would not have to do that again in order to begin the healing process.

It has been through this process of healing by the sea that I was reassured of the fact that I knew all along I needed to come back to it to find safety as a way of integrating. I followed a deep bodily knowing that I needed to cultivate a relationship with the sea and to express my anger, my pain, and my grief to it, so that it could act as a placeholder and hold the emotions I could not express to my perpetrators. By following the wisdom of my body that has always sought to protect me, I found healing.

Pete Walker describes 'angering' as a grieving process. As he writes,

> survivors need to anger – sometimes rage – about the intimidation, humiliation, and neglect that was passed off to them as nurturance in their childhoods. As they become adept at grieving, they anger out their healthy resentment at their family's pervasive lack of safety.
>
> (Walker, 2013, p.222)

Through my healing process, with the help of a very caring therapist, support group, and friends, I found that beneath my anger lay my grief, the 'yin' to the 'yang' of angering as Walker suggests (2013, p.225). This grief was a gut-wrenching emotion that sought to tear me open and let all the harsh experiences pour out of me. The grief was lonely, drew me into myself, and gently asked me to love myself, to let myself be who I was, not denying or minimising the trauma I experienced. Expressing my anger made way for the grief to tumble out of me, surrendering to the vast power of the sea and all it can hold.

Walker (2013) explains how grieving is mourning the losses incurred in childhood through which a survivor fully comprehends how the abuse and the subsequent coping mechanisms and self-abandonment were not their fault. This grief taught me how loveable I am, how sacred my vulnerabilities are and how my capacity for joy co-exists with my capacity to feel my grief. As Piepzna-Samarasinha, a queer survivor of colour, asks (2021, p.234): what would it be like if we 'believed that grief was sacred and valuable, a source of life-giving knowledge?'

With the rituals of screaming, I started to scream with friends. This turned into documented performances. These were sometimes spontaneous, sometimes planned, on the beach with or without public walking by. We would drive out to different beaches or set up on the beach at the end of my road. Sometimes we would record on our phones or with a camera. Over time, this ritual became a performative practice, slipping between planned and intuitive, often inviting others to witness or join in.

As this screaming evolved from something I did privately to something I was documenting and bringing others into, I began to think about our collective relationship to expressing grief and anger. I was using the sea as a vehicle to bring the community together to witness, share feelings, and heal collectively. In an auto-theoretical piece I wrote about our modernised relationship with the sea in the UK, I move between my personal relationship to the grieving and angering with the sea as a survivor and trans person, and the possible collective grieving and angering that could occur because of global issues related to the sea, such as climate change and Brexit:

> How do we begin to heal our relationship to the sea? How do we heal our relationship to the ecologies that live in the sea that we harm? How do we heal our relationship to the sea and the lives that have been lost and a refusal to let people find safety when they are just trying to build better lives for themselves and their families? Whose responsibility is it to heal this? How do I take personal responsibility to heal this and acknowledge my specific relationship with the sea?
>
> (Sharp, 2022b)

During this time, I considered how there are a multitude of traumas associated with the sea, both globally and locally, such as pollution, global warming, overfishing, and the transatlantic slave trade including the pre-meditated

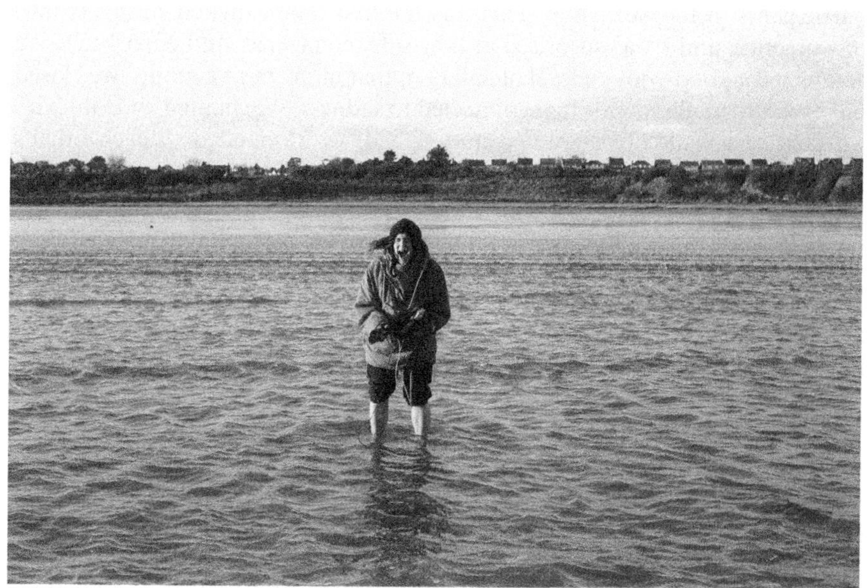

Figure 12.1 Performance at Hovercraft Harbour, Pegwell Bay, 2021
© Greta Sharp

murder of thousands of people such as the Zong massacre (1781). Learning more about these historical and present-day traumas made me realise how much healing there is to be done collectively with and through the sea. Although, like my own trauma, the sea did not cause these, I wanted to see if I could create spaces where individuals could come together and begin a relationship with the sea. Maybe the sea could hold our grief, and maybe by getting really angry at it, we could hold one another, hear what others have to say and find ways to heal as a community.

Public Workshop

In January 2022, I ran a public workshop in collaboration with singer and vocal coach, Naomi Hammerton. The purpose was to create a space for people to scream in an emotionally and physically safe and structured way. Naomi's involvement was to teach us how to scream without straining our vocal chords, so that this practice would be physically safe. We began with familiar and easy vocal and movement exercises, such as passing a sound or movement around a circle. As we became more familiar with one another and more comfortable in our bodies in this environment, Naomi led us through exercises to explore how we could make different sounds with our breathing, body, and mouth shapes. Through making these sounds, we engaged more mindfully with the physicality of sound making, breathing into our stomachs and opening our mouths wide. During the meditation exercise that consisted of connecting to our feelings of joy and sadness, a new embodied experience occurred for me in relation to the participants in the workshop. This was the first time I invited strangers into this practice, and I was surprised at how safe, connected, and open I felt. We co-created a good-enough level of safety in that moment as a group. We closed our eyes and made sounds that connected to sadness. We chanted and 'ahhh'd', we sang and wailed, we grunted and sighed, we responded to each other's sounds, we added to the sounds we were hearing, we started new sounds, and we paused to listen. It was an incredibly powerful experience whereby our bodies in the same space connected through the sounds we could make, rather than words.

When we walked down to the beach, I didn't need to give much instruction at this point as our previous exercises had created a very held and safe environment for everyone. With the sea behind me, I read a poem I wrote about anger. This poem, which opens this chapter, evidences the journey I made from anger, as a repressed and hardened emotion stuck inside me, to using my voice and my body to express it in a safe way. I found out in my recovery that 'old' emotions were triggered when a familiar dynamic was played out. By creating spaces for those old emotions to be expressed safely, I was able to increasingly tend to and be in the present.

We created a space for releasing whatever sounds were needed, as loud as we wanted them to be – shouts, screams, wails, or cries. One scream would encourage another one as safety was found in a collective expression that enabled individuals to make whatever sounds they needed to. When a scream would stop, another one would start soon after, revealing more sounds that needed to be expressed. All screams were unique in the way in which they expressed rage, wails of grief, or cries of joy. What I had felt on my own – this ritualistic, spiritual pilgrimage to the sea, the sense of release and of being held – was amplified with the group. This lasted for about 30 minutes, until just as with the meditation, our collective experience found a shared ending.

To close the workshop, we held space for sharing and reflections. I was struck by how moved the participants were and how connected they felt. If they were not sure about being able to scream before the group started, they found it much easier afterwards. I discovered how closely connected joy and grief were. If my screams were of anger and grief, for others they were joyous and an expression and celebration of themselves.

The workshop confirmed for me the need to create safe spaces for people to come together, feel and express emotions that often are not acceptable in our culture, particularly for those socialised as women. Participants reflected on a common experience of how screaming and shouting offered a sense of release that was not possible in ordinary life. The performative environment and the safety that myself and my co-facilitator were able to create allowed for a different atmosphere where individuals were able to go beyond their comfort zone and experience something new. Following this, I began to research the impact of trauma on the body and on the nervous system to contextualise what I had learned in the workshop within a wider conversation on trauma and healing.

Healing in Relationship

Our Social Engagement System

Polyvagal Theory, developed by neuroscientist Stephen W. Porges, explains why our autonomic nervous system is highly important when it comes to understanding the body's responses to danger and trauma, and how we learn to identify cues of safety with others and within environments (Porges, 2017). Through the study of the vagus nerve, Porges discovered that, whilst it assists in lowering our heart rate and acts as a 'brake' to create a calm state, it is also capable of stopping the heart entirely in response to life-threatening events. Polyvagal Theory makes a distinction between our freeze response (dorsal vagal) and our social engagement (ventral vagal) within the parasympathetic nervous system. With Polyvagal Theory, we understand that in response to danger, our sympathetic nervous system becomes activated into a fight/flight response or shuts down because of 'a massive down-regulation of autonomic function by an ancient pathway of the parasympathetic nervous system' (Porges, 2017, p.54).

For those who have experienced severe and prolonged trauma, it is common that one of the trauma responses becomes 'overdeveloped' in that it is used so often and so effectively that we get 'stuck' there (Walker, 2013, p.13). Relationships become places where we feel a threat of danger, and so relating to others from our social engagement system, from a place of curiosity and playfulness, is very difficult. Previously, I detailed how this manifests as compulsive behaviours and dysfunctional relationship patterns:

> We are easy to anger, abandon relationships prematurely, busy ourselves at work, numb out on sex, drugs, alcohol, and TV, abandon ourselves in relationships, and a myriad of other things. Forming safe and secure relationships is insanely difficult if every time a friend takes a few days to text you back, you ditch the friendship, or if every time your boundaries are crossed, you lash out in rage, or if you stay in relationships that are abusive because that is what is familiar to you. But these behaviours are signs of a traumatised nervous system that is struggling to find safety and comfort from relationships. Forming a community, which consists of individual intimate relationships with others, is near impossible. But these relationships are exactly what we need to heal as humans are social animals that need others.
>
> (Sharp, 2022a)

With developmental trauma, the trauma is relational, in that it occurs when a child is so overwhelmed at the continual disconnection from a parent or caregiver whilst remaining dependent on them to survive (Walker, 2013). The trauma ultimately causes a disconnection from oneself, which adds to the levels of distress experienced in all relationships because of the absence of an internal secure base and gauge on boundaries and needs. Whilst this trauma occurs in relationships, it is ultimately healed through relationships, including the relationship to oneself (Walker, 2013). However, the act of receiving care is complex and faced with many internal barriers and protective mechanisms that have been crucial for survival within families but also institutions. As Piepzna-Samarasinha (2021, p.132) reminds us,

> Many people I know and love have a hard time receiving care because 'care' has always been conditional or violent – the invasion of social workers or Child Protective Services, or psychiatrists with the power to lock you up. I think about the need for care that can be accessed when you are isolated, disliked, and without social capital – which many disabled people are.

A key point of Polyvagal Theory is that our feeling of safety is dependent on vocal and facial cues from others (Porges, 2017). When our social engagement system is activated, it supports the development of safe relationships and the ability to give and receive care. It helps understand why we can feel stuck in patterns of abuse, violence, or unsafe situations, and how we can find safety in ourselves through our relationships with others, and vice versa, in others through our relationship with ourselves.

I recently took part in a grief tending ritual. As I usually do when sharing or expressing my feelings, I look away from the people around me. When the facilitator invited me in my grieving state to look up and see that the group was with me, the connection felt overwhelming. I later realised that the facial expressions of those in the group were signalling cues of safety and, as a result, helped me to feel safe and to share my feelings. In being held in my vulnerability and in connecting through my grief, I was able to let go of something I had been holding on to for a long time and experienced something truly transformational. It is a powerful experience to be lovingly witnessed in our grief, especially for those who experienced abuse and grew up unable to share their feelings with those who were meant to protect them because they were also those who harmed them. Sophy Banks (2023), grief tending facilitator, has described how the group has been, throughout human history, a sacred place for healing, particularly in Indigenous cultures, not only for individuals, but as a way of keeping the village or community healthy. This experience of grief tending affirmed for me the power of community healing.

The Voice and Nervous System Healing

A conversation with the artist and DJ Melika Ngombe Kolongo introduced me to the idea that sounds and the voice can affect our nervous system and ultimately support healing. Through a group listening exercise, we discussed how sounds, at a physical level, are just vibrations, and how our body receives these vibrations and makes sense of them as sounds. So not only do we hear music, we also feel the vibrations of the sound on a physiological level. Equally, we also create sounds through vibrations in our body, such as with the larynx – our 'voice box'.

If Bessel van der Kolk (2014) pioneered our understanding of the way trauma is stored in the body, researchers have begun to consider how, as muscles tighten in response to trauma, this can also include our vocal chords and the muscles in our jaws to create a detectable change in our voices (Brown et al., 2020). Heleen Grooten (Brown et al., 2020), a speech and language therapist, describes how the voice and hearing play an integral part in our fight/flight response to danger, for example, in the survival strategy of not making a sound. I experienced intense hyperarousal around hearing sensitivity, becoming extremely distressed by subtle background noises that those around me were able to tune out automatically.

In conversations with other survivors, I found that many who experienced abuse became attuned, as children, to subtle changes in their parents' or caregivers' voices. For example, I found that it was a common experience for individuals to listen out for any detectable signs indicating that their parents would break out into a rageful attack. When living in a constant state of potential threat, one becomes very good at detecting small signs that something bad is going to happen. From these conversations, I also found that many, as children, instinctively monitored their expression of emotions through their facial expressions and voices, so that they could attempt to control the response of their parents or caregivers and therefore limit any abuse. Engaging with the senses – hearing and creating sound – becomes an obvious place to turn to to soothe the nervous system. An important point to note regarding sound making and its relation to healing is that Polyvagal Theory has shown how we can downregulate our mobilisation defence system (fight/flight) and activate our social engagement system through the breath: slow and deep exhalations, singing, playing a wind instrument, or slowing down speech (Porges, 2017).

Diane Austin (2008) has incorporated the voice and singing into her clinical practice since the 1980s. Over the course of 20 years, she developed Vocal Psychotherapy, which uses, as Reynolds (2022) explains, 'the breath and natural vocal sounds, vocal improvisation, songs and dialogue to facilitate interpersonal growth and change for the client'. This model seeks to facilitate a connection between the mind and body to enable the client to get in touch with unconscious feelings and memories held in the body, and recreate through the relationship between client and therapist important developmental needs such as the capacity to self-regulate. For those who have experienced developmental trauma, the ability to self-regulate hasn't had the chance to fully develop because of deficits in co-regulation from caregivers. In that respect, experiencing co-regulation as an adult is extremely important to develop the capacity to self-regulate (Walker, 2013). Reynolds (2022) describes how the Vocal Psychotherapist uses singing and the voice to create a symbiotic relationship with the client in order to attune and meet important developmental needs. For example, this could be achieved through an exercise where a client sings their own melodic line and the therapist repeats it back to them, 'mirroring' the client and their voice. Mirroring provides reassurance and validation and meets important developmental needs to help become our 'true' selves. Another example is singing in harmony, which represents the beginning of separation and supports a client to gain more independence. It is important for these developmental stages to be recreated and for needs to be met for clients who have never had a close emotional relationship with their caregivers.

Singing and making sounds with the voice creates an immensely powerful experience as something exquisitely unique as music is made through our own bodies. It is immensely powerful to find that *our body*, the body with which we experience the world, has a wondrous ability to create sounds that can also regulate our nervous system. Equally, when we sing with others, we are co-creating, receiving, and immersed in music through which we are able to co-regulate with those involved in that experience. As Austin (2008, p.20) outlines,

> Our voices resonate inwards to help us connect to our bodies and express our emotions, and they resonate outwards to help us connect to others. Internally resonating vibrations break up and release blockages of energy, releasing feelings and allowing a natural flow of vitality and a state of equilibrium to return to the body. These benefits are particularly relevant to clients who have frozen, numbed off areas in the body that hold traumatic experiences.

It is interesting to note here how the vibrations created by sound can enable a release or unblocking of feelings and responses held in the body. McQuistin (2020), soprano and singing teacher, describes how the entire body is used to sing and how, most importantly, the breath is utilised. However, for survivors whose body is the very source of pain and fear, the body's protective measures can prevent them from connecting to their breath to the point that 'the very act of feeling the body's vibrations and sensations, to use them as markers, is disproportionately difficult' (McQuistin, 2020, p.425). The act of singing requires an individual to give up some control over their bodies and sounds to create resonance with their voice. McQuistin heeds caution of the importance of a safe container for survivors to connect to their body and the energy that is released through the voice, whilst also acknowledging the profoundly healing effects of reclaiming and connecting to one's voice because it supports survivors to connect to their bodies.

I have found that through using my voice in different ways, I can alter my physiological state through nervous system activation. As previously outlined, singing, with its long exhales, can activate our social engagement system, whilst shouting or screaming is a sympathetic nervous system 'fight' activation. As I described at the beginning of this chapter, screaming was a way for me to release the anger held in my body as the vocal sounds released a long overdue 'fight' response to abuse – my rightful anger about what happened. With internal and external safety, screaming releases a 'stuck' sympathetic fight response that was unable to be expressed at the time when the trauma(s) took place. With Polyvagal Theory and the body's different automatic responses to threat, we can understand that the 'freeze' (dorsal vagal) autonomic nervous system response happens when 'fight/flight' fails or is too dangerous – which is most commonly the case with childhood abuse where fighting or running away from the perpetrator is rarely an option because of a dependence on them for survival. Accessing the voice in this way helps us move 'up' from a freeze/dorsal vagal response where we experience helplessness, dissociation, and immobility as the body 'shuts down' in order to survive.

When we facilitated a group vocal meditation for the 'Screaming at The Sea' public workshop, the aim was to create a powerful and connecting experience that would help facilitate a level of comfort and emotional safety for the participants. Through meditative group singing exercises, we co-created safety as a group and were able to activate our social engagement system. With this sense of safety and through both self- and co-regulation, we moved on to screaming, shouting, and wailing, and were able to actively mobilise collectively, supporting one another in expressing our anger and rage.

In Conclusion: Community, Healing, and Performance

When we enter a stage of healing that involves learning how to be safe in relationship with others, we begin to experience seeing and being seen. As Shayda Kafai explains regarding Sins Invalid performance events that are run by and for disabled, queer, and transgender people of colour: 'When in community, we feel our way back to ourselves and away from the ableist belief that we are inherently broken and unworthy of celebration and love' (2022, p.50).

Kafai (p.44) describes how 'crip centric liberated zones' have helped them 'arrive at a place of abundance and rootedness' because they found their disabled, queer, or colour community. They view this community building as a 'somatic experience' where they could feel the joyous embodied sensation of being seen, as opposed to feeling the physical effects of being disconnected from themselves and the community.

Performances, workshops, and other alternative group spaces can play an important role in the healing journey as they allow for collective experiences, and for individuals to situate themselves within a 'we' – to be a part of something larger than themselves. For those who experienced developmental abuse, the ability to trust and feel safe with others has been actively diminished. Creating spaces for community healing can be essential to practice feeling safe with others. As Porges writes, 'this feeling of safety *is* the treatment' (2017, p.187).

Writing about the role that performance plays in supporting these safe enough spaces where healing can happen, authors have considered how socially engaged performance can 'move beyond social utility and position performance as a mode of care that exists somewhere in-between art and social practice' (Fisher, 2020, p.7). The workshop described in this chapter functioned as a form of alternative community space, sitting between an exploration of healing and artistic practice to bring into question our individual and collective relationship to the sea and the voice. In developing the workshop with my co-facilitator and opening up possibilities for the participants, I was able to create and facilitate an interdependent practice that demonstrates how there is much experiential wisdom to be gained through community-focussed work to heal trauma. I learned so much by sharing my practice and inviting others into it as it sparked an in-depth journey into embodied healing. The public workshop demonstrates how we can draw effectively on trauma-informed therapeutic models and on the knowledge of the impact of trauma on the nervous system, body, and voice to explore ways of creating spaces for healing in groups.

As we understand the nervous system, we understand how being in community can have such profound effects on feeling valued and connected, how it counters the silencing of emotions characteristic of trauma, and how it is a healing practice in itself. It seems vital to create such safe spaces in community where it becomes possible to speak out, express our feelings, and share our experiences.

References

Austin, D. (2008). *The theory and practice of vocal psychotherapy: Songs of the self.* Jessica Kingsley Publishers.

Banks, S. (2023, February 15). *The shoulders on which we stand.* Retrieved from https://grieftending.org/about-us/

Brown, A., Grooten, H., & Rosen, D. (2020). *Voice and trauma: Where are we at?* Online panel discussion hosted by The Voice and Trauma Group. Retrieved from https://vimeo.com/459684682

Fisher, A. S. (2020). Introduction: Caring performance, performing care. In A. S. Fisher & J. Thompson (Eds.), *Performing care: New perspectives on socially engaged performance.* (pp. 1–17). Manchester University Press.

Kafai, S. (2022). *Crip kinship: The disability justice & art activism of Sins Invalid.* Arsenal Pulp Press.

Levine, P. (1997). *Walking the tiger.* North Atlantic Books.

McQuistin, L. (2020). The effects of childhood sexual abuse on singers. *Journal of Singing,* March/April 2020, 76(4), pp. 423–428.

Piepzna-Samarasinha, L. L. (2021). *Care work: Dreaming disability justice.* Arsenal Pulp Press.

Porges, S. (2017). *The pocket guide to the polyvagal theory: The transformative power of feeling safe.* W. W. Norton & Company.

Price, M. (2015). The bodymind problem and the possibilities of pain. *Hypatia,* 30(1), Winter 2015, pp. 268–284.

Reynolds, A. (2022). *Introduction to vocal psychotherapy.* Online Zoom talk hosted by The Voice and Trauma Group. Retrieved from https://vimeo.com/674498661

Schwartz, R. (2021). *No bad parts: Healing trauma and resorting wholeness.* Sounds True.

van der Kolk, B. A. (2014). *The body keeps the score*. Penguin Books.
Sharp, G. (2021). *Anger*. Sticky Fingers Publishing.
Sharp, G. (2022a). *(Re)Claiming agency: Care trauma and the medical institution*. Self-published zine.
Sharp, G. (2022b). *Screaming at the sea: Rage and grief*. Self-published zine.
Walker, P. (2013). *Complex PTSD: From surviving to thriving*. Azure Coyote.

Chapter 13

Embodied Theatre Practice Towards the Creation of New Meaning

Ailin Conant

Introduction

This chapter interrogates the way that new meanings are created through embodied theatre practice which responds to trauma. It is centred around a practice-as-research project on embodied meaning-making in theatre, considered through the dual lens of trauma theory and cognitive studies. My research sought to develop a directorial practice which facilitated the embodied creation of meaning. This was explored through a cross-community participatory theatre production in Derry, Northern Ireland, which examined personal and collective memories of the Troubles.

Meaning-making can include several dimensions depending on the interpretative paradigms of researchers (Waters et al., 2013). Trauma therapies include several approaches including verbal narrative (Zaleski, 2018), creative expressive (Sajnani & Johnson, 2014; Tuval-Mashiach et al., 2018), and embodied (Levine, 2010; van der Kolk, 2015). While the entry point into the psyche differs across these, they largely agree in the way they articulate trauma as a dissociation or splitting of different self-parts, and an inability for meanings to cohere across them (Bohleber, 2007; Crossley, 2000; Laub, 2005; Sewell & Williams, 2002). In the face of trauma, 'new meanings' are needed to reframe or buffer the traumatic experience, and to restore stability and coherence to a person's identity and worldview.

As a devising physical and visual theatre director trained in Lecoq pedagogy, I have developed a practical understanding of the way that meaning is constructed multimodally[1] through theatre. When working in contexts of trauma, I have seen how transformative the embodied, visual, and symbolic elements of a play can be, for audiences and creators alike. This has been apparent even when non-verbal aesthetic forms were emphasised over fidelity to a literal truth or a verbal story. Despite this, I have struggled to find precise language within the field of performance and trauma which articulates the specific mechanisms of meaning-construction in my theatre practice, finding more alignment with the discussions of multimodal meaning-making taking place in cognitive studies and cognitive trauma theory. These discussions offer new

DOI: 10.4324/9781003322375-17

insight into the specific ways that the generative models which organise meanings are constructed and updated through embodied action (Clark, 2015; Murphy, 2018). Critically, research in cognitive studies evidences the way that embodied processes feed into more abstract symbolic and verbal processes to produce models of self and world that are grounded in and informed by our primary embodied experience.

Cognitive linguist Barbara Dancygier (2016, p. 39) writes:

> Multimodality of theatre is the source of not only its meaning potential, but also of its complexity. The interaction between the material, the embodied and the linguistic is intricate, and relies on a number of dimensions: visual perception, frame evocation, conceptualization of the human body, understanding of space and, last but not least, the language.

Dancygier highlights the difficulty in tracking the complex interplay between modalities. My research attempts to pinpoint the specific and iterative ways that meanings are multimodally constructed through theatre. Key to untangling this is understanding the role that body and environments play in its construction. In this chapter, I will interrogate some of the ways that I used theatrical techniques from Lecoq pedagogy to construct 'meaning' in theatre that responds to trauma, analysing these techniques through an embodied and schema-based model of meaning-making drawn from cognitive science.

My overview of the critical context is divided into two areas. In the first, I present articulations of multimodal cognition as it relates to meaning-making in trauma and performance studies, tracing the way that Freudian conceptions of non-rational abreaction and rational meaning-construction are still central to current debates. Through this discussion, I will identify a need for performance and trauma scholarship that engages with non-rational and non-verbal modes of new meaning creation. In the second, I highlight key theatre making techniques from my Lecoq training and devising directing practice, connecting these to recent developments in cognitive studies which have been particularly useful for considering how meaning is constructed multimodally through theatre which responds to trauma.

The enquiry described in this chapter has been conducted through Robin Nelson's (2013) multimode practice-as-research methodology, adapted to an epistemological frame grounded in ecological theory (Gibson, 1977) and a participatory research paradigm (Heron & Reason, 1997). The specific practice at the centre of the research, *First Response*, was created with eight retired first responders who worked through the Troubles, and eight University of Ulster drama students. The piece was presented in Northern Ireland in February and March 2020, playing to 800+ audiences across six performances in Derry and Coleraine. In this article, I will share some of the key learnings from this production.

Critical Context

Early Trauma Theories and Multimodal Meaning-Making in Trauma and Performance

Differentiated brain function was not a mainstream idea at the time that psychological trauma was originally articulated. Freud and his contemporaries connected the somatic and symbolic expressions in the wake of trauma to a subconscious part of the psyche (Freud, 1912). This, they theorised, had to be abreacted or outwardly expressed in order to be integrated into conscious narrative memory, which they considered to be in the remit of the verbal and rational sphere (Breuer & Freud, 1955, 2009). Some early ideas around differentiated brain process did, however, emerge in this period. Jung's work (1915, 2014) was especially foundational in articulating the ways that our brains can construct meaning in multimodal ways, especially through metaphor and symbol. He drew on the thinking of William James (1890, 1994) to differentiate between 'fantasy thinking' and 'directed thinking'. The former is imagistic and associative, while the latter is logical, analytical, and scientific (Jung, 2014). Sandor Ferenczi sustained a line of inquiry rooted in the embodied experience and processing of trauma, writing: 'When the psychic system fails, the organism begins to think' (Ferenczi, 1995, p.5). A critical difference between Freud and Ferenczi's theory of trauma was that Freud came to believe that traumatic memories were actively repressed, whereas Ferenczi believed that 'no memory traces of [traumatic] impressions remain, even in the unconscious, and thus the causes of the trauma cannot be recalled from memory traces' (Ferenczi, 2019, p.240). This led to widely different theories around how to access traumas to reintegrate them later, with Ferenczi emphasising the importance of accessing the trauma through embodied repetition. Ferenczi brought this physical thinking directly into his practice, pioneering a therapeutic methodology which emphasised the need for the therapist to take an empathetic approach to client relationship, physically being the reparative attachment figure instead of just analytically discussing the client's psyche (Mucci, 2017; Rachman, 1997).

These nascent articulations of multimodality, and their cognitively different access points through which to integrate trauma, are reflected in the way that approaches to trauma therapy are broadly divided today, with most approaches falling into 'top-down' (rational/narrative), 'side-door' (symbolic/metaphorical), or 'bottom-up' (somatic/embodied) categories. Theatre is notable in its construction of meaning across all of these domains, combining embodied action, symbolic expression, and spoken text into new theatrical narratives. Despite this, performance theory that investigates trauma tends to draw heavily on literary trauma theory, which in turn is grounded in Freud's top-down view of trauma integration (Schönfelder, 2013). As Balaev (2008, p.151) writes, the formulations of trauma and memory

> based on the abreactive model and informed primarily by Freud, have become an important source for the theorization of literary trauma studies [...] This form of literary trauma theory makes several important claims about trauma, stating that traumatic experience is repetitious, timeless, unspeakable, yet, it is also a literal, contagious, and mummified event.

This theoretical foundation results in a schism in the way that meaning-making is theorised across rational, symbolising, and embodied modes of meaning-creation in performance and trauma. Verbal or articulable meanings are linked to integration and healing on the one hand (Sepinuck, 2013) or to a falsely imposed, inauthentic coherence on the other (Little, 2015; Schneider, 2001); while somatic and symbolic meanings are linked to pathological rupture on the one hand, or the 'authenticity' of the traumatic representation on the other (Duggan, 2018; Stuart Fisher, 2011; Haughton, 2018).

In *Performance in Place of War*, Thompson et al. (2009) define traumatic memory as something that a survivor must 'transform into narrative memory', asserting that the implied treatment that emerges from this definition – 'speaking about or talking through their past' – can be connected to 'a range of cultural practices such as testimonial performance or storytelling' (p.33). The authors point to the efficacy of non-verbal multimodal performance approaches like 'songs, dances, laments and games' (p.34), using this to critique what they call the 'trauma/healing paradigm' as insufficiently broad to include these multimodal expressive forms. This critique is illustrative of the way that trauma and healing are often connected to verbal narrative forms of treatment within theatre and performance scholarship.

Theatre scholars who do include non-linear and non-verbal dramaturgies within their consideration of the trauma/healing paradigm are still informed by the abreactive model, highlighting the authenticity of non-verbal expressive forms, and critiquing the documentary narrative approach as inadequate and inauthentic in its (re)presentation of trauma. Suzanne Little (2015, p.48) argues that 'editing and arranging the individual testimonial accounts to fit within a causal linear narrative produces a coherence that belies traumatic experience'. Little finds more promise in an approach to dramaturgical representations of trauma which reflect the form of traumatic experience itself. This is echoed by Duggan (2018) who argues that – contrary to Peggy Phelan's (2003) assertion that trauma cannot be represented – trauma can be represented through the non-rational form of traumatic expressions themselves. He proposes that 'a more accurate reading may be to suggest that trauma is beyond representation outside of the representational trauma-symptoms' (Duggan, 2018, p.27). This leads to his definition of trauma-tragedy (p.174):

> Trauma-tragedy does not imply a performance of violence or shocking imagery, although this may be part of it, but rather it is a mode of performance which attends to trauma through one or many of its key terms, for example: cyclical/repetitious, paradoxical, dichotomous, polysemic, uncomfortable, visceral, emotional, kinaesthetic, uncanny, 'real'.

Duggan's definition of trauma-tragedy includes key terms that are connected to the repeated intrusions and ruminations of trauma, like 'cyclical/repetitious', and trauma's dissociation and psychic splitting, like 'dichotomous' and 'paradoxical'. However, it also includes terms that are connected to everyday non-traumatic multimodal cognition like 'visceral', 'emotional', and 'kinaesthetic'. His definition highlights the association that currently exists in the dominant discussions in the field of performance and trauma, where non-rational representational modes are closely connected to the paradoxical and unresolved expressions of a stuck trauma, and are therefore overlooked as potential avenues for new meaning-production. Metaphorical and poetic theatrical modes are conflated with trauma-tragedy, which 'does not propose a world view which could be identified as a resolution, or way to achieve resolution, of traumatic schism' (Duggan, 2018, p.174). This implies that resolution and transformation can only occur through a direct connection to a decathected traumatic experience, or from the critical reflection that this encounter facilitates, as opposed to the creation of new meaning through embodied or metaphoric process. There is a gap in the existing trauma and performance literature with regards to the potential of multimodal theatrical forms to integrate trauma through new meanings, especially of those which are non-verbal and non-rational. To bridge this gap, I turn to the ways that multimodal meaning construction is theorised in cognitive science, connecting this to specific tools used in my own theatre making practice.

Multimodal Meaning-Making in Theatre and Cognition

In the relatively newer field of theatre and cognition, trauma is not explicitly theorised, but the nature of meaning as well as its multimodal construction is. Theatre and cognition scholars point to the way that cognition (and therefore meaning-making) is embodied, embedded, and distributed, co-created by people and their environments (Kemp & McConachie, 2019). Murphy (2018, p.11), who explores Lecoq-based practice through an enactivist lens, writes: 'In terms of Lecoq pedagogy, as an actor begins an exercise, she is simultaneously forging her own identity as an actor-creator and creating a matrix of meanings for it'.

This idea of a 'matrix of meanings' is consistent with Andy Clark's (2015) predictive processing (PP) framework which proposes that the brain is organised in dynamic and hierarchically structured networks, each involved in predictively representing models of ourselves and our environments at different levels of specificity across space and time in order to shape perception and drive action (Clark, 2015; Seth, 2014, 2021). Meaning-making within this framework is not relegated to the rational sphere. It is a creative process which draws on multimodal models, or schemas, which are grounded in and iteratively connected to our embodied process. This means that our embodied experience informs our so-called rational narratives and meaning structures, just as our rational thoughts help form our embodied experience.

Through my research, I identified four key theatre making techniques which are important to the production of new meaning in response to trauma. In this section, I will discuss these in relation to cognitive science research which helps to explain the underlying cognitive mechanisms that they are describing.

Embodiment

In Lecoq pedagogy, language, and thought are considered in relation to movement and physicality. Rick Kemp (2019) presents a case study from a Lecoq class to illustrate the embodied nature of language. Students from different countries are grouped by their native language and asked to create a simple gesture that illustrates the phrase 'je prends' ('I take'). Each actor's experience of a word or concept is grounded in their own unique physiology and lived experience to produce a slightly different felt sense connected to it. This is consistent with the embodied basis of conceptualisation, the idea within cognitive studies that we understand objects and concepts in direct relation to the way that we experience them through our body. All concepts, even at the level of language are 'modal' insofar as they are understood in connection to sensorimotor information (Barsalou et al., 2003). Lakoff and Johnson (1999, 2008) extend this idea to argue that all conceptualisations are bootstrapped from embodied modal experiences, like 'up', 'take', or 'far', which are used as scaffolding to construct increasingly complex ideas.

In order to engage the body, actors in Lecoq training use techniques of imagination and repetition. These exercises are designed to augment a performer's sensorimotor activation in connection with the text. Theatre and cognition scholars often highlight the modality of language in order to challenge mind-body binaries in theatre practice. Rhonda Blair (2010, p.11) points out how terms like 'be in your body' or 'get out of your head' are useful as they help increase the degree of embodiment, but also problematic as they perpetuate false binaries. In acknowledging their utility but also the problem in separating body and head, Blair suggests that the sensorimotor activation connected to language is – as Lakoff and Johnson theorised – ever-present, but also – as Lecoq implies – *variable*, and that, as theatre makers, we have tools to increase or decrease it. This is particularly relevant in the context of working with survivors of trauma who may be able to engage with narrative text around their trauma in a distal way, but may struggle with hyperarousal when asked to increase their level of embodiment – or somatosensory activation – in connection to this language.

Transposition

Transposition involves the mapping of qualities from one cognitive model to another. It is a foundation element of Lecoq training. In animal study, we borrow from the known attributes of something non-human, to 'humanise an element of an animal' (Lecoq, 2000, p.45). The same is done with elements like water, air, and clay. This connects to the concept in cognitive science of 'cross-modal abstraction', which is the direct mapping of features from one modality onto a new one. If we were building a character around 'air' for example, the lightness of air – which we connect to a sense of weightlessness in movement – may translate into a high wafty voice, cross-modally abstracting embodied movement information to give it a value in terms of pitch and resonance. Transposition also involves cross-modal association, which is the correlation of non-redundant information across different modalities (Ramachandran, 2012). As our predictive pattern-seeking models make sense of the world through the correlation and clustering of traits that tend to go together, cross-modal abstractions can bring further cross-modal associations. In our example, the wafty voice may in turn evoke an association with 'hippie', connecting this character to a slew of new meaning structures which organise behaviours, character traits, and psychology. Transposition expands the multimodal complexity of an idea, object, or character, augmenting its existing meaning structures. In so doing, it offers us new multimodal avenues through which to play and engage with them.

Play

For Lecoq, the power of transposition exists in its ability to generate meaning through the body at a metaphorical or poetic level directly through embodied play, or 'le jeu' (Lecoq, 2000). As Mark Evans writes in his introduction to *The Moving Body*:

> The idea of the poetic body and the idea of play are deeply entwined [...] Play is strongly related to the body's potential for transposition and for transformation, to the role of the body in our ability to understand and to make sense of the world around us.
>
> (Evans, 2000, pp.xvi–xxxv)

Play in this way is conceived as an engagement between actor and environment and is considered a creative act. This description is consistent with the idea that cognition is embedded, insofar as our embodied cognitive processes are constrained by – and therefore partly constituted by – the environments that our organisms are embedded in. Gibson (1977) further nuanced this with his theory of 'affordances' and the idea that objects and environments are understood through what we – with our own body and its specific limitations – can actively do with them. Gibson's principle of affordances theoretically grounds the idea that play is creative by illustrating the way that explorative physical play can lead to both meaning production and knowledge acquisition. If our understanding of an object or environment is grounded in what we can physically do with it, then the way to change or increase our knowledge of it is to explore it in an embodied way. When combined with Lakoff and Johnson's (2008) ideas around cognitive scaffolding, this concept suggests that meaning at more abstract levels of cognition can also be generated through embodied play.

Theatrical Juxtaposition

In addition to the Lecoq-specific techniques, a fourth idea from cognitive science emerged as particularly relevant to the research. The notion of 'conceptual blending', as defined by Fauconnier and Turner (2008), is a deep cognitive activity that combines words, images, and ideas in a network of mental spaces to make new meanings out of old. The mind, they propose, is capable of containing multiple conceptual models. The process of blending these results in the creation of an emergent structure which has new and more information than the original blended inputs. This is connected to the theatrical technique of juxtaposition which describes ways in which different elements are presented together, in order to emphasise differences, reveal similarities, or explore a unique relationship between them. Cook (2007) describes the way that blending theory provides a method to understand how resonant connections and new meanings emerge through multimodal practice. Conceptual blending also helps nuance the predictive processing (PP) model of meaning (Clark, 2015) because it demonstrates the way that multiple generative models can coexist, actively updating and informing one another. Bruce McConachie (2012) and Rhonda Blair (2009) have highlighted the way that this process is employed explicitly by actors in their blended conceptualisation of self and role. The playing of a role requires actors to engage the character's experience imaginatively, while at the same time maintaining a sense of self that is separate from the character. These conceptualisations are 'blended' because at moments they share connections, and the simultaneous existence of both brings new meanings and new possibilities to each.

Research and Methodology in *First Response*

In the remaining half of this chapter, I will present reflections on the practice-as-research project *First Response* through the lens of the critical context and the four theatrical techniques outlined above. I will focus my analysis on the way these techniques were variously employed, as well as the specific obstacles that I encountered in my practice, and the learning that I took from these.

The aim of my research is to investigate how new meaning is created through multimodal theatre making which responds to and works in contexts of trauma. It is centred around the development of a directorial practice that is informed by both trauma theory and cognitive science, and is able to dynamically respond to the challenges and opportunities specific to a post-traumatic context.

The research is built on the participatory inquiry paradigm put forth by Heron and Reason (1997). As an ecological and co-creative epistemology, it is aligned with enactivism and the embodied cognition movement. It is also congruous with the Predictive Processing framework put forth by Clark (2015), highlighting the way that meanings and knowledge are embedded, embodied, and distributed.

The investigation is arts-led and its methodology is grounded in Robin Nelson's Practice as Research in the Arts model (Nelson, 2013), adapted according to Heron and Reason's (1997) extended epistemology. This methodology allowed me to consider experiential, performative, and embodied forms of knowing. This is useful as it differentiates between experiential, symbolising, and embodied modes of cognition, all of which function in unique ways and are considered separately in my research.

Research Design

First Response was a theatre project devised during a six-month residency in Derry[2], Northern Ireland, as part of a two-year Theatre and Peacebuilding Academy commissioned by the Derry Playhouse and funded by PEACE IV, an EU programme designed to support peace and reconciliation in Northern Ireland and the border region. My role was to direct a cross-community play with a retired group of first responders – frontline workers such as police officers, firefighters, nurses, and paramedics – who worked through the Troubles.

For the production I recruited eight first responders, two artists, and nine drama students. The first responders were chosen for a number of factors including but not limited to their enthusiasm for multimodal theatre devising, their specific lived experiences during the Troubles, their gender, their profession, their community affiliation, their overall mental stability and fitness to engage with the project. The University of Ulster students were selected according to their course modules and availability for the project. Through 30+ interviews, 10 workshops and rehearsal process of 18 days, we created a 75-minute devised piece grounded in short personal anecdotes and stories. The production featured a mix of stories from the past, told by the first responders, and intergenerational dialogues about the present, interrogating the place of these stories in contemporary Northern Irish society. The production engaged 800+ audience over six performances in Derry and Coleraine. A post-show panel was held at each performance.

A video of the production can be viewed here: https://vimeo.com/810948124/afdcf7ee41

Ethical Considerations

As a devising director making theatre in post-conflict settings, my work is trauma-informed and seeks to be psychologically safe. In my practice-as-research, I employ techniques designed to amplify the valence and increase the modality of text, movement, and images. The aspects of a person's story that may be most significant or theatrical for an audience may also be retraumatising for a participant-performer, or triggering for audiences or other participants, especially in cross-community post-conflict projects. In light of this, the most important ethical consideration in my dual role as an artist-facilitator was an ongoing reflexivity and 'situational ethics' (Guillemin & Gillam, 2004) to guide my practice moment-to-moment. This meant that my ethical framework was bespoke to each situation and grounded in moral relativism, so that each situation was taken into account, before deciding on absolute rules to determine what was right and wrong for the context. This was supported by procedural ethics through the University of Essex[3], where participant consent was obtained for the dissemination of my research, and Derry Playhouse Safeguarding measures which included ongoing risk assessment and the attachment of a project therapist. Additional considerations and measures put in place included a script-veto policy if performers needed to change or adapt their text, and a unified decision not to include any creative team surnames on show print and marketing material. First names were used in the production and also in this chapter. Participants gave their consent for this. The project was also externally evaluated by researchers at the University of Ulster as part of its condition for funding.

Discussion

In my discussion I will share some of the ways that we used the techniques of embodiment, transposition, play, and juxtaposition to create new meanings, highlighting where this was successful and where we encountered obstacles.

New Meanings Through Transposition and Embodied Play

I found that the project was most multimodally successful in engaging in aspects of trauma that were shared across the whole group, as this was where we were able to use our collective time to engage more deeply with specific objects and images. In early recruitment interviews for *First Response*, several of the cast often referred to their own memories – and the phenomenological felt sense of inhibition which surrounded them – as 'boxed up' or 'shut away'. They expressed a deep ambivalence in their relationship with these 'memory boxes' as they were unsure whether to engage with them ('open them') or stay dissociated (keep them 'boxed up'). As one retired firefighter explained, throughout his career the adrenaline of each successive incident allowed him to box up his memories and move on to the next event, but the mound of boxed-up memories loomed threateningly in his psyche towards the end of his career: 'As I approached retirement, I knew those boxes were still going to be there … and I just wanted so much to forget about them, and I couldn't'.

Responding to this, I brought small makeshift boxes filled with objects into very early workshops, and later worked with the set designer to create a stage that was comprised entirely of boxes.

By transposing 'memories' into 'boxes' and making them the core visual and physical element on the stage, a central question emerged as to what to do with these boxed-up memories. The physical boxes expanded the multimodality of the abstract box-images, bringing them into a material world, which opened up a new set of physical affordances in relation to them (Gibson, 1977). This allowed us to physically play with the boxes – and through them, the more abstract concept of repressed memories – in ways that we might not have been able if working cerebrally. The boxes could still be opened and closed to reveal the objects – and their associated memories – but they could also be cast aside, passed around, shared, hidden, stepped on, stepped over, sat upon, wrestled with, and so on. Critically, this physical action of playing generated a new sense of possibility and agency for the first responders vis-à-vis their memories,

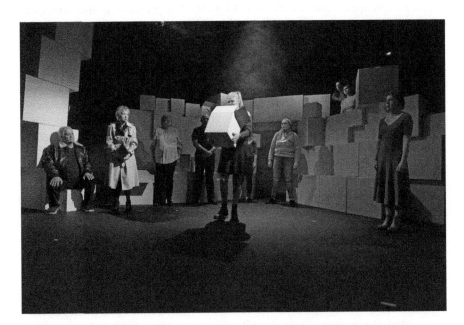

Figure 13.1 A cast member peers into a box, the symbolic space of a memory

© 2020 Gav Connolly

updating their own metaphorical understanding of their internal landscape via their embodied play. The external evaluators for Playhouse noted this in their final report:

> An example given by one of the participants illustrates the visceral power of this symbolism. How heavily or lightly he set down a box in which a hidden story was held was entirely dependent on his emotional state in that moment of performance.
>
> (Grant & Durrer, 2020, p.25)

In this way, the relationship between the physical construction of a metaphor and the performers' subsequent playing could be iterative, with the objects affording the performers a way of engaging and relating directly with intangible meaning structures, like the concept of repressed memories. This extends Lakoff and Johnson's assertion that high-order concepts are scaffolded onto primary embodied metaphors (Lakoff & Johnson, 2008). Theatrical transposition and embodied play allow actors to reengage with the primary metaphors to create new meanings. By bringing the high-order concept of 'boxed-up memory' into the material embodied world of objects, the cast were afforded the change to physically play with them, and through this play update their relationship to the concept of 'memory' directly through their bodies.

What follows is an extract from my rehearsal diary that describes a spontaneous reaction from a cast member, which subsequently was transposed into a theatrical score. This entry is followed by a link to an excerpt of the performance showing that transposition.

> *Jim begins what I recognise as one of his more difficult-to-process experiences: "A little old lady who looked like everyone's favourite granny, with her blue rinse… No." The "No" is a visceral reflex, he pushes the recorder away and I immediately stop recording. With Jim's abrupt "no" we all feel the door to his memory slamming shut. With the recorder off, Jim is able to slowly walk us through some of the imagery that is most difficult for him. He explains why the physical position that the granny was left in by the impact of a vehicle was an assault on her dignity. He explains why he struggles to this day with the image of a pork fillet. He describes certain smells which he associates with road traffic accidents.*
>
> *Jim's definitive "no" is theatricalised as the ensemble urge him to confront his memories, carrying a succession of boxes towards him. "A little old lady with blue rinse…"; "Torn and twisted metal…"; "The smell of burnt flesh…" Jim shoves each box away with a firm "No", until finally one cast member gently coaxes him to open one. An LED light has been placed inside of the box, so when he opens it, Jim's pensive face is illuminated as he peers into the space of his memory. "I think… I think that's a pork fillet".*

Link to the performance: https://vimeo.com/811093003/cc21200b0e

The movement score offered Jim an opportunity to physicalise his initial 'no' and to nuance this rejection through physical choices like quality of touch, directionality and degree of force. These actions created new meaning in the moment, actively transforming his own relationship to these memories – and his own rejection of them – throughout the rehearsal and performance period. The choreography of Jim peering inside the box without explaining what he was seeing, was one that was arrived at through a long discussion about the ethics of what is and isn't said in the play. The affordances offered by the box helped to solve this debate by offering a more nuanced set of possible actions than the 'tell/don't tell' binary of asking someone to share a memory onstage.

The set design allowed to refer to the many hundreds of unopened boxes – and unshared stories – that the cast contained between them. As these boxes weren't transformed by the end of the piece, I felt that we had managed to pose a significant question – 'what should be done with these memories?' – through the use of transposition. However, the fact that the boxes remained in the same fixed position throughout the piece indicated that we hadn't managed to make use of this same technique to answer it. The norms and timescales for technical production meant that the boxes arrived *after* the script had been created, meaning that we could not physically play with them to create a dramaturgically significant ending. In addition, only a few of these boxes were structurally reinforced and secure. This meant that we could only propose the existential question of what to do with the pile of memories in a cerebral and abstract way. On reflection, it would have been useful to have started the process with a room full of reinforced boxes on the first day of rehearsal, allowing the company to physically 'solve' the dramatic question of how this image could transform or change by the end of the piece. This could have been done through a process of physical exploration and play, instead of sitting around a table discussing possible ways of transforming the set.

Trauma and Aesthetic Limitations

There were several transpositions that we played with in the workshop process that never made it into the production, because within the timescale and multi-participant format that we were working in, it didn't feel appropriate to ask people to engage with potentially traumatising images in an embodied way. The increased sensorimotor activation of engaging with these images physically brought with them the potential to cause physiological arousal and distress, meaning that more time was needed to work with them in a way that was sensitive and ethical.

This complexity shaped many aspects of the rehearsal process, and ultimately had aesthetic implications on the production. For example, when we worked with a movement artist to explore the vocabularies of movement from the first responders' careers, an ambulance person experienced physiological freezing and distress when he considered a situation in which he was lying prone as he responded to a shooting. The same participant had been able to tell the story of the shooting verbally on several occasions without exhibiting any distress, but when asked to physically place himself in the position he had been in during the event, he physically froze and responded that he couldn't take the position.

We faced a similar difficulty when working with text-based theatrical techniques designed to essentialise or distil the narrative meaning of events through poetic writing. Poetic techniques like repetition can condense time and selectively amplify aspects of someone's experience. Coupled with the theatrical imperative to speak text in an embodied way, spoken poetic text can work to amplify both affective arousal and somatosensory engagement in relation to an image or theme. In one rehearsal, I worked with the idea of 'lists' with the hopes of creating a multi-layered and poetic vocal soundscape. A member of the group who had lost several professional colleagues during their career was reading out a list of fallen comrades. In her list, she included the methods of death – most of her colleagues had been killed by IRA shootings or bombs. Another member of the group interjected and asked for proof that this list was verifiable. They felt that the IRA actions were being presented unfairly and out of context, and that including this list in the production would present an unbalanced view. This event led to a major disagreement which split the group and took several days to resolve. This incident illustrates the way that increasing the affective and somatosensory effect of text or images can be volatile in a post-conflict setting, especially when working with cross-community groups who are likely to have upsetting, personally significant, and conflicting meaning structures connected to these words and images.

Despite my pedagogical and artistic commitment to non-verbal and embodied forms of meaning construction, a literal and linear form of fact-based storytelling became one of the most utilised aesthetic languages in the piece. Theatre techniques which were specifically designed to promote symbolic expression, affective arousal, and embodiment were at times too volatile, complicated, or uncomfortable for us to pursue within the limited timescale and in the ensemble format of rehearsal. Storytelling, on the other hand, borrowed on skills that the participants were already familiar with, and called upon pre-formed narratives that the participants had already rehearsed and honed through past conversation. As such, it was the theatrical style that was most easily and ethically employed when working to generate material quickly with a large cohort of people who had all lived through different specific traumas. The fact that these confidently spoken narratives had the potential to cause distress when explored through an embodied or symbolic approach is an indication that 'integration' is not easily connected to the simple ability to form a coherent verbal story. The participants in *First Response* showed an incredible ability to keep the somatosensory activation and hyperarousal connected to the meanings of their words at bay, as long as they were not asked to increase this activation through transposition, embodiment, and play.

Conceptual Blends and Complex Emergent Meanings

For narrative reasons, I was interested to incorporate into the larger piece the story of today's young people in Northern Ireland, to ground the production in the lasting effects of the Troubles, and bring the thrust of the action to the present moment. I also had a presentational desire for the embodied and visceral immediacy that young, mobile actors could bring to the stories that were shared. This is what led me to collaborate with students from the University of Ulster Drama Department.

What was notable about the young performers was that even if they weren't the young people most affected by the conflict, onstage they nevertheless became a clear embodiment of Northern Ireland's affected next generation, and greatly increased the opportunities to explore and create new narrative meanings both rationally and symbolically. As physical performers, they were able to create embodied imagery that brought new dimensions to the First Responders' stories, as can be seen in the following excerpt: https://vimeo.com/811115744

As collaborators, the young people were able to bring a fresh perspective into the rehearsal process, and – when given the space to do so – to gently challenge the centrality of the 'war stories' in the production and, by extension, in Northern Irish society as a whole. This challenge was supported by the transposed boxes, as seeing the young people surrounded by the older generations' memories made it viscerally clear how much space these stories take up, affecting all generations of Northern Irish society. A scene illustrating this challenge can be seen in the following excerpt: https://vimeo.com/811110760/a01aa10914

However, the most interesting meanings did not emerge from the young people 'being' themselves or 'being' the first responders, but from their simultaneous ability to inhabit a blended space between the two. It was in this ambiguous space of complex and colliding schemas that some of the most affecting and interesting new meanings were able to unfold. In this blended space, we saw the older generation imagining their own histories played out in these young lives, or seeing themselves in their memories as the extremely young people that they were at the time. Here was a more subtle form of interrogation, investigation, and challenge from the young performers who fumbled to perform the first responder's movements. In the end, it was this complex dialogue between older and younger generation that was identified as the most meaningful aspect of the production by cast and audience alike.

Conclusion

This research has highlighted the iterative relationship between abstract concepts and embodied experience, and has demonstrated how the tools of transposition and embodied play can be used to generate new multimodal meanings through theatre. The work with the boxes demonstrated theatre's ability to use transposition to map complex concepts onto objects that could be played with in a direct embodied way, creating new physically grounded and conceptually complex meanings. In addition, the research has shown that theatrical forms like poetic repetition and embodiment which were designed to increase sensorimotor engagement and affective arousal took more time to work with sensitively, meaning that logistical constraints including limited time and large cohort size could limit the aesthetic possibility. In our production, this meant that the more familiar aesthetic forms – like storytelling – were privileged over other forms like poetic repetition and working with transposed movement and images. The research also showed that creative choices made for aesthetic reasons – like the inclusion of a young ensemble who could create interesting visual images – could bring new dimensions of meaning to the piece, in unexpected or novel ways. Some of the most interesting meanings emerged from the complex relational space of blended schemas, where different perspectives and meaning structures could dialogue and inform one another in nuanced ways.

A central limitation of this research was the inability to explore individual traumas and traumatic images in great depth, due largely to the collective cross-community model of the project and the sensitivities of working with traumatised people who had very different experiences of the conflict. A lack of time was also a major limitation. As a cross-disciplinary, multimodal research project, the inquiry required a broad focus throughout, limiting the time available to pursue specific avenues more deeply, even as clear opportunities for further exploration became clear.

There are two key areas of study in particular that deserve deeper exploration. The first would be working in a deeper multimodal way with one individual, or a group of professionals supporting one participant, to explore their personal traumatic images. The second would be working with a group to collectively create new complex conceptual meanings through material action and play. This could be done through a collective engagement with a transposed object (like the boxes), working together physically to find an embodied, non-rational solution to a metaphorical problem.

Overall, this research has drawn on cognitive science to demonstrate how new meaning was created in a post-conflict project through embodied theatre techniques that were not strictly verbal or rational. While as an artist my practice is centred on meaning-construction and not trauma integration, my hope is that theatre artists and dramatherapists alike can build on these findings, and continue to explore the multimodal ways that new meanings can be created in theatre that responds to trauma.

Notes

1 Multimodality refers to the various theatrical vocabularies used in the expression and communication of meaning (movement, sound, symbol, text, visual design, etc.) in terms of how they relate holistically. This is in keeping with Leigh and Brown's (2021, p.30) definition of multimodality as 'multiple means of making meaning', and Jewitt et al.'s (2016) assertion that meanings must be considered as a 'multimodal whole'.

2 Derry is a small town with a vibrant arts community on the border of Northern Ireland and Ireland. It was the sight of several notable incidents during the recent 30-year civil conflict, including the Battle of the Bogside in 1969 (widely regarded as the beginning of "the Troubles") and Bloody Sunday (1972). National focus on the stories of Derry in the past four decades have including two formal inquiries into Bloody Sunday: the 1972 Widgery Inquiry and the 1998 Saville Inquiry.
3 The research was conducted as part of a practice-as-research PhD at East 15, University of Essex.

References

Balaev, M. (2008). Trends in literary trauma theory. *Mosaic: A Journal for the Interdisciplinary Study of Literature*, 149–166.

Barsalou, L. W., Niedenthal, P. M., Barbey, A. K., & Ruppert, J. A. (2003). Social embodiment. In B. H. Ross (Ed.), *The psychology of learning and motivation: Advances in research and theory*, 43(1), 43–92. Elsevier Science.

Blair, R. (2009). Cognitive neuroscience and acting: Imagination, conceptual blending, and empathy. *The Drama Review*, 53(4), 93–103.

Blair, R. (2010). Acting, embodiment, and text: *Hedda Gabler* and possible uses of cognitive science. *Theatre Topics*, 20(1), 11–21. https://doi.org/10.1353/tt.0.0087

Bohleber, W. (2007). Remembrance, trauma and collective memory: The battle for memory in psychoanalysis. *The International Journal of Psychoanalysis*, 88(2), 329–352.

Breuer, J. & Freud, S. (1955). On the psychical mechanism of hysterical phenomena: Preliminary communication from studies on hysteria. In *The standard edition of the complete psychological works of Sigmund Freud, Volume II (1893–1895): Studies on hysteria* (pp. 1–17). Hogarth Press.

Breuer, J. & Freud, S. (2009). *Studies on hysteria*. Hachette UK.

Clark, A. (2015). *Surfing uncertainty: Prediction, action, and the embodied mind*. Oxford University Press.

Cook, A. (2007). Interplay: The method and potential of a cognitive scientific approach to theatre. *Theatre Journal*, 59(4), 579–594. https://doi.org/10.1353/tj.2008.0015

Crossley, M. L. (2000). *Introducing narrative psychology: Self, trauma and the construction of meaning*. Open University Press

Dancygier, B. (2016). Multimodality and theater: Material objects, bodies and language. *Theatre, Performance and Cognition: Languages, Bodies and Ecologies*, 21–39.

Duggan, P. (2018). *Trauma-Tragedy: Symptoms of contemporary performance*. Manchester University Press.

Evans, M. (2000). Introduction. In J. Lecoq (Ed.), *The moving body: Teaching creative theatre* (pp. xvi–xxxv). Bloomsbury Publishing.

Fauconnier, G. & Turner, M. (2008). *The way we think: Conceptual blending and the mind's hidden complexities*. Basic books.

Ferenczi, S. (1995). *The clinical diary of Sándor Ferenczi*. Harvard University Press.

Ferenczi, S. (2019). *Final contributions to the problems and methods of psycho-analysis*. Taylor and Francis.

Freud, S. (1912). *Selected papers on hysteria and other psychoneuroses*. Journal of Nervous and Mental Disease Publishing Company.

Gibson, J. J. (1977). *The theory of affordances*. Erlbaum Associates.

Grant, D. & Durrer, V. (2020). *'Living and learning': An evaluation of the Playhouse Theatre & Peacebuilding Academy*. Retrieved from https://pureadmin.qub.ac.uk/ws/portalfiles/portal/222746356/PLAYHOUSE_PEACE_ACADEMY_REPORT_Final_.pdf

Guillemin, M. & Gillam, L. (2004). Ethics, reflexivity, and 'ethically important moments' in research. *Qualitative Inquiry*, 10(2), 261–280.

Haughton, M. (2018). *Staging trauma: Bodies in shadow*. Springer.

Heron, J. & Reason, P. (1997). A participatory inquiry paradigm. *Qualitative Inquiry*, 3(3), 274–294.

James, W. (1890). *The principles of psychology*. Henry Holt and Company.

James, W. (1994). The physical basis of emotion. *Psychological Review*, 101(2), 205–210. https://doi.org/10.1037/0033-295X.101.2.205

Jewitt, C., Bezemer, J., & O'Halloran, K. (2016). *Introducing multimodality*. Routledge.

Jung, C. G. (1915). *Psychology of the unconscious*. Kegan Paul.

Jung, C. G. (2014). *Collected works of CG Jung, Volume 5: Symbols of transformation* (Vol. 7). Princeton University Press.

Kemp, R. (2019). Acting technique, Jacques Lecoq and embodied meaning. In R. Kemp & B. A. McConachie (Eds.), *The Routledge companion to theatre, performance, and cognitive science* (pp. 177–190). Routledge.

Kemp, R. & McConachie, B. A. (2019). *The Routledge companion to theatre, performance, and cognitive science*. Routledge.

Lakoff, G. & Johnson, M. (1999). *Philosophy in the flesh: The embodied mind and its challenge to western thought*. Basic books.

Lakoff, G. & Johnson, M. (2008). *Metaphors we live by*. University of Chicago press.

Laub, D. (2005). Traumatic shutdown of narrative and symbolization: A death instinct derivative? *Contemporary Psychoanalysis*, 41(2), 307–326.

Lecoq, J. (2000). *The moving body: Teaching creative theatre*. Bloomsbury Publishing.

Leigh, J. & Brown, N. (2021). *Embodied inquiry: Research methods*. Bloomsbury Publishing.

Levine, P. A. (2010). *In an unspoken voice: How the body releases trauma and restores goodness*. North Atlantic Books.

Little, S. (2015). Repeating repetition: Trauma and performance. *Performance Research*, 20(5), 44–50.

McConachie, B. (2012). *Theatre and mind*. Macmillan International Higher Education.

Mucci, C. (2017). Ferenczi's revolutionary therapeutic approach. *The American Journal of Psychoanalysis*, 77(3), 239–254.

Murphy, M. (2018). *Enacting Lecoq: Movement in theatre, cognition, and life*. Springer.

Nelson, R. (2013). *Practice as research in the arts: Principles, protocols, pedagogies, resistances*. Springer.

Phelan, P. (2003). *Unmarked: The politics of performance*. Routledge.

Rachman, A. W. (1997). *Sándor Ferenczi: The psychotherapist of tenderness and passion*. Jason Aronson.

Ramachandran, V. S. (2012). *The tell-tale brain: Unlocking the mystery of human nature*. Random House.

Sajnani, N. & Johnson, D. R. (2014). *Trauma-informed drama therapy: Transforming clinics, classrooms, and communities*. Charles C Thomas Publisher.

Schneider, R. (2001). Performance remains. *Performance Research*, 6(2), 100–108.

Schönfelder, C. (2013). *Wounds and words : Childhood and family trauma in romantic and postmodern fiction*. Transcript Verlag. https://doi.org/10.26530/oapen_627792

Sepinuck, T. (2013). *Theatre of witness: Finding the medicine in stories of suffering, transformation, and peace*. Jessica Kingsley Publishers.

Seth, A. K. (2014). The cybernetic bayesian brain – from interoceptive inference to sensorimotor contingencies. *Open MIND*, 35, 1–24. https://doi.org/10.15502/9783958570108

Seth, A. (2021). *Being you: A new science of consciousness*. Penguin.

Sewell, K. W. & Williams, A. M. (2002). Broken narratives: Trauma, metaconstructive gaps, and the audience of psychotherapy. *Journal of Constructivist Psychology*, 15(3), 205–218. https://doi.org/10.1080/10720530290100442

Stuart Fisher, A. (2011). Trauma, authenticity and the limits of verbatim. *Performance Research*, 16(1), 112–122. https://doi.org/10.1080/13528165.2011.561683

Thompson, J., Balfour, M., & Hughes, J. (2009). *Performance in place of war*. Seagull Books Pvt Ltd.

Tuval-Mashiach, R., Patton, B. W., & Drebing, C. (2018). 'When you make a movie, and you see your story there, you can hold it': Qualitative exploration of collaborative filmmaking as a therapeutic tool for veterans. *Frontiers in Psychology*, 9, Article 1954. https://doi.org/10.3389/fpsyg.2018.01954

van der Kolk, B. A. (2015). *The body keeps the score: Brain, mind, and body in the healing of trauma*. Penguin Books.

Waters, T. E. A., Shallcross, J. F., & Fivush, R. (2013). The many facets of meaning making: Comparing multiple measures of meaning making and their relations to psychological distress. *Memory*, 21(1), 111–124.

Zaleski, K. (2018). *Understanding and treating military sexual trauma*. Springer.

Chapter 14

The Harmless Ghost

A Mythopoetic Approach to Trauma

Shruti Garg

Introduction

This chapter is a self-reflective account and analysis of my own lived experiences with childhood trauma while growing up as a woman and a queer identifying individual in India. The intention of this chapter is to explore trauma from a mythopoetic lens in order to actively engage in understanding the role of myths, symbols, and embodied rituals in healing, and to give a unique language of expression to one's distinct experience of trauma. I will examine different roles of mine throughout the chapter as a former student of drama-therapy[1], client in therapy, and practising drama-therapist.

The term 'mythopoetic' can be understood as a derivation from the term 'mythopoeic' which is defined as pertaining to the making or giving rise to myths (HarperCollins, 2023). I will be exploring how myths get composed in the dreams of the victims of childhood trauma and in the client–therapist relationship in psychotherapy, giving rise to a mythopoetic language or imagery. The coming together of the two terms 'myth' and 'poem' in the word 'mythopoetic' can be enlightened by what Joseph Campbell writes about myths: 'reread them [myths] as poems and they become luminous' (Campbell, 2012, p.9). Therefore, while engaging with my lived experiences, I will be looking at the universality of symbols and rituals, alongside their individual meaning held in my poetic imagination. I hope to argue how this mythopoetic language can act as a container for the memories, thoughts, emotions, ideas, and healing resources that might be unavailable to conscious awareness due to traumatic experiences. Engaging with stories, myths, rituals, or symbols is engaging with the lost resources of emotions, memories, and wisdom present in the body.

I will be exploring a mythopoetic approach to trauma, not only with reference to the unconscious psyche, but also in relation to an embodied felt experience. I wish to achieve this not just through 'what' I am writing but also 'how' I am writing about it. For instance, while exploring my experiences of the countertransference/transference relationship in therapy, I will be looking at it not just in terms of projections of the unconscious psyche, but also as an archetypal event, where myths (both private and collective) get re-enacted

DOI: 10.4324/9781003322375-18

through the embodiment of roles or archetypes within the client–therapist relationship. I hope to argue that, through the use of many unique creative tools in its theory and practice, drama-therapy effectively addresses mind and body simultaneously to facilitate embodied healing for individuals and groups.

I have been able to explore and document my experiences through different media: self-reflective essays, daily journal entries, record of my dreams over a period of two years, and personal memories. Memories can be deceiving. Working with trauma as a therapist, I remind myself that it is not so much about the accuracy of the content of the traumatic memories of the clients but about the meaning we made of them together. In this writing too, I focus upon the meaning-making of memories. Exploring one's own very vulnerable experiences has the potential to be evocative, painful, and triggering. I therefore would like to acknowledge the support systems and containers I had in the person of my therapists, supervisors, friends, and colleagues.

Social Location and Cultural Considerations

Since I will be exploring cultural and religious symbols, it is essential to name and acknowledge my social location. I grew up as a Savarna Hindu woman in a Hindi-Haryanvi speaking upper middle-class family of urban Northern India, where we had the privilege to practise our religious beliefs and rituals without any socio-political barriers.

Though I will be giving voice to some of the experiences that might be unique to the context of India, I would like to put a point of caution here for the reader to not treat my experiences as the universal experience of all the different communities and groups of India. Especially because many Western and Hindu upper caste theorists have, over the decades, promoted and assumed 'the Hindu' context as 'the Indian' context. Hinduism is one of the many religions practised on the country's diverse land. The reality of caste and ethnicity-based oppression and differences makes it imperative to be mindful of the different individual and collective meanings attached to symbols and rituals before taking them into a therapeutic setting. Multiple cultural voices of India continue to remain missing from the vast drama-therapy literature, conversations, and practices because of many systemic barriers.

The role of culture in trauma and healing in the Indian context can be understood by reflecting on the ideas and beliefs around good and evil, guilt and shame, love, sexuality, human suffering, healing, god, religion, and myths held by individuals and groups. It can be useful to be reminded of what the Indian psychoanalyst Kakar (1982) writes about the complexities of the traditions of healing in the Indian context:

> Indians have long been involved in constructing explanatory systems for psychic distress and evolving techniques for its alleviation. [...] There are the traditional physicians – the vaids of the Hindu Ayurveda and Siddha

> systems and the hakim of the Islamic unani tradition – many of whom also practice what we today call psychological medicine. In addition, there are palmists, horoscope specialists, herbalists, diviners, sorcerers and a variety of shamans, whose therapeutic efforts combine elements from classical Indian astrology, medicine, alchemy and magic, with beliefs and practices from the folk and popular traditions. And then, the ubiquitous sadhus, swamis, maharajs, babas, matas and bhagwans, who [...] claim to specialize in what in the West [...] used to be called 'soul health' – the restoration of moral and spiritual well-being.
>
> (Kakar, 1982, p.1)

We understand from this how the religious, ritualistic, or mythopoetic dimensions of understanding healing and suffering have traditionally been part of the Indian landscape. These dimensions will be explored as a vital aspect of drama-therapy to make it a unique modality for therapy that can bridge, through the embodiment of metaphors, symbols, rituals, and stories, traditional healing practices and psychotherapy in the field of trauma.

Explaining Trauma

There is not one single definition of trauma. Through this writing, I have engaged with different definitions relevant to the inquiry of this chapter. I refer to the literature in the fields of psychodynamic and analytical (Jungian) schools of thought, alongside trauma-informed care, drama-therapy and expressive arts therapies (Kalsched, 1996; Sajnani & Johnson, 2014; Herman, 1992; Malchiodi, 2020). Herman's (1992, p.33) definition of trauma stands close to my experiences:

> Psychological trauma is an affiliation of the powerless. At the moment of trauma, the victim is rendered helpless by overwhelming force. When the force is that of nature, we speak of disasters. When the force is that of other human beings, we speak of atrocities. Traumatic events overwhelm the ordinary systems of care that give people a sense of control, connection, and meaning.

Seen from an intercultural lens, Krimayer (2007) shares a concern about defining trauma. While discussing the term 'trauma' as a metaphor, they suggest that it might include certain human experiences but exclude others. For example, trauma brings attention to a psychological wound caused by discrete events such as violence or sudden loss. However, it takes the focus away from the human struggles that may be prevalent in some cultural contexts. This requires an awareness of several intercultural issues, especially in the understanding of the idioms of suffering used by different theorists when explaining trauma. I have borrowed from these different perspectives to give one language to my own experiences. Certainly, my interpretation and understanding of these different languages of trauma have been influenced by my own socio-cultural lens.

Furthermore, I am aware that saying one has experienced trauma could seem vague as there is no defined set of events that can be labelled as traumatic. For it is not in the content of these events but in the nature of the impact of these events upon an individual that we can locate trauma. In order to provide the reader with a context for the rest of the chapter, I would like to mention that I will be engaging with the experiences described as Complex Post Traumatic Stress in relation to childhood abuse and trauma.

Ghost in My Dreams

> This is from the time when I was a drama-therapy trainee in London. It was a cold December night when I saw 'it' for the first time. I saw a huge ghost-like figure entering my room. It shifted some stuff that stood on the study table by the side of my bed and disappeared. As it became recurrent, dream after dream, the image started coming closer to me, penetrating my physical boundaries that felt like violation and abuse. I would be left with the bodily sensations of having been touched. I could see a clear archetypal image that looked like a ghost and felt an energy, like a force of the wind, touching my body. As the dreams continued, there were multiple implications upon my physical and mental wellbeing in the form of disturbed sleep, reduced appetite, anxiousness, feelings of numbness, helplessness, fearfulness, and persistent fatigue.

I have struggled to give one name to this image. However, for this chapter, I find it useful to call it a 'ghost' as I have used this term intuitively since I saw it. The Hindi word for ghost is *bhoot*. It is not a surprise that it also means 'past' when seen in relation to trauma. In his book *The Inner World of Trauma*, Kalsched (1996) calls such a figure a 'diabolical trickster' (p.16). His explanation of this term stands nearest to my experience. He uses this term to describe the persecutory figures found in the dreams of his patients who have suffered unbearable life experiences including sexual abuse and violations. These figures were found invading their physical boundaries, cutting their body or raping the victim.

Kalsched (1996) describes trauma in childhood or early infancy as any experience that causes the child unbearable psychic pain or anxiety, and that overwhelms their defensive resources. Such anxiety causes the annihilation of the human personality and the destruction of the personal spirit. To avoid this, a protective mechanism, or in Kalsched's words 'a second line of defences' (p.1), comes into play, which gets created in the inner world through unconscious fantasies and dreams. He argues that traditionally these fantasies and dreams have been viewed as dissociative or primitive, neglecting their life-saving capacities and rich archetypal meaning. Therefore, he suggests in the context of clinical practice that:

> If we study the impact of trauma on the psyche with one eye on traumatic outer events and one eye on dreams and other spontaneous fantasy-products that occur *in response* to outer trauma, we discover the remarkable mythopoetic imagery that makes up the inner world of trauma.
>
> (Kalsched, 1996, p.2)

To explain and express the overwhelming and elusive nature of the impact of trauma on the human psyche and the body, multiple authors have used the term 'ghost' as a symbol, metaphor, or image. In their book *Ghosts in the consulting room: Echoes of Trauma in Psychoanalysis*, Harris et al. (2016, p.1) write that:

> Ghosts emerge from war and catastrophes that cannot easily be assimilated in the surrounding cultures and communities or in the minds and bodies of individuals. The body may be the absorber and also the communicator of ghosts. We draw on the term 'ghosts' to capture the sense of objects that are neither internal nor external solely, that may disturb the atmosphere, the soma, the mind, temporality, and the surrounding fields.

In a classic paper *Ghosts in the nursery*, Fraiberg et al. (2018) use the term 'ghosts' to represent the repressed traumatic experiences and emotions that parents can pass on to their children. These experiences and emotions continue to haunt them like ghosts in dreams and behaviours. It is interesting to note that the dramatic mythical language of 'ghosts', 'haunted', or 'daimonic' is used alongside a more common language of 'inner objects' or 'dissociation' (Harris et al., 2016). This is maybe to capture the intensity and unknown nature of the impact of trauma on the psyche and body alike.

Other authors who haven't necessarily used the term 'ghost' have also in their own way acknowledged its presence. For example, Pitre, while exploring the modality of Developmental Transformations (DvT) from an attachment perspective, talks about the principle of 'forced accommodation' (2014, p.244) in the life of the victims of childhood abuse. She describes it as the perpetrator dominating and controlling the life of the victim. She illustrates it through an example of an abusive uncle who is ever-present for a child long after the abuse happened, and who resides within sensory reminders such as a colour, a sound, or a smell. This abusive uncle looks no different from our ghost.

The way I felt in the dream upon seeing the ghost could be described as reflecting a state of 'immobility' or 'freezing', as Peter Levine would describe it (1997, p.25). He argues that traumatic symptoms are not caused by the 'triggering' event itself but by the frozen residue of energy that has not been resolved or released. This residue remains trapped in the nervous system and can dysregulate body and spirit. Confronting the ghost in my dreams created a pathway for me to sense this residue energy within my body.

Entry of the Trickster Hero: Hanuman

> Soon after in my dreams, when the ghost attacked me, a trickster hero would enter. This trickster hero was the Hindu Monkey God, Hanuman. I would recite 'Hanuman Chalisa' (which is one of the most popular Hindu devotional hymns in praise of Hanuman) and the ghost would run away. Interestingly in these dreams, I saw myself in a much younger form as a child. When the ghost attacked the child, I would feel helpless and paralysed in my body. Whereas when the child remembered Hanuman, I would feel some power and movement within my body.

Growing up, I learnt about the ritual of Hanuman Chalisa by observing my family and most importantly while reading and watching horror stories where the protagonist would overcome the ghosts by reciting the chant. Although I considered myself to be an atheist during my teenage years, these stories still impacted my psyche. It is popularly believed in Hinduism that reading Hanuman Chalisa helps get rid of evil spirits and demons.

In the famous Hindu mythology, Ramayana, Hanuman plays the role of a mediator between Ram and Sita, between gods and demons. In my dream, he played the role of a 'third' between the innocent child and the persecutory ghost. The role of trickster heroes in myths is to bring down the arrogant and to save the innocent child (McNeely, 2011). Jung (1965) talked about the trickster archetype as a container of paradoxes, and about its role in myths as one who is both a trouble-maker and a trouble-solver. These two opposite roles were taken up in my dreams by the diabolical trickster ghost and the trickster hero, Hanuman.

Kalsched (1996) describes the word 'diabolical' as the one who dis-integrates. Interestingly, he observes that the antonym of diabolic is 'symbolic', meaning to 'throw together' (p.17). After investigating the nature of dreams in his patients who experienced trauma, he suggested that the negotiation between these opposites is carried out by the psyche's self-care system consisting of mythological and archetypal imagery that can be expressed through dreams. In my dreams, while the diabolical trickster ghost was violently dis-integrating my mind and body, the archetype of the trickster hero Hanuman held me together. While the ghost put me in touch with my vulnerabilities, the monkey-god helped me experience and embody resilience.

Drama-Therapy and Dreams as Private Myths

The famous mythologist Joseph Campbell (1993) often described dreams as private myths. The myth composed in my dreams gave me a language to describe my experience when the memory of the actual event had not come to conscious awareness and when my ability to symbolise was impaired. In relation to trauma, both Kalsched (1996) and Jones (2011), have emphasised the importance of the symbolisation of the unconscious mind. Across many theorists, descriptions of trauma refer to words such as 'split', 'fragmentation', and 'loss of soul' (Kalsched, 1996; Mogenson, 1989; Garland, 1998). It is fascinating to see how our inner world can produce these fragments in the form of images that come together to form one dramatic myth.

The relationship between myths composed in dreams and trauma has been explored through Mogenson's perspective in his book *God is a Trauma* (1989). He identifies the two terms 'God' and 'trauma' to explore the spiritual dimension of the psychology of trauma. As he writes (p.115),

> Overwhelming events which cannot be incorporated into the life we have imagined for ourselves, cause the soul to bend back on itself [...]. Like the festering process which removes the silver from a wound, the traumatised imagination works and re-works its metaphors until the events which have pierced it can be viewed in a more benign fashion. The traumatised soul is a theologizing soul.

Staying with the symbols and images from my dreams without interpreting or pathologising them facilitated a personal journey where I could eventually be more in touch with the loss of emotional and creative resources, and parts of myself.

I believe that the exposure in my training to pre-verbal and non-verbal forms of expression, such as fairy tales and myths (that I was devoid of when growing up), allowed some repressed unconscious memories, affects, and images to emerge. Carl Jung (1965) defined the personal unconscious as consisting of the forgotten, repressed, or subliminally perceived images, thoughts, and feelings from one's personal life. He described the collective unconscious as the unconscious shared by the whole human race, consisting of archetypes and ancestral memories that get expressed in fairy tales, literature, religion, and universal themes in various cultures. The use of myths and rituals in drama-therapy facilitates a space where these archetypes, images, and themes can be embodied, performed, and witnessed. Through play and creative expression, individuals can get to relive and re-work their experiences in an imaginative space, when the mind and the body might not be available to be conscious of the literal events. Drama-therapy and other arts therapies can be compared to conscious dreaming (Jennings, 1990), as they view dreams as personal myths that can actively be embodied or played with. Reflecting on this, Jones (2015) concludes that drama-therapy enables trauma to be communicated and actively engaged with through images and enacted improvisations. As he writes (2015, p.8), 'In dramatherapy, the dream cannot just be the road to expression and communication but to change: the enactments give a language of encounter and of potential help within the therapeutic relationship'.

Healing Through Rituals

Knowing about my health concerns, my aunt, who trained in traditional healing practices, asked me if I experienced 'bad dreams', as she called them. I had found someone who listened to my dreams, believed in the ghosts, and gave me a story to make meaning of an overwhelming experience. Moreover, they also offered me a way to heal through certain rituals that I could practise, and that stemmed from various sacred healing practices. The rituals involved repetitive actions of creating a boundary around myself and pushing away the ghost. They involved both imagination and physical actions. To my utter surprise at the time, my health started to improve as I started to get better sleep, felt more control, power, and agency within my body.

I had no literal recollection of the overwhelming events from the past but working with the rituals served as a canvas where I could lay the actual story. One can participate in a ritual without knowing the literal story or the mythology behind it and still find it meaningful as, Harman writes (1992, p.68), 'a ritual has a life of its own'. I continued using theatre rituals in my personal drama-therapy as I worked with imagining a bubble around me, moving with a partner in the role of a ghost, and creating physical boundaries with art material. Writing about rituals, Schrader (2012, pp.38–39) beautifully observes,

> The symbols and metaphors expressed in ritual theatre, experienced at an emotional and unconscious level, may touch into the participant's suppressed unconscious material. They may not understand why they are feeling that way but at the same time healing is happening. Unconscious emotion is being released.

Talking about childhood sexual abuse and trauma, several authors (Kalsched, 1996; Sanderson, 2013) have pointed out that, due to not being able to see the abusive carer as bad, victims can perceive themselves as dirty, faulty, evil, or possessed. Rituals can provide a chance to externalise this evil and shift the blame from the victim to the abuser. In my case, the ritual served as a container for my dreams. It helped me weave them into one embodied story that I could find meaning in. This meaning-making process and connection to the body were significant as they transcended the experience of overwhelming suffering and pain.

Rituals and the Issue of Superstition

As a drama-therapist, whenever I share my experiences of rituals and healing, I find myself being cautious and hesitant. This, I think, stems from the awareness of the intentional exploitation of many vulnerable people through superstitions. It is a real problem that cannot be overlooked. Besides the issue of superstition, the socio-political context of individuals can greatly impact on how they see and associate with different rituals and symbols. What might be a symbol of healing for one individual could be a symbol of oppression for another. In the context of India, I have found that many mental health professionals, including myself, advocate for professional help as opposed to the idea of going to a priest to get 'jhaad-phoonk'[2] done to get rid of evil spirits. This raises the question of how to and why integrate faith, beliefs, myths, and rituals in the therapy room. As a drama-therapist, I keep struggling to navigate these thin lines. On the other hand, drama-therapy in its form offered me a safe container where I could integrate faith and religion in healing without the fear of judgement or exploitation. As long as we remain aware of intercultural issues, drama-therapy holds the potential to be inclusive of experiences that may reflect local cultural practices and stories.

It might be useful to look at drama-therapy as a bridge between traditional healing practices and clinical practices. Clinical perspectives may fail to acknowledge the religious symbols produced by the psyche, and traditional healing practices may not facilitate the integration of stories of abuse, such as in the case of incest, that society may prefer to ignore. Drama-therapy combines the use of rituals with the rich knowledge of human psychology. It trains us to use the traditional art of healing rituals and myths while being grounded in the scientific understanding of the human mind. This is important as trauma impacts the mind, body, and spirit alike, and as healing may consist in bringing these together. This also allows for an understanding of the different roots of trauma in political violence, social oppression and discrimination, and childhood neglect and abuse.

Myths Composed in the Client–Therapist Relationship

The ghost followed me to my therapy sessions. I imagined my analyst as a ghost attacking me by throwing 'arrows' at me and making me fall ill. Being from a collectivist society in India where authority figures were obeyed unconditionally, I could not find words to express my disagreements to my analyst on Western soil. I felt that my unique cultural experiences were being misunderstood. I did not have words to describe the discomfort I felt within my body. I was not aware of how cultural differences or my relationship with authority figures were being played out in therapy, but I could intuitively develop the metaphor of arrows being thrown at me to capture the feelings of helplessness and invasion. I grew up watching the stories of Ramayana and Mahabharata where arrows were depicted as a weapon used by the invaders to attack the enemy's body from a distance.

Arrows can be viewed as projectiles which can symbolise projection (Von Franz, 1995). Jung (1965) defined projection as an act of forming an image about another individual based on personal unconscious impulses, fears, or desires. I felt that the therapist was projecting onto me the narrow streams of cultural stereotypes and strict reductionist interpretations. The sense of fragmentation and disconnection from one's body or the sense of loss of self that an individual can experience as a result of trauma may get mirrored through these interpretations that fail to see an individual as a whole. The authority and power held by or projected onto the therapist might re-create the experience of a lack of agency and autonomy experienced during the actual event. As Harris et al. write (2016, p.9),

> Ghosts haunt analyst and analysand, participating in impasses and uncanny experiences in the countertransference and in the transference, while more traditional spiritual practices involving hauntings seek to expel ghosts and demons. It is intriguing and important to us to stress that psychoanalysis and psychotherapies – drawing on trauma work – rather seek to have ghosts readmitted and repatriated.

Therapists can stereotype clients when they are insecure about their knowledge and power in the relationship (Casement, 1990). The analyst acted out my projections onto them, of the persecutory caretaker or the internalised bad object. The trickster, which is both a creator and a destroyer, can often create disruptions for its own pleasure (Radin, 1972). Trauma awakens something archaic in both the therapist and the client which results in an enactment of roles from their inner world (Mann & Cunningham, 2009). I could not say a 'no' to the ghost in the actual traumatic event, but I was able to say a 'no' to the ghost in therapy.

The Birth of the Harmless Ghost

Going to a new analyst felt like going to the ghost (bad object) again. Due to repetition compulsion in trauma victims, the child in me knew that the ghost could again invade my boundaries and leave me uncontained (Kalsched, 1996). But this time, the child met the 'harmless ghost' who did not throw arrows but rather held a vessel in which the traumatised soul could safely place its shattered parts. The analyst became a container for my projections. Negative transference and resistance were met in an open and non-interpretive fashion, where there was space for play and imagination. I found healing through faith in the self-regulating and self-healing capacity of the psyche that allowed metaphors and symbols to breathe, as opposed to interpretations or confrontations (Pearson, 1996). The destructive ghost from my dreams and the embodied felt experiences upon encountering it were seen and held in a safe space. The therapeutic relationship gave birth to the harmless ghost. While the persecutory ghost overwhelmed and dis-regulated my mind and body, the harmless ghost was more approachable and digestible. The metaphor of the harmless ghost helped me capture the complexity and paradoxical nature of my experiences. It brought together the ghost and Hanuman, the good and bad, the safe and unsafe, and the scary and playful. This helped me to acknowledge my vulnerable and resilient parts that were disowned in the past.

Subsequently, I participated in a drama-therapy workshop in India which aimed at building self-awareness and reflective practice for therapists. In that, we were asked to embody our successful selves and to find masks to represent these. I wore a mask of a ghost who jumped around trees like Hanuman. The metaphor of the harmless ghost helped me integrate the disruptive and the creative trickster energies in an integrated whole. The embodiment of archetypes helps connect to the archetypal energies which may be living a 'shadow' existence in the psyche (Sidoli, 2000). Acting with the mind and body together is of value when working with trauma, as the body and its feelings might have been disowned to survive the traumatic event (Miller, 1987).

Conclusion

Trauma-informed work encourages us to address both mind and the body through a growing knowledge of their connection. However, there are several ways of facilitating this that can vary depending on the professional, the individual client, and the cultural context. In this chapter, I have focused on one of those: the mythopoetic way. I have shown how trauma expresses itself in a mythopoetic form and language through the means of dreams, metaphors, and the client–therapist's relational enactment. Listening to this mythopoetic language enables a deep listening of the body. This complex and elusive language can be captured through play, imagination, and creative expression in dramatherapy. Besides, the engagement with archetypal energies, myths, and rituals facilitates a simultaneous engagement with the mind and the body at a deeper level. From a trauma-informed lens, this is valuable as an individual might not remember or share the literal traumatic details of an event but could still explore its impact on their inner world within the safe container of symbols, stories, images, or role-play that can also enable a connection with one's cultural wisdom, inner resources, and resilience.

In this chapter, I have not explicitly discussed the clinical applications of the mythopoetic approach. This is something that I invite practitioners to reflect on. Equally, this chapter only constitutes one account of the approach and of its contribution to embodied healing, which the reader may have found difficult to relate to their practice or context. However, as the field of dramatherapy is growing around the world as an intercultural practice, I would like to invite the reader to begin reflecting on the myths, stories, fairy tales, and rituals unique to the experiences of their clients. This cultural resource acts as a container not just for the clients but also for the therapists to be able to offer their imagination and empathy to the varied experiences of human suffering and resilience. Like I found Hanuman, others may be discovering a Coyote, Hermes, Anansi, Loki, or a Raven in other corners of the world.

Notes

1 Drama-therapy is spelled with a hyphen (-) throughout the chapter. Drama Therapy India (India's first and only registered association for drama-therapy) came up with the idea of using this unique spelling. This was used for the first time in Drama Therapy India's newsletter published in March 2021.

2 Jhaad-phoonk is a Hindi term for exorcism. The term is popularly used in northern India to refer to the rituals performed by a priest to help get rid of evil spirits.

References

Campbell, J. (1993). *Myths to live by*. Penguin/Arkana.

Campbell, J. (2012). *Myths of light: Eastern metaphors of the eternal*. New World Library.

Casement, P. (1990). *Further learning from the patient*. Routledge.

Fraiberg, S., Adelson, E., & Shapiro, V. (2018). Ghosts in the nursery: A psychoanalytic approach to the problems of impaired infant–mother relationships. *Parent-Infant Psychodynamics*, 87–117. https://doi.org/10.4324/9780429478154-10

Garland, C. (1998). *Understanding trauma: A psychoanalytical approach*. Duckworth.

Harman, W. (1992). *The sacred marriage of Hindu goddess*. Indiana Press.

HarperCollins Publishers Ltd. (2023, May 6). *Mythopoetic definition and meaning: Collins English Dictionary*. Retrieved from www.collinsdictionary.com/dictionary/english/mythopoetic

Harris, A., Kalb, M., & Klebanoff, S. (2016). *Ghosts in the consulting room echoes of trauma in psychoanlysis*. Routledge, Taylor & Francis Group.

Herman, J. (1992). *Trauma and recovery*. Pandora.

Jennings, S. (1990). *Dramatherapy with individuals and groups*. Jessica Kingsley Publishers.

Jones, P. (2015). Trauma and dramatherapy: Dreams, play and the social construction of culture. *South African Theatre Journal*, 28(1), 4–16. https://doi.org/10.1080/10137548.2015.1011897

Jones, R. A. (2011). *Body, mind and healing after Jung*. Routledge.

Jung, C. G. (1965). *Memories, dreams, reflections* (trans. R. C. Winston). Fontana Press.

Kakar, S. (1982). *Shamans, mystics, and doctors: A psychological inquiry into India and its healing traditions*. Oxford.

Kalsched, D. (1996). *The inner world of trauma: Archetypal defences of the personal spirit*. Routledge.

Krimayer, L. J. (2007). Foreword. In B. Drozdek & J. P. Wilson (Eds.), *Voices of trauma: Treating psychological trauma across cultures* (pp. v–vii). Springer.

Levine, P. A. (1997). *Waking the tiger: Healing trauma: The innate capacity to transform overwhelming experiences*. North Atlantic Books.

Malchiodi, C. A. (2020). *Trauma and expressive arts therapy: Brain, body, and imagination in the healing process*. The Guilford Press.

Mann, D. & Cunningham, V. (Eds.) (2009). *The past in the present: Therapy enactments and the return of trauma*. Routledge.

McNeely, D. A. (2011). *Mercury rising: Women, evil and the trickster gods*. Fisher King Press.

Miller, A. (1987). *The drama of being a child*. Virago Press.

Mogenson, G. (1989). *God is a trauma: Vicarious religion and soul-making*. Spring Publications.

Pearson, J. (1996). *Discovering the self through drama and movement*. Jessica Kingsley Publishers.

Pitre, R. (2014). Extracting the perpetrator: Fostering parent/child attachment with developmental transformations. In N. Sajnani & R. Johnson (Eds.), *Trauma-Informed drama therapy: Transforming clinics, classrooms, and communities* (pp. 243–269). Charles Thomas Publishers.

Radin, P. (1972). *The trickster: A study in American Indian mythology*. Schocken Books Inc.

Sajnani, N. & Johnson, R. (Eds.) (2014). *Trauma-Informed drama therapy: Transforming clinics, classrooms, and communities*. Charles Thomas Publishers.

Sanderson, C. (2013). *Counselling skills for working with trauma: Healing from child sexual abuse, sexual violence and domestic abuse*. Jessica Kingsley Publishers.

Schrader, C. (2012). *Ritual theatre the power of dramatic ritual in personal development groups and clinical practice*. Jessica Kingsley Publishers.

Sidoli, M. (2000). *When the body speaks: The archetypes in the body*. Routledge.

Von Franz, M. L. (1995). *Projection and recollection in Jungian psychology*. Open Court Publishing House.

Chapter 15

Healing the Intergenerational Trauma of Enslavement

The Enactment of Historical Documents with Afro-Colombian Youth

Angelo Miramonti

Introduction

Colombia has one of the largest Afro-descendant[1] populations in Latin America. According to the UN, 25% of the Colombian population (13 million) is Afro-descendant (Human Rights Council, 2011). This population is concentrated on the Pacific coast where Afro-Colombians reach 90% of the population, and the Atlantic coast where they are 60% (Bratspies, 2018).

This chapter presents the results of a drama-based participatory research I conducted with a group of Afro-descendant youth affected by the armed conflict on the Pacific coast of Colombia. My purpose was to explore how performance-based drama therapy using the embodiment of historical and autobiographical documents could help heal the multidimensional trauma of Afro-Colombians whose bodies carry the legacy of past enslavement and deportation, combined with the impact of present-day systemic racism and armed conflict. In particular, I discuss the place and role of embodiment and performance of historical materials as a distinctively unique form of healing intergenerational trauma. I show that the multidimensional trauma of Afro-descendants needs a multidimensional therapy that addresses the belonging of the individual to an intergenerational and collective body, and opens spaces of reconnection of the individual with a shared identity and memory. This research extends the knowledge in the field of trauma and embodied healing because it adapts the standard Autobiographical Therapeutic Performance method (Pendzik et al., 2016) to intergenerational trauma, and shows that this specific form of performance-based drama therapy can help groups affected by intergenerational trauma to co-create a cohesive narrative of the self, and embody a collective memory and sense of belonging to a shared identity and legacy.

Intergenerational Trauma: A Brief Review

Recent research on trauma stresses its intersubjective dimension (Herman, 2015; Wilde, 2019) and shifts the focus from trauma as an individual psychopathological affliction to a collective and socio-historical experience, especially

DOI: 10.4324/9781003322375-19

when traumatic events affect significant portions of a population – as in the case of natural disasters – and persist for decades – as in armed conflicts (Volkas, 2009). Moreover, transcultural psychology highlights the importance of inscribing trauma both in brain psychophysiology and in cultures (Kirmayer et al., 2007, 2014). Maercker et al. (2019) advocate for the adoption of transcultural perspectives in the conceptualization of trauma and Post-Traumatic Stress Disorder, while Rousseau and Drapeau (1998) show the role of culture in the transmission of trauma. Besides, studies on historically marginalized groups have documented the intergenerational transmission of trauma (Kaufman & Zigler, 1989; Solkoff, 1992). Focusing on the intergenerational trauma of enslavement and deportation of Afro-descendants, recent research emphasizes that institutionalized, physical, and symbolic violence of enslavement and systemic racism can have long-term effects on mental health, including severe depression and depression-associated disabilities (Hankerson et al., 2022). Jackson et al. (2018) analyze the psychopathological aspects of trauma in African American patients and find evidence of a link between intergenerational epigenetic trauma and environmental stimulations. These authors document the existence of feedback loops between prolonged environmental stimuli, human genomes, and behaviours, especially in the case of Afro-descendants 'as a consequence of intergenerational exposures to 250 years of chattel slavery followed by 150 years of systemic discrimination' (Jackson et al., 2018, p.1), amounting to approximately 16 generations of exposure to traumatizing factors. Henderson et al. (2021) apply the notion of historical trauma to African Americans and emphasize the need for intergenerational healing. Finally, a recent article in *The Lancet* highlights the health consequences of past enslavement and systemic racism, and urges the measurement of progress on racial equity in global public health and medicine (Khan et al., 2022).

While the literature on the intergenerational trauma of Afro-descendants focuses mainly on North American cases, Cardenas et al. (2020) show that a similar situation applies to Afro-Colombians. The first enslaved persons were deported to the present-day Colombian territory at the beginning of 16th century and the slave trade continued until its official abolition in 1851 (Lohse, 2001). Afro-Colombians were exposed to over 300 years of institutionalized slavery and the subsequent 170 years of institutionalized discrimination. Data on access to education and employment show evidence of institutionalized racism in present-day Colombia (Cardenas et al., 2020). Furthermore, Afro-Colombians have been exposed to an additional traumatizing factor: the armed conflict. The report of Colombia's Truth Commission found that Indigenous and Afro-Colombian people were disproportionately affected by the armed conflict in the last five decades. The report also documented the perduring institutionalized racism against these groups and shows that the areas with the highest prevalence of Afro-Colombian population have been throughout the conflict among the most affected by displacement, forced recruitment, extrajudicial executions, and disappearances (Comisión de la Verdad, 2022a).

Performance and Intergenerational Trauma

Drama therapy research has been investigating the healing potential of embodiment and dramatization to work with traumatized individuals and communities (Sajnani & Johnson, 2014; Snow, 2009), and documented the effectiveness of performance-based drama therapy and Autobiographical Therapeutic Performance to heal the long-term effects of trauma (Emunah, 2015; Miramonti & Millán, 2022; Pendzik 2021). Emunah (2015) finds that 'embodied stories' based on autobiography have the potential to generate or strengthen constructive self-narratives in traumatized individuals, while Ray and Pendzik (2021) analyse the impact of Autobiographical Therapeutic Performance on brain functioning and show that embodiment and performance can help reshape and rewire the neuronal architectures of individuals affected by traumatic stress. Focusing on performance and intergenerational trauma, St. Germain (2015) explores how drama therapy can heal the trauma of Aboriginal youth in Canada and stresses the significance of its contribution to the creation of spaces of dialogue, while Hammes (2021) analyses the use of therapeutic performance in the Northern Ireland armed conflict and finds that it can be effective in addressing historic trauma by providing individuals with agency in the narration of their collective story. Investigating the Latin American context, Taylor (2020) shows that performance can make visible the intergenerational roots of collective trauma. In a different study, Capitaine (2017) investigates the case of Indian residential schools in Canada and shows that performance can help construct intergenerational solidarity around the identity of the survivor. Drama therapy research converges in conceptualizing psychological trauma as an embodied, collective, intergenerational, and culture-bound experience, and stresses the potential role of embodiment and performance to help individuals and communities work through their lived traumatic experiences.

However, Pendzik et al. (2016) note that most of the literature on performance-based autobiographical drama therapy comes from Europe and North America, whereas similar experiences from other contexts remain significantly under-documented. Moreover, while the therapeutic role of embodiment and performance is well established in the literature, specific research on this approach to heal intergenerational trauma outside of Europe and North America remains limited. This chapter addresses this gap and presents research where the embodiment and performance of historical documents is analysed as a specific somatic intervention to heal the intergenerational trauma of enslavement of Afro-Colombians affected by the armed conflict.

The Context: The Impact of the Colombian Conflict on Afro-Descendant Communities

The Colombian armed conflict is an ongoing low-intensity war started in the mid-1960s. It involves the Colombian state and various armed groups (guerrillas, paramilitaries, drug traffickers, and unidentified militias). The root causes of the conflict are complex and lie in the structural inequalities of the country. It is fuelled by the revenues generated by illegal mining, narcotrafficking, and land grabbing (Yaffe, 2011). The victims of the conflict are estimated to be over 250,000, of which approximately 80% are civilians (Steele, 2018). According to the UNHCR (2022), the conflict forced 7.6 million people to leave their homes, making Colombia the second country in the world for internally displaced people.

One of the regions most affected by the armed conflict are the territories of the Afro-descendant communities of the Colombian Pacific coast, which are rich in natural resources and constitute a strategic corridor for narcotraffickers to connect the production areas in Latin America with main consumption zones in North America (Chalk, 2011). The Colombian Pacific coast has been affected by military operations of guerrillas, paramilitaries, narcotraffickers, and the Colombian army in the last 60 years (Comisión de la Verdad, 2022b). Despite having been exposed to decades of violence, forced recruitment, displacement, and cultural uprooting, the Afro-descendant communities on the Pacific coast have managed to develop grassroot resistance strategies. In some cases, their efforts have been effectively coordinated with local governments and international actors to protect their territory from the infiltration of armed groups (Gretchen, 2006). The self-reliance and resilience of Afro-descendant communities against the infiltration of armed forces has attracted the interest of research institutions and peacebuilding practitioners to understand how those affected by protracted conflicts, combined with the traumatic legacy of enslavement, have collectively developed strategies to cope with systemic violence.

Research Project

The project '*Mingar la Paz: Teachings of Yurumanguí to Think of Territorial Reparation and Peace Building in the Colombian Pacific Coast*' was a research initiative of the Faculty of Law and Political Sciences of the National University of Colombia in Bogota, started in 2017 (Universidad Nacional de Bogotá, 2022). The objective of this project was to explore the relationship of the Afro-descendant communities of the Yurumanguí River (situated on the Colombian pacific coast) to their shared memories, systems of beliefs, and territory. This project sought to strengthen the grassroot peace-building processes of the Afro-Colombian communities, and to investigate how their world visions play an important role in shaping their resistance strategies against violence and marginalization (Aguilar Gómez, 2022). To achieve this goal the project partnered with the *Proceso de Comunidades Negras* (Black Communities Process), a network of Afro-Colombian organizations whose aim is to advocate for the rights of Afro-descendant communities in Colombia.

This network made contact with the Yurumanguí River (hereinafter called 'the River') authorities and agreed a partnership with the research team (hereinafter called 'the Team') to implement the research. In 2018, the

Team identified a family archive in Popayán (south-west of Colombia) containing historical letters dating from 1743 to 1766 (Arroyo, 2017). The letters were written by an enslaved foreman working in a gold mine on the Yurumanguí River and addressed to the slave master who lived in Popayán. The letters provided details of the extractive activity and the daily lives of the enslaved people in the mine, including episodes of rebellion, repression, and resilience. They also contained extensive lists of names of the slaves who were almost certainly the biological ancestors of the population currently living along the River. The Team decided to pilot the dramatization of episodes contained in the letters as an art-based method of inquiry and a form of collective healing. Based on a previous collaboration we had (Miramonti, 2021), the Team contacted me as the coordinator of the Arts for Reconciliation research project (Miramonti, 2019) and invited me to design and conduct a theatre workshop based on the letters for a group of youth of the River. The purpose of the workshop was to explore how embodiment and performance of episodes recounted in the letters could help heal the trauma of enslavement and enhance the youths' self-perception and sense of belonging to a shared identity and history. Following consultations with the representatives of the River's communities, we agreed on the following strategy.

Research Strategy

The aim of the research was to investigate how the embodiment and performance of historical and autobiographical materials could be a distinctively unique approach to the healing of the intergenerational trauma of enslavement, systemic racism, and the protracted armed conflict affecting Afro-Colombians. To generate data, I designed and conducted drama-based participatory research (Grierson & Brearley, 2009; McIntyre, 2008). The first step was to design a workshop based on the different stages of devising Autobiographical Therapeutic Performance (Pendzik, 2020, 2021):

1 storytelling of autobiographical experiences;
2 embodiment of the narratives;
3 performance in front of an external audience;
4 individual and group reflection.

I modified the first stage to instead take as the main dramaturgical source the episodes described in the letters and link these to the autobiographical experiences of the performers. The key steps in data collection were to:

- conduct a theatre workshop focusing on the enactment of episodes described in the letters and related to the autobiographical experiences of the youth;

- have the youth perform in front of an external audience and interact with the audience;
- invite the performers to reflect on the whole experience and add my self-reflections as a facilitator.

I analysed the data using the categorical aggregation method which involves reviewing the verbal and behavioural data seeking common themes, and using them to produce relevant meaning related to the research aims (Creswell, 2007; Moustakas, 1990). During the consultations with the representatives of the River's communities, we agreed that they were going to identify a group of seven to eight gender-balanced participants satisfying the criteria of being born and raised on the River, aged between 18 and 35, and engaged in resilience activities on the River. Three women and four men were identified, mainly through self-selection. Another three participants were selected by the Team to provide support in the workshop and performance. The total number of participants was ten (five women and five men)[2]. Before the workshop, the Team pre-selected and transcribed six letters from the historical archive, according to two criteria: they provided information on the everyday life of the enslaved ancestors (especially episodes of resistance and resilience) and described events that could be dramatized.

The theatre workshop leading to the performance lasted three consecutive days for a total of 24 hours of creative work. The workshop agenda followed four steps. Firstly, I conducted group foundation games to create a space of non-judgment and deep listening among the participants. Secondly, I invited the participants to read the transcriptions of the six pre-selected letters and choose three episodes that strongly resonated with them. Thirdly, I asked the participants to discuss if and how the mechanisms of physical and symbolic violence described in the letters were affecting their lives in the present. Three situations occurring in their communities were identified that they felt replicated the same oppressive mechanisms faced by their ancestors. Finally, I invited the participants to analyze the resilience strategies that their ancestors adopted and to reflect on whether they could be applied to their present-day oppressions. The three-day workshop ended with the performance of the play *Memoria y Presente* (Memory and Present), composed of three historical scenes based on the letters and three scenes happening in the present.

Performance

Four weeks later, the group presented the play in front an audience of about 60 members of the Black Communities Process in Buenaventura, Colombia. At the beginning, a performer read a letter in which the foreman listed the slaves working in the mine. The performer invited by name the spirits of all the enslaved ancestors to join the performance, witness the re-enactment of their

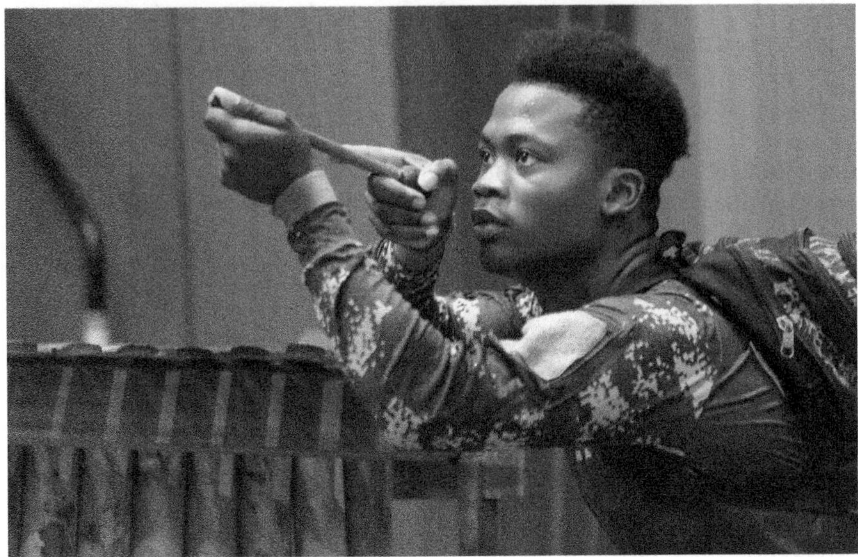

Figure 15.1 A young man is forced to fight with a group of narcotraffickers

lives, and inspire the audience with their struggles. After this ritual evocation, the play started.

In the first scene, an enslaved man manages to escape from the gold mine and reach a *palenque*, a community of run-away slaves in the deep forest inaccessible to the slave masters. The corresponding present-day episode depicts the forced recruitment of youth perpetrated by armed groups operating in the River, which is a new form of deportation and enslavement.

In the second scene, an enslaved man who attempted to kill the foreman is discovered and punished. The corresponding episode in the present is the assassination of Afro-descendant leaders perpetrated by narcotraffickers as a new form of punishment of the communities who resist the exploitation by armed groups. The resistance strategy consisted in avoiding infiltrations of armed groups in the River and rejecting any form of collaboration.

In the third scene, an elderly enslaved man manages to purchase freedom from the slave master with the mediation of a Catholic priest and an enslaved woman. The corresponding episode in the present depicts how community leaders are being threatened and assassinated by narcotraffickers to gain control of territory and use it as a drug trade corridor, while also illegally exploiting mines in the River. The resistance strategy consists in strengthening collaboration with NGOs and international actors to help community leaders leave the country and raise awareness of the ongoing human rights' violations in the River.

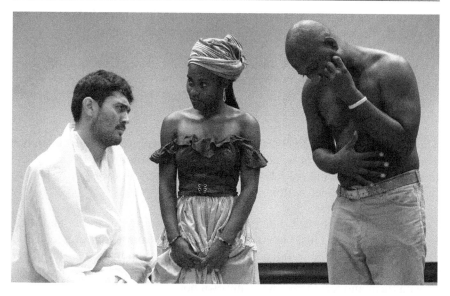

Figure 15.2 An enslaved woman asking a Catholic priest to mediate with the slave master for the purchase of the freedom of an elderly enslaved man

Discussion

In this section, I discuss how this performance-based approach to healing can intentionally address the multidimensional nature of the trauma of Afro-Colombians, combining past enslavement with present-day systemic racism and the armed conflict.

Re-Storying History: Shifting the Narrative of the Self and the Group

In the first part of the creative process, the participants accessed an invisible fragment of their collective history that had been ignored by hegemonic historiography and unintendedly transmitted by the colonial power. The enslaved foreman who wrote the letters did not mean to empower his descendants to resist cultural uprooting and discrimination, nor did the slave master who requested those letters imagine that they would become, more than two centuries later, a source of healing and resilience for the descendants of his slaves. This unintended function of the letters shows how documents not meant to tell the stories of exploited groups can indirectly play a role in decolonizing the narratives of the self in marginalized groups, and bring visibility to the stories of people neglected by official historiography. Discovering new aspects of their past allowed the youth to acknowledge that the lived experiences of Afro-Colombians belonged to human history, although many aspects of their stories were still to be told. As one of the research participants stated in the post-performance reflection:

> We often feel ashamed of our Afro-descendant identify, because the story of our enslaved ancestors was not told in the books with the same level of detail than the story of those who enslaved them. Now I feel that the people described in the letters are part of myself.

This acquisition of new knowledge was not only cognitive and individual, but also mediated by the group and the bodies on stage. Another performer highlighted how embodying collective memory was part of a process of reshaping his identity and self-perception:

> Before the workshop, I didn't know much about my ancestors and their living conditions. I just knew they were deported from Africa and forced to work in the gold mines of our River. The workshop made me feel in my body what they lived and how they felt. It made me physically re-connect with them and feel them alive in my own body.

However, performing Afro-descendant history was not enough for healing. It was equally important to re-write that history, moving from a narrative of victimization and defeat to one of resistance and preservation of the Afro-descendant culture. The body became the primary material on which a fragment of Afro-descendant history was written but could also be re-written and connected to the present. The names of enslaved persons who so far had not deserved the attention of official historiography were read out loud on stage and invited to come back to life in the dramatic space. While discovering the letters, the participants re-signified them according to the urgencies of their present. Embodying the stories told in the letters, the performers encountered the remnants of their past and at the same time created meaning to interpret their present (Jacques, 2020). This highlights an important aspect of this approach. The historical documents we used were authentic and there was no reason to doubt the truthfulness of their accounts, but they were re-signified in the dramaturgical work of the performers and charged with the subjective meaning they created in their collective dramaturgy (Lynn & Sides, 2003). The letters became the dramaturgical starting point to connect historical and autobiographical memory. A participant highlighted the strong link between the enactment of history and a shift in the understanding of his present situation, showing how the performance reshaped how the subject saw and interpreted his own present:

> Before the workshop, I had never thought about the recruitment of youth in the armed group as a new form of enslavement or the forced displacement we experience as a new way of uprooting and deportation. What we rehearsed

> made me see my own reality with new eyes, made me give new names to situations I have been experiencing since my childhood. I feel slavery is not over and the fight against it continues today, in me, in my community.

In conclusion, this first stage of re-storying history and attaching personal significance to it allowed for a shift in the narrative of Afro-descendant history, a first step in healing the intergenerational Afro-descendant body.

Embodying History: Playing New Roles

The collective dramaturgy was strongly linked to the embodiment of the stories. The participants were not asked to re-write the history of their ancestors on paper, but to tell and perform it on stage through their bodies. This expanded the perception of the performers' bodies beyond the individual. When they imagined the situation that could correspond to the episode of an enslaved person who found shelter in a community of escaped slaves, the performer noted that the *palenque* was both a physical and a symbolic space of freedom, where their individual body was woven into a collective of liberated bodies. The thought of joining a *palenque* could be envisaged as a present-day liberation strategy. The participants felt that the *palenque* was a metaphor of a society of runaways and saw in the River's diaspora an example of such society, where people escaping current forms of enslavement could find protection, preserve their cultural beliefs and transmit them to their descendants. The embodiment step of this process not only meant a shift from the individual to the collective Afro-descendant body, but also an experience of the use of the voice as part of the embodiment of the stories. The performers called out loud the names of those who were silenced. During the reflection, a participant shared that:

> When I invocated the name of real people who passed-away and invited them to come on stage with me, I felt deeply touched. These people really suffered enslavement and gave me life. I am here because they managed to survive and give birth to their descendants. They passed on life, they passed on their struggle to me. I would not be here without them. When I read that long list of names, I wondered when exactly I pronounced the name of my grand-grandparents. I wondered who, in that long list, was my biological ancestor.

Furthermore, the embodiment of historical characters avoided fixing each participant in one role and intentionally pursued the assumption of new roles through performance. Each participant played the role of different characters, in both the historical and present-day scenes. This strategy allowed them to build empathic understanding of the subjective motivations and world view of each character, without necessarily justifying their behaviours. Through embodying new roles, the performers transcended the 'doer–done to' dynamic, experiencing in their bodies the postures and attitudes of all characters. This allowed them to become aware of how their traumatic experiences shaped their postures and attitudes across generations. Embodying all the characters also helped the integration of collective memory in the individual self (Taylor, 2003; van der Kolk & van der Hart, 1995), and further contributed to healing the traumatic consequences of the invisibilized history of Afro-descendants. Some participants felt that playing all the roles was useful to re-signify the past and imagine a future beyond the exploiter–exploited binary opposition. As one of the participants reflected:

> I feel that in this workshop we connected the written history of the coloniser with the embodied and performative history of the colonised, and in this way, we dreamt and built a new future, without the exploited nor the exploiter.

Performing History: The Ancestors as Witnesses

The participants performed the play in front of an audience of representatives of various Afro-descendant communities of the Colombian Pacific coast who represented their elders. Having Afro-descendant youth perform the ancestors in front of their elders added a new layer of healing and reconnection. As a participant reflected:

> I feel my body evoked the ancestors for them [the witnesses] and our elders validated me while I was connecting with the ancestors. In a way, I feel I helped them to do the same reconnection, without coming on stage.

During the post-performance dialogue, the audience highlighted how they appreciated learning about the letters through an aesthetic dialogue that linked the youth, the ancestors, and the elders. This dialogue embodied their shared memory in the collective Afro-descendant body, symbolically connecting the youth and the elders with the ancestors. The elders highlighted how important it was to learn about their past not through scholarly historiography but through witnessing a performance and sensorily identifying with the ancestors. The bodies of the witnesses were engaged in the performance through both the senses and cognition. During the reflection, an audience member highlighted that hearing the names of his ancestors pronounced loudly and publicly had an important healing effect for him:

> When I heard the names of our real ancestors being called, I had goosebumps. I think nobody else had called their names loudly in the last two centuries. Even those who discovered this letter in the archives, probably

> never read these names aloud. It was like suddenly breaking two centuries of silence.

Another spectator highlighted that witnessing the performance made him feel that his history reconnected to the body of human history:

> We, Afro-descendants, sometimes feel we do not have a history because the written history of our people was written by western historians. This exercise of historical theatre makes us feel that we do belong to history, because we write history with our bodies, feelings and words.

Finally, the identification with the characters on stage represented a strong call to action for both the performers and the witnesses. For the performers, having embodied the oppressive historical conditions and the resistance strategies of their biological ancestors was a strong motivator to cope with the challenges they were currently facing. The certainty of having the stories of their biological ancestors in the letters increased their determination:

> I was impressed when I felt that those persons were really being my great-grandfathers and mothers. When they asked me if this was still happening to me, I immediately made the connection to what is happening in the River and felt motivated to connect with my fellow participants and fight. I feel that, if you do not have deep roots in our history, you cannot sustain the high branches of our fight.

On the same issue, an audience member commented:

> When I saw the violence of repression and the courage to resist of our ancestors unintendedly documented by our oppressors, I felt a physical need to stand up and fight. I wanted to go on stage and help the protagonist struggle and survive.

The dramatic space of performance proved to be a time and space machine where different generations of historical and current characters inhabited the bodies of the performers and were witnessed by the elders. The ancestors' lived experiences documented in the letters provided the dramaturgical source of the play and the names of the ancestors were evoked at the beginning of the play to join the elders and witness the re-enactment of their lived experiences. During the performance, performers and witnesses established a mutual interaction that conferred meaning to the experience of both. The triadic relation between the ancestors-characters, the performers, and the witnesses enabled the reconnection of generations, a reciprocal validation and the shift from a narrative of victimization to one of dignity and resilience.

The Outsider's Mirror: Self-Reflections

Throughout this research I reflected on the situatedness of my body in the research and on the intercultural implications of working with intergenerational trauma. I wondered how my body appearance, embodied attitudes, and cognitive biases influenced how the participants perceived me and how this influenced their reaction to what I proposed. I was perceived as a middle-aged European White man with experience in applied theatre, coming from a university in a big city to facilitate a group of young Afro-descendant men and women coming from rural communities affected by decades of armed conflict. The participants perceived me as an outsider, with very limited knowledge of their context, but willing to listen and give them the role of experts, while also bringing an expertise in collective dramaturgy and theatre direction. This prompted the participants to explain in more detail their present-day stories and led them to question experiences they had normalized. This further helped critical thinking and dialogue that resulted in the search for a common narrative to explain their experiences to an outsider. I also observed that the perception of my 'not knowing' contributed to re-signifying the performers as experts. This positively impacted on their self-perception and enabled a deconstruction of the hegemonic idea that my colour, age, gender, and nationality identified me as the expert.

My outsider positioning not only influenced how the performers subjectively perceived me, but also determined how I subjectively collected and analyzed data. The notes I took and the relevance I gave to certain categories of analysis reflected my theoretical background as a drama therapist and applied theatre practitioner. The research is therefore the result of an outsider's perspective intersecting with the multiple views of a relatively homogeneous group.

After reflecting on how my body influenced the research, I believe it is equally important to reflect on how this embodied process impacted me as a human being. Throughout this process, I have been wondering about who my ancestors were in the 18th century and whether they were oppressed, like the people in the letters. They were probably peasants living in southern Europe. I wondered how my body keeps carrying their legacy. In the post-performance reflections, I shared with the participants that I had never had the opportunity to reconnect with my ancestors in the same embodied and performative way, and that witnessing them doing it motivated me to honour my intergenerational roots and reconnect with their stories.

I believe that one of the key findings of the research shows that multidimensional trauma needs an intentionally multidimensional form of therapeutic intervention. When trauma is inscribed in the collective and intergenerational body, therapy has to address the belonging of the individual to a body of ancestors, and open spaces of aesthetic dialogue and embodied reconnection across generations. In this study, the synergic interaction of collective dramaturgy based on history, autobiography, embodiment, and performance constitutes a therapeutic space in which the healing of intergenerational trauma is possible.

Conclusion

This research showed that discovering and re-writing Afro-descendant history and performing it in front of significant witnesses was a distinctively unique form of healing that helped the co-creation of a cohesive narrative of the self, and a sense of belonging to a collective and intergenerational legacy and identity. As Siegel showed (2003), embodiment and performance contribute to building cohesive narratives, including the creation of an integrated storyline of collective memory, present struggles, and shared future. This approach prompted the participants to experience their individual bodies as belonging to the Afro-descendant body as an intersubjective and historical entity. The process of storying personal and collective memories to make them communicable to others was a first step in generating a cohesive narrative of the self. In addition, the embodiment and role playing of different characters (including the exploiters) contributed to an expansion of this narrative, transcending the binary exploiter–exploited opposition and aspiring to a new society based on inclusion. Performing and being witnessed allowed for the validation and imprint of the newly created narrative in the Afro-descendant body.

The collective and intergenerational trauma inscribed in the Afro-descendant body needs somatic, collective, intergenerational, and culture sensitive healing. The approach I piloted synergically addressed all these aspects using a modified version of Autobiographical Therapeutic Performance. This approach explored the multidimensional nature of Afro-descendants' trauma, healing its historical roots and its transmission across generations. The embodiment and performance of collective memory helped inscribe new narratives of Afro-descendant history and reconnect the lived experiences of individuals to a textile of intergenerational stories. The perception of the body as a network of belongings across the social space and history constitutes a specific theoretical contribution of this study to somatic therapies, and questions individualistic approaches to the healing of collective trauma. This specific way of working with the traumatized Afro-descendant body constitutes an original approach to intergenerational trauma healing that complements other somatic and art-based approaches.

This research has some limitations to bear in mind. The in-depth exploration of how the politics of the Afro-descendant body and memory can heal or perpetuate trauma (Juárez Rodríguez, 2022) is left for future research. I also intentionally did not focus on the relation between the Afro-descendant body and the Afro-descendants' territories of the Colombian pacific coast (Miramonti, 2021), and the role of geographies of identity and resistance (Mollett, 2020) in trauma healing.

However, the research described in this chapter enables me to suggest a number of recommendations for drama therapy practice and research. Regarding practice, I recommend that, when working with groups that have been structurally and intergenerationally discriminated, drama therapy intentionally focus on the history of the collective body and open spaces of dialogue between generations. I also recommend that drama-based approaches become part of mental health and psychosocial support programmes targeting communities affected by multidimensional trauma, such as historical discrimination and armed conflicts (IOM, 2021; Miramonti, 2020; Premaratna, 2018). Regarding future research, I recommend systematic inquiry on the therapeutic impact of performance of historical materials on populations affected by multidimensional traumas and how performance can reshape collective memory in traumatized groups. Finally, I recommend more scholarly valorization of experiences from non-Western cultures. This cultural and geographical refocus should be paired with the valorization of approaches that question the epistemological and political hegemony of Western culture in the production of knowledge representations, as a way to decolonize drama therapy theory, practice, and research.

Acknowledgements

I would like to thank:

1 My university, Bellas Artes, Institución Universitaria del Valle (Colombia) for financially supporting this research as part of my 'Arts for Reconciliation' research project;
2 The *Mingar la Paz* project and the *Colectivo Guía Nómada* of the National University of Bogotá for the invitation to carry out this research;
3 The *Proceso de Comunidades Negras* in Buenaventura for actively supporting the research;
4 The Yurumanguí River communities and in particular the three young women and four young men who participated in the workshop and shared their lived experiences of resilience and dignity.

Notes

1 For the purpose of this research, we adopt the definition of Afro-descendant established in the Regional Conference of the Americas, held in preparation for the Third World Conference against Racism, Racial Discrimination, Xenophobia and Related Intolerance in the city of Santiago, Chile (2000): 'Afro-descendant is the person of African origin who lives in the Americas and in the region of the African Diaspora as a result of slavery, who have been denied the exercise of their fundamental rights' (Rojas Dávila, 2018). This definition shows that the defining characteristic of this group is a collective and intergenerational violation of their rights: nearly three

centuries of enslavement, cultural uprooting, and present-day marginalization. In this chapter, I use the term 'Afro-Colombian' to refer to Afro-descendants who lived a significant part of their life within the borders of present-day Colombia.

2 The participants presented in this chapter gave their consent for their verbal productions, photos, and videos taken during the workshop and performance to be analysed and published for research purposes.

References

Aguilar Gómez, D. (Ed.) (2022). *Mingar la paz: Enseñanzas de Yurumanguí para pensar la construcción de paz en los territorios del Pacífico Sur colombiano*, Universidad Nacional de Colombia, Bogotá.

Arroyo, M. A. (2017). *La vida cotidiana en los reales de minas de Yurumanguí y Juntas de la Soledad (Raposo), 1743–1766*. Unpublished Bachelor thesis, Universidad del Cauca, Colombia.

Bratspies, R. (2018). 'Territory is everything': Afro-Colombian communities, human rights and illegal land grabs. *HRLR ONLINE*, 291–323.

Capitaine, B. (2017). Telling a story and performing the truth: The Indian residential school as cultural trauma. In B. Capitaine & K. Vanthuyne (Eds.), *Power through testimony: Reframing residential schools in the age of reconciliation* (pp. 50–73). UBC Press.

Cardenas, R., Mina Rojas, C., Restrepo, E., & Rosero, E. (2020). Afro-descendants in Colombia, anti-racist struggle and the accomplishments and limits of multiculturalism. In J. Hooker (Ed.), *Black and indigenous resistance in the Americas: From multiculturalism to racist backlash* (pp. 93–122). Lexington Books.

Chalk, P. (2011). *The Latin American drug trade: Scope, dimensions, impact, and response*. RAND Corporation.

Comisión de la Verdad (2022a). *Informe Final. Resistir no es aguantar. Violencias y daños contra los pueblos étnicos de Colombia*. Retrieved from www.comisiondelaverdad.co/sites/default/files/descargables/2022-08/CEV_ETNICO_DIGITAL_2022.pdf

Comisión de la Verdad (2022b). *Colombia adentro. Relatos territoriales sobre el conflicto armado*. Retrieved from www.comisiondelaverdad.co/colombia-adentro-1

Creswell, J. W. (2007). *Qualitative inquiry and research design: Choosing among five approaches*. Thousand Oaks.

Emunah, R. (2015). Self-revelatory performance, a form of drama therapy and theatre. *Drama Therapy Review*, 1(1), 71–85.

Gretchen, A. (2006). Colombian peace communities: The role of NGOs in supporting resistance to violence and oppression. *Development in Practice*, 16(3/4), 278–291.

Grierson, E. & Brearley, L. (2009). *Creative art research: Narratives of methodologies and practices*. RMIT.

Hammes, L. (2021). Stories to be told: A literature review of therapeutic performance theatre and historic trauma in Ireland. Lesley University. Retrieved from https://core.ac.uk/display/427079976?source=2

Hankerson, S. H., Moise, N., Wilson, D., Waller, B. Y., Arnold, K. T., Duarte, C., Lugo-Candelas, C., Weissman, M. M., Wainberg, M., Yehuda, R., & Shim, R., (2022). The intergenerational impact of structural racism and cumulative trauma on depression. *American Journal of Psychiatry*, 179(6), 434–440. https://doi.org/10.1176/appi.ajp.21101000

Henderson, Z. R., Stephens, T. N., Ortega-Williams, A., & Walton, Q. L. (2021). Conceptualizing healing through the African American experience of historical trauma. *American Journal of Orthopsychiatry*, 91(6), 763–775. https://doi.org/10.1037/ort0000578

Herman, J. (2015). *Trauma and recovery: The aftermath of violence. From domestic abuse to political terror*. Basic Books.

Human Rights Council (2011). *Report of the independent expert on minority issues, Gay McDougall*. Addendum. Mission to Colombia. U.N. Doc. A/HCR/16/45/Add.1.

IOM (2021). *Manual on community-based mental health and psychosocial support (MHPSS) in emergencies and displacement*. International Organisation for Migrations.

Jackson, L., Jackson, Z., & Jackson, F. (2018). Intergenerational resilience in response to the stress and trauma of enslavement and chronic exposure to institutionalized racism. *Journal of Clinical Epigenetics*, 4(3). https://doi.org/10.21767/2472-1158.1000100

Jacques, J. F. (2020). Investigation into the production of meaning in autobiographical performance in dramatherapy. *The Arts in Psychotherapy*, 69. https://doi.org/10.1016/j.aip.2020.101659

Juárez Rodríguez, B. (2022). Black women's geographies of resistance and the Afro-Ecuadorian Ancestral Territory of Imbabura and Carchi. *Latin American and Caribbean Ethnic Studies*, 17. https://doi.org/10.1080/17442222.2022.2156259

Kaufman, J. & Zigler, E. (1989). The intergenerational transmission of child abuse. In D. Cicchetti & V. Carlson (Eds.), *Child maltreatment: Theory and research on the causes and consequences of child abuse and neglect* (pp. 129–150). Cambridge UP.

Khan, M. S., Guinto, R. R., Boro, E., Rahman-Shepherd, A. & Erondu, N. A. (2022). The need for metrics to measure progress on racial equity in global public health and medicine. *The Lancet*, Vol 400. https://doi.org/10.1016/S0140-6736(22)02464-3

Kirmayer, L., Lemelson, R., & Barad, M. (2007). Introduction: Inscribing trauma in culture, brain, and body. In L. Kirmayer, R. Lemelson, & M. Barad (Eds.), *Understanding trauma: Integrating biological, clinical, and cultural perspectives* (pp. 1–20). Cambridge UP.

Kirmayer, L., Guzder, J., & Rousseau, C. (2014). *Cultural consultation: Encountering the other in mental health care*. Springer.

Lohse, R. (2001). Reconciling freedom with the rights of property: Slave emancipation in Colombia, 1821–1852, with special reference to La Plata. *The Journal of Negro History*, 86, 3, 203–227. https://doi.org/10.2307/1562445

Lynn, K. & Sides, S. (2003). Collective dramaturgy: A co-consideration of the dramaturgical role in collaborative creation. *Theatre Topics*, 13(1), 111–115. https://muse.jhu.edu/article/40836/pdf

Maercker, A., Heim, E., & Kirmayer, L. J. (2019). *Cultural clinical psychology and PTSD*. Hogrefe Publishing.

McIntyre, A. (2008). *Participatory action research*. Sage Publications.

Miramonti, A. (2019). Healing and transformation through art: Theatre for reconciliation. *Educazione Aperta*, 6.

Miramonti, A. (2020). Stories of wounds, paths of healing: Theatre of Witness with victims of the Colombian conflict. *Educazione Aperta*, 8.

Miramonti, A. (2021). Bodies, memory, territories. A testimonial theatre experience with Colombian Afro-descendant Women, *Educazione Aperta*, 9. https://zenodo.org/record/5163990#.Y8Ps3nbP25c

Miramonti, A. & Millán, K. (2022). Scarred dancer. Autobiographic Therapeutic Performance with a woman in the psychiatric system. *Educazione Aperta*, 11. https://zenodo.org/record/6854776#.Y8PtEHbP25c

Mollett, S. (2020). Hemispheric, relational, and intersectional political ecologies of race: Centring land-body entanglements in the Americas. *Antipode, a Radical Journal of Geography*. 53(3), 810–830. https://doi.org/10.1111/anti.12696

Moustakas, C. (1990). *Heuristic research: Design, methodology, and applications*. Sage.

Pendzik, S. (2020). *Autobiographical therapeutic performance in drama therapy*. In D. Johnson & R. Emunah (Eds.), *Current approaches in drama therapy*, 3rd Edition (pp. 338–361). Charles C Thomas.

Pendzik, S. (2021). Performance-based drama therapy: Autobiographical performance as a therapeutic intervention. *PÓS: Revista do Programa de Pós-graduação em Artes da EBA/UFMG*, *11*(23). https://doi.org/10.35699/2237-5864.2021.36301

Pendzik, S., Emunah, R., & Johnson, D. R. (Eds.) (2016). *The self in performance – autobiographical, self-revelatory, and autoethnographic forms of therapeutic theatre*. Palgrave Macmillan.

Premaratna, N. (2018). *Theatre for peacebuilding. The role of arts in conflict transformation in south Asia*. Palgrave Macmillan.

Ray, P. & Pendzik, S. (2021). Autobiographical Therapeutic Performance as a means of improving executive functioning in traumatized adults. *Frontiers in Psychology*, 12, 1–6. https://doi.org/10.3389/fpsyg.2021.599914

Rojas Dávila, R. (2018). Afro-descendants as subjects of rights in international human rights law. *International Journal on Human Rights*, 28, 151–164.

Rousseau, C. & Drapeau, A. (1998). The impact of culture on the transmission of trauma. Refugees' stories and silence embodied in their children's lives. In Y. Danieli (Ed.), *International handbook of multigenerational legacies of trauma* (pp. 465–486). Plenum Press.

St. Germain, M. (2015). *Opening the conversation: An investigation into the interface of drama therapy, intergenerational trauma, and aboriginal youth of Canada*. Concordia University Graduate Projects. Unpublished. Retrieved from https://spectrum.library.concordia.ca/id/eprint/980527/

Sajnani, N. & Johnson, D. R. (Eds.) (2014). *Trauma-informed drama therapy: Transforming clinics, classrooms, and communities*. Charles C Thomas Pub Ltd.

Siegel, D. J. (2003). An interpersonal neurobiology of psychotherapy: The developing mind and the resolution of trauma. In M. F. Solomon & D. J. Siegel (Eds.), *Healing trauma: Attachment, mind, body and brain* (pp. 1–56). Norton.

Snow, S. (2009). Ritual/theatre/therapy. In D. R. Johnson & R. Emunah (Eds.), *Current approaches in drama therapy* (pp. 117–144). Charles C Thomas.

Solkoff, N. (1992). Children of survivors of the Nazi Holocaust: A critical review of the literature. *American Journal of Orthopsychiatry*, 62(3), 342–358. https://doi.org/10.1037/h0079348

Steele, A. (2018). *Democracy and displacement in Colombia's civil war*. Cornell University Press.

Taylor, D. (2003). *The Archive and the repertoire: Performing cultural memory in the Americas*. Duke UP.

Taylor, D. (2020). Trauma and performance: Lessons from Latin America, *PMLA*, 121(5), 1674–1677. http://www.jstor.org/stable/25501645

UNHCR (2022). *Colombia*. Retrieved from www.unhcr.org/colombia.html

Universidad Nacional de Bogotá (2022). *Mingar la paz: enseñanzas de Yurumanguí para pensar la reparación territorial y la construcción de paz en las comunidades negras del pacifico colombiano.* Retrieved from www.hermes.unal.edu.co/pages/Consultas/Proyecto.xhtml?idProyecto=40634&tipo=0

van der Kolk, B. & van der Hart, O. (1995). The intrusive past: The flexibility of memory and the engraving of trauma. In C. Caruth (Ed.), *Trauma: Explorations in memory*. (pp. 158–182). Johns Hopkins UP.

Volkas, A. (2009). Healing the wounds of history, drama therapy in collective trauma and intercultural conflict resolution. In D. Johnson & R. Emunah (Eds.), *Current approaches in drama therapy* (pp. 145–171). Charles and Thomas.

Wilde, L. (2019). Trauma and intersubjectivity: The phenomenology of empathy in PTSD. *Medicine, Health Care and Philosophy*, 22, 141–145. https://doi.org/10.1007/s11019-018-9854-x

Yaffe, L. (2011). Armed conflict in Colombia: Analyzing the economic, social, and institutional causes of violent opposition. *CS*, 8, 187–208. https://doi.org/10.18046/recs.i8.1133

Index

Pages in *italics* refer to figures, pages in **bold** refer to tables, and pages followed by "n" refer to notes.

For Product Safety Concerns and Information please contact our EU representative GPSR@taylorandfrancis.com Taylor & Francis Verlag GmbH, Kaufingerstraße 24, 80331 München, Germany

Printed and bound by CPI Group (UK) Ltd, Croydon, CR0 4YY

08/06/2025

01897002-0015